HEALTH AND HATHA YOGA

With sections on Kundalini,
Swara Yoga, Brahmacharya
and Meditation

Other books in this series:

Sivananda: Biography of a Modern Sage
Karma Yoga
Raja Yoga: The Yoga System of Patanjali
Bhakti Yoga
Vedanta
Mind: Its Mysteries and Control
Sure Ways for Success in Life and God-realisation
Sivananda Day to Day

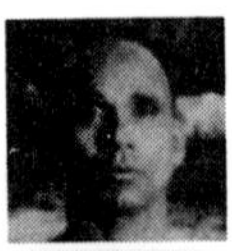

Photographs of Swami Krishna courtesy of Divine Life Society, Rishikesh.

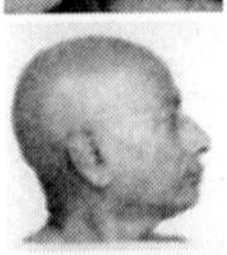

Photographs of Swami Venkatesananda courtesy of Chiltern Yoga Trust (Aust).

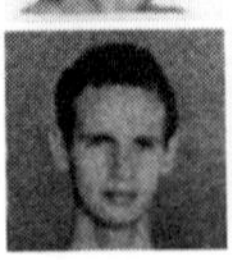
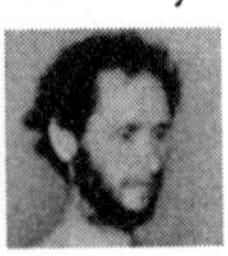

Photographs of Narayan and Graeme by Photowork, Fremantle.

HEALTH AND

Hatha Yoga

Life and Works of Swami Sivananda

Volume 2

Published by

THE DIVINE LIFE SOCIETY

P.O. SHIVANANDANAGAR—249 192

Tehri-Garhwal, Uttarakhand, Himalayas, India

www.sivanandaonline.org, www.dlshq.org

First Edition: 1985
Second Edition: 2007
Third Edition: 2019
Fourth Edition: 2021

[1,000 Copies]

ISBN 81-7052-217-X
EO 67

PRICE: ₹235/-

Published by Swami Padmanabhananda for
The Divine Life Society, Shivanandanagar, and
printed by him at the Yoga Vedanta Forest Academy
Press, P.O. Shivanandanagar, Distt. Tehri-Garhwal,
Uttarakhand, Himalayas, India
For online orders and Catalogue visit : dlsbooks.org

CONTENTS

Section II
HATHA YOGA

Section III
KUNDALINI

Section IV
SWARA YOGA

Section V
BRAHMACHARYA

Section VI
CONCENTRATION AND MEDITATION

ACKNOWLEDGEMENTS

We are indebted to:

H.H. Sri Swami Venkatesanandaji Maharaj, whose mammoth task was to compile and edit almost 300 of Holy Master Sri Swami Sivanandaji's books into 19 volumes, in spite of his demanding programmes and failing health.

Swami Lakshmi Ananda for the final editing.

—The Publishers

Section I

Health

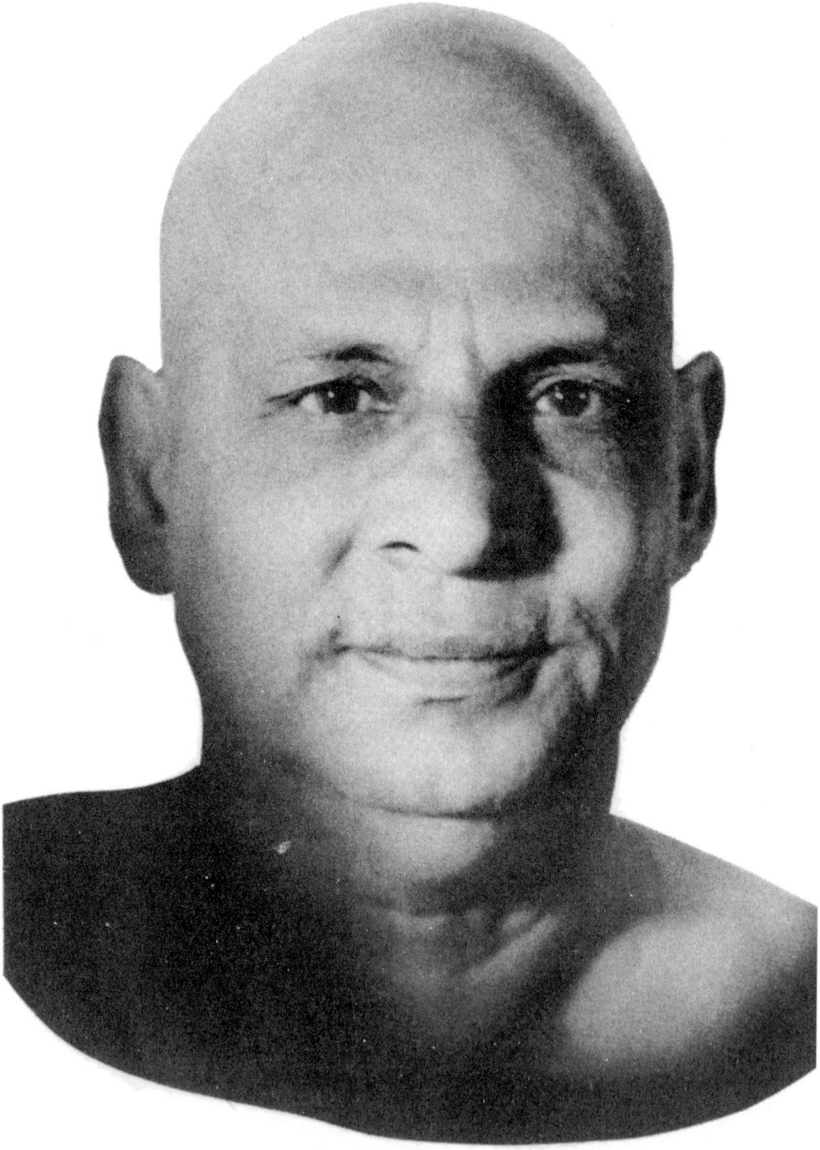

There was an extraordinary radiance about Swami Sivananda

SECRET OF HEALTH AND LONG LIFE

What is Health?

Health is that condition of the body in which all its functions are efficiently performed without any difficulty. It is the condition of comfort, ease, ability to eat, move and perform other functions of life. It is the state which results from the harmonious performance of the various functions of the bodily organs. It is the condition of the body when every organ or part of it is sound and performs without pain or suffering the functions or duties assigned to it.

If the stomach or bowels possess all their natural strength and efficiently discharge their duties in the digestion of food-stuffs; if the heart and its blood vessels are in good order and circulate the blood properly and satisfactorily; if the lungs work properly in allowing the blood to receive its due supply of oxygen; if the brain performs all its functions and if the skin carries off the perspiration normally, the chief conditions of health are observed. We then do not experience any uneasiness or painful sensation and are able to attend to all our appointed duties. To be in this state is to enjoy one of the greatest blessings. It has been provided by our beneficient Creator that all the organs and parts of our frame should continue in their original soundness (if we only take care not to injure them) and that wc should consequently be healthy. But if we do not take care to keep them sound, it is impossible that we can be healthy.

Health is that state of equilibrium of the three humours of the body viz. vatha, pitha and kapha (wind, bile and phlegm), wherein the mind and all the organs of the body work in harmony and concord, man enjoys peace and happiness and performs his duties of life with comfort and ease. It is that condition in which man sleeps well, has good digestion and appetite, normal breathing and a normal pulse, good quantity of pure blood, strong nerves and a calm mind, a free movement of the bowels, normal state of urine, rosy cheeks, shining face and sparkling eyes. It is that state in which a man jumps, sings, smiles, laughs, whistles and moves about with joy and ecstacy. It is that condition in which he can think, speak and act properly.

A life with good health is a great blessing indeed. What is the earthly use of wealth and possessions if a man cannot eat well on account of a disease of the stomach, if he cannot walk on account of rheumatism or paralysis, if he cannot see the beautiful sceneries of nature on account of cataract or defective vision? Life without good health is a miserable condition, even if one is lord of the whole earth.

Health is joy; health is wealth, health is the elixir of life. Without health there is no enjoyment. Without health one cannot earn well; without health one cannot attain one's desired objects; without health one cannot put in strenuous effort; without health there is no earnestness in work; without health life becomes a burden. Foremost attention should therefore be given towards keeping perfect health.

Without good health you cannot achieve anything in the material or the spiritual line. Good health is the most coveted possession of all. Therefore preserve good health by natural ways of living.

Health is a positive state. It is not simply negation of disease. A healthy man can turn out more physical and mental work than an unhealthy man. He can practise good meditation for a long time. A healthy man need not necessarily be strong and robust; a strong and robust man need not necessarily be healthy. Health is a gift from Mother Nature or the Lord who is the power behind all life. Health is your birthright, and not disease. It is as natural to be well as it is to be born.

Health is above gold and infinite wealth and treasures. It enlarges the soul and opens all its powers to receive instructions and relish virtues. "This Atman cannot be attained by a weak and unhealthy man," is the emphatic declaration of the *Upanishads*.

Emerson says, "The first wealth is health. Give me health and a day, I will make the pomp of emperors ridiculous." He who has good health has nothing more to wish for. He is really a blessed man.

Health depends upon karma. A virtuous man enjoys long life and good health. A wicked man is unhealthy. Patanjali Maharishi says in his *Yoga Sutras*: "Span of life, caste, enjoyment, all depend upon one's own karma." Therefore perform virtuous actions. Shun evil deeds. Body, mind and spirit constitute the whole man. There is an intimate relationship between body and mind. Mental health is more vital than physical health. All diseases originate in the mind first and then affect the body.

Health is the foundation of your career, in fact of your life. To be completely healthy is to live fully — body, mind and spirit performing their tasks efficiently and working together as a harmonious whole. When you are healthy you enjoy your food, sleep soundly, work hard and tackle your difficulties with courage.

We should have good health to achieve the four aims of life viz., dharma, artha, kama and moksha (righteousness, wealth, enjoyment and liberation). Without good health you cannot achieve anything. Without good health you cannot perform any selfless service. Without good health you cannot pray and meditate. Without good health you cannot do asanas and pranayama. That is the reason why scriptures declare that this body is a boat to cross the ocean of worldly existence. It is an instrument for doing virtuous deeds and attaining liberation from the cycle of birth and death.

The chief conditions required for maintaining a man in natural sound health are these:

1. The place where he lives must be dry. His house must be clean, and fresh air must be allowed to circulate through it by night as well as by day.
2. He must never sit for a single minute in damp clothes or in a room where a cold draught of wind is passing.
3. He must frequently wash the whole surface of his body.
4. Each day he must take not less than twenty-four ounces of solid food. He must avoid too great a sameness in his food, and also too great a variety at one meal. He must avoid indulgence in spirituous and fermented liquors.
5. He must spend an hour at least, and as much more of his time as possible, every day in the open air.
6. He must have some occupation to give him bodily and mental exercise, and which may engage his attention eight or ten hours every day.

7. He must spend some part of the leisure time of every day in japa, kirtan, meditation and study of religious books.
8. He must be careful to avoid great anxiety of mind, and endeavour to sustain his fortitude against sorrow which arises from misfortune.
9. He must sleep for a minimum of six hours daily.

If all men were to live in accordance with these rules, disease would, in time, be little known on earth, and human happiness would be increased to a degree of which we cannot now form any notion.

Unnatural life shortens existence and leads to ill health and various sorts of diseases. Unfortunately man goes astray from nature in order to gratify his perverted propensities and passions.

Disease

You should have a clear idea of what disease is and how it is caused. Then you will be able to prevent disease. Disease can be averted if you understand the biological laws which govern life, the rules of health and hygiene and the importance of cleanliness. A more general knowledge of the laws of health would help considerably to prevent sickness and death and improve the health of the people.

Disease is only being 'dis' — 'ease' i.e. not at ease. It is the opposite state to comfort, ease and ability to perform the avocations of life. Disorder or deviation from health is a response to the retardation of some vital process; it is the state which follows the rupture of the harmonious performance of the various functions of the bodily organs. It ordinarily involves pain and discomfort, and it is generally dreaded in proportion to the degree it is painful.

Disease is the result of a violation of some laws of nature. Nature wants every one to be healthy and strong. If you are weak it indicates that your organs or the various cells of your body are not functioning properly. Remove the cause of the disease. Do not play with the symptoms. It is simpler to prevent than to cure.

To treat the cause is the rational method of treatment of any disease or impaired health. There is no use in suppressing the symptoms. If the root-cause is not eradicated and if the symptoms are suppressed for the time being, the disease will assume an aggravated chronic form. The only rational method of treatment is that which takes into consideration the causes, and directs all its efforts towards the restoration of normal functioning throughout the whole system. For instance, habitually taking too much food, or food of an injurious kind, is sure to hurt the stomach. A draught of cold air upon the skin when it is hot closes up the pores, so that it is no longer able to carry off the perspiration. Each organ is liable to be thus hurt or deranged in its function by some erroneous course of conduct or some accident that may befall it — and the consequence is disease which, in its worst form, often occasions death.

Of every hundred deaths occurring in India, Europe and other countries, sixty are said to be due to disease which can be prevented to a very large extent, if people are only wise and will take those measures advocated by sanitary science.

All chronic, long-standing and functional derangements or ailments are invariably associated with definite abnormal conditions in the mechanism, tissues and organs of the body.

Before the age of machinery a man's life was more natural. The people of the past generations were more healthy and strong. In this twentieth century, life has become (and is becoming) more artificial. Hence there is much deterioration in health and strength in spite of innumerable doctors and various medical discoveries. Although we have no control over present conditions, we can adapt and control ourselves to a certain extent if we follow the rules of health. We can then keep up fairly good health and lead a joyful life.

The human body is the weakest piece of mechanism on earth, likely to go out of order without a moment's notice. Its parts are made not of steel or brass, but of the flimsiest materials imaginable, which cannot be replaced if deranged or worn out. What a blessing it would be if the dyspeptic could cast off his feeble old stomach and replace it by a strong and sound new one, and if the man of weak nerves could tear off his shattered old stuff and put on a grand new system of ramified, throbbing, vigorous nerves! That unfortunately cannot be done. The human machine however, unlike machines of steel and brass, is provided with a circulatory system by which properly chosen nourishment is imparted to the remotest portion of the body and the damaged and worn out tissues repaired.

The chief causes which impair the human machine are as follows:

1. Pessimistic thoughts.
2. Fear of disease.

3. Lack of the proper kind of food.
4. Overwork.
5. Working late at night.
6. Various kinds of anxieties and worries.

All these causes upset the digestive organs, and so constipation and other diseases of the digestive system result. When the digestion becomes impaired, all other diseases follow in its train.

Most diseases take their origin in over-eating, sexual excess and outbursts of anger and hatred. Energy is depleted by fits of anger. The cells and tissues are filled with morbid, poisonous material when one loses one's temper and entertains deep hatred. Various sorts of physical ailments crop up. Various sorts of nervous diseases are attributable to excessive loss of seminal energy and frequent fits of explosive anger or wrath.

If the mind is kept cool and calm at all times, you will have wonderful health, strength and vitality. Develop the powers of endurance and resistance. Strengthen your body, mind and nerves. Take plenty of exercise in the open air, substantial nutritious food, medicated oil baths and plenty of rest. Have mental and physical recreation. Lead a well-regulated life. Be moderate in food, drink and enjoyments. Lead a spiritual life. All diseases will leave your body by themselves. All microbes will die when your vitality, vigour and strength are at a flood tide. This is the secret of health and happiness.

Do not be carried away by the pompous advertisements made by quacks and charlatans. Lead a simple natural life. You will become alright soon. Do not spend any money in purchasing so-called patent medicines and specifics. They are worthless. Quacks try to exploit the credulous and the ignorant. Beware. Do not go to doctors very often. Endeavour to qualify yourself as your own doctor. Understand the laws of nature and the principles of hygiene and health. Do not trespass against the laws of health.

Bask in the sun. Expose your body to the rays of the sun for a short time daily. This is heliotherapy or sun-treatment. Sun is the source of energy and power. You will derive energy and power from the sun.

Rest in bed is necessary. Adjust your diet. Take simple wholesome, easily digestible, bland and non-irritating food. Give up hot, pungent curries, chutneys and chillies. Rest the stomach and the small bowels by taking recourse to fasts. If you can fast for a whole day, it is all the better. Fasting eliminates poisons and overhauls the system thoroughly. You can take sago and milk, barley water and fruits like sweet orange, grapes, etc. If you are thirsty, you can take lemon or orange juice with sugar-candy.

Observe celibacy. Get up at 4 a.m. and practise japa of 'Hari Om' or any mantra and also meditation for one hour. The name of the Lord is the best medicine or tonic in the world. You should have intense faith in the power of the names of the Lord. Incurable diseases are cured by japa or by singing the Lord's name. Meditation creates new, healthy vibrations in all the cells of the body and removes any kind of disease. All the tissues are bathed in the nectar that flows during meditation. All germs that cause diseases are destroyed. (The rationale of this kind of yoga or spiritual treatment is not yet fully known to the medical profession.)

Why do you unnecessarily introduce foreign drugs into the system? Resort to Nature-cure. Practise regularly breathing exercises, asanas, concentration and meditation. This is the ideal treatment.

Do not think too much of the disease and too much of the body. Too much thinking of the disease will intensify the malady. Keep the mind fully occupied in some way or the other. This is very important. Take away the mind from the body and think of the diseaseless Atman or soul within, the bed-rock or substratum for the body and mind. Friend, cultivate this kind of Atma-chintana (thinking of the Atman) and attain the painless state, or immortal Brahman.

Cheer yourself up. Have a cheerful countenance always. Meditate on OM*. Think of OM. Sing OM. OM is thy real name. OM is the best tonic, specific or sheet anchor, panacea or cure-all, 'pick-me-up' or sovereign remedy for all diseases. Smile and laugh. Thou art bodiless, undying Soul. Never, never forget this.

May God bless you with perfect health, high standard of vigour, strength, vitality and longevity. May you prosper gloriously! Om Shanti!

Karma and Laws of Nature

Man gets good health on account of good karma (actions) done in his previous birth. He who had done meritorious services in his previous incarnation, he who had shared what he had with others, he

---

*See *Raja Yoga: The Yoga System of Patanjali*

who had helped the poor and the needy, he who had done worship, meditation, yogic kriyas and pranayama in his previous births, enjoys sound health in this birth. The law of causation is inexorable and unrelenting.

Without cause there is no effect, so there is no sickness without violation of the laws of nature. Nature always tries to keep up health, but we bring on sickness by continuous violation of its laws. Of course the natural laws are relentless. There is no mercy.

There is seldom any sickness amongst the animal kingdom. They do not violate laws of nature and therefore they seldom require any medical help. Only rarely a few domesticated animals require some medical help as they cannot lead a natural life.

Some people inherit diseases from their parents. There are also diseases which are spread by infection or contagions (that is to say the air carries them, or they are imparted from one person to another by touch); these diseases consequently seize many persons who had no concern in originating them. Nevertheless, in such cases as in all others, the malady can be traced to human error, however innocent a particular victim may be. The parents, grandparents or some other ancestors must have contracted the disease by imprudence. Infectious and contagious diseases invariably take their rise from people dwelling in unhealthy places like marshes, or in the close and filthy parts of large cities, or from their not taking wholesome and sufficient food, or from not keeping themselves and their houses clean.

The whole universe, from the mightiest sun to the tiniest atom, is controlled by a supreme law. There is perfect order everywhere. The sun performs its duties quite regularly. It rises at the proper time and sets at the proper time. The stars and planets revolve in an orderly manner. They are governed by laws. There are laws in the mental plane. There are laws of physics, of astronomy, of mathematics. There are laws of hygiene and health which govern our being. In the vast universe man is the only breaker of laws and violater of rules. He is the single example of lawlessness and discord. He wilfully disregards the laws of health, leads a life of dissipation and then wonders why he suffers from diseases and disharmony. He deliberately ignores the rules of hygiene and right living and then weeps when he is ailing from an incurable, dire malady.

God has provided for you defensive forces in the body to act against the invaders, viz. the germs. The leucocytes or white cells in the blood fight with the germs and kill them. The lymphatic glands serve as strong fortresses. Further, an antidote called bacteriolysin is formed in the blood. This destroys the germs. How merciful is the Lord! He takes care of you in all possible ways. But you have forgotten Him. You have become ungrateful in not remembering Him. Let the past be buried. Try to remember Him from now and attain eternal bliss and immortality.

Spiritual Materia Medica

Anger: Generates poison in the blood and heat in the blood, brain, liver and the whole body; produces fever, depression, etc.

Hatred: Causes nervous weakness, uneasiness, restlessness, cough, fever, loss of blood, indigestion, etc.

Fear: Causes low blood pressure, weakness, destroys red blood cells, makes the face pale, affects the heart, liver and stomach, produces indigestion, diarrhoea or constipation and impotency.

Renunciation: Removes a host of ailments, such as dyspepsia, rheumatism, diabetes, diseases of the liver and the intestines, and blood pressure, and strengthens the heart, brain and nerves.

Pure Love: Produces joy, peace of mind and harmonious function of the bodily organs, increases the blood qualitatively and quantitatively and turns the mind towards God. It is the best antidote for hatred.

Truth: Strengthens the heart and mind, brings happiness, peace of mind, inner calmness and spiritual strength, and fearlessness. It is the best antidote for fear. It removes all diseases caused by fear.

Meditation: Wonderful tonic, tones all systems and organs, renovates the cells, enriches the cells of the blood, removes all diseases, checks the development of diseases, generates two miraculous health-giving, energy-producing, soul-elevating, kundalini-awakening principles — 'divinin' and 'puritin' — of marvellous potency, which transform man into divinity. 'Puritin' helps the meditator to enter into savikalpa samadhi. 'Divinin' helps him to attain nirvikalpa samadhi.

May you all be endowed with good health and long life! May you all be free from all kinds of diseases! May you all be established in that diseaseless, immortal Atman, through silent and ceaseless meditation!

How to Become a Centenarian

Do not worry, never be in a hurry. Do not eat what you call quick lunches. Take nutritious food. Never fool with doctors and do not go into a drug-store except to get a stamp or to consult the directory. (When you reach the age of ninety years you may do as you please!)

Wear loose collars, because tight collars present obstacles to the free circulation of the blood through the thyroid gland. Take large quantities of milk, this being the extract of various glands. Remain as much as possible in the open air and especially in the sunshine, and take plenty of exercise, taking care to breathe deeply and regularly. Take a bath daily, and in addition once a week or every two weeks take a Turkish or vapour bath. Wear porous clothing, light headdress and low shoes.

Go early to bed and rise early. 'Early to bed and early to rise makes a man healthy, wealthy and wise.' Sleep in a very dark, very quiet room with a window open, and do not sleep less than six or more than seven and a half hours. Give up alcohol. Be temperate in the use of tea or coffee. Avoid places that are overheated, especially by steam, and badly ventilated.

With advancing age toxicity is inevitable. If that is arrested, illnesses due to advancing age can be arrested. Toxicity due to advancing age can be overcome by combining the following:

*Viparita karani, not less than one hour both morning and evening.

Then, bandha traya in the following order — jalandhara bandha, uddiyana bandha and mulabandha.

If the above be combined with kevala kumbhaka, old age onset can be arrested.

---

*See Hatha Yoga Section

SCIENCE OF RELAXATION

Life has become very complex in these days. The struggle for existence is very acute and keen. There is unhealthy competition in every walk of life. There is unemployment everywhere. Brilliant young men with extraordinary qualifications and recommendations alone get a job in these days. Therefore a great deal of continuous mental and physical strain is imposed on modern humanity by its deadening daily work and unhealthy mode of life.

Man has acquired many artificial habits and has allowed nature's original habits to lapse. He has brought tension in many muscles and nerves through incorrect posture. He has forgotten the first principles of relaxation. He will have to learn lessons from the cat, dog and the infant in the science of relaxation.

If you practise relaxation no energy will be wasted. You will be very active and energetic. During relaxation the muscles and nerves are at rest. The prana or energy is stored up and conserved. The vast majority of persons who have no comprehensive understanding of this beautiful science of relaxation simply waste their energies by creating unnecessary movements of muscles and by putting the muscles and nerves under great strain. Some persons shake their legs unnecessarily while sitting. Some drum with their fingers on the table when their minds are idle or vacant. Some whistle. Some shake their heads. Some tap their chests or abdomen with their fingers. Energy is thus dissipated through unnecessary movements of the different parts of the body on account of lack of knowledge of the elementary principles of the science of relaxation.

Fatigue is due to the overworking of some part of the body. It may be the brain if you study too much or do much mental work or it may be bodily wear and tear when you rush about all day long, because you use up nervous energy as well. If something exciting happens you react and are soon tired when the thrill is over. You must at intervals relax and be restful during the day as well as at night.

When the brain gets tired the first sign is that you cannot keep your attention fixed on what you are doing, no matter how hard you try. The brain demands rest, relaxation. If you give your full attention to any kind of work or game it will be very interesting. You will have no feeling of tiredness.

Exercise is necessary for health. Relaxation is equally necessary. You get complete relaxation in sleep. Disturbed sleep or dreamy sleep does not give full relaxation. The person feels tired and exhausted when waking in spite of the sleep.

You can maintain good health by alternating exercise with relaxation. Only then the tissues of the body utilise the blood fully, absorb nutrition, grow, repair and throw off the waste material.

Remember well that laziness or indolence is quite different from relaxation. Do not mistake laziness for relaxation. The lazy man is inactive. He has no inclination for work. He is full of lethargy and inertia, whereas a man who practises relaxation has vigour, strength, vitality and endurance. He never allows even a small amount of energy to trickle away. He accomplishes wonderful work, gracefully, in a minimum amount of time.

When you feel sleepy it indicates that your system is in need of rest. Give the needed rest to the brain and body at once. A few minutes rest and relaxation serve as a great restorer and refreshener. You will be quite fit for doing further work efficiently. Develop the habit of sleeping at will at any time.

You can get relaxation even when you are awake or working. All the parts of the body do not work at the same time. When certain parts or tissues are working you can give rest and relaxation to other parts. You must know well the science of relaxation.

The quality of relaxation depends on the mental poise of the person. A man who has a worrying habit cannot relax well. He always gets disturbed, dreamy sleep.

Relaxation comes through discipline. Busy people such as doctors and lawyers should know the science of relaxation. They should practise it daily. They can relax the mind and take rest also in the waiting rooms of railway stations and bar rooms as well. They will thus be quite fit for further activity in the courts or the dispensary. Relaxation refreshes a man completely.

Yogis know this science well. They are perfect masters of this useful science. Those who practise relaxation can conserve their physical and mental energy and utilise it to their best advantage. They will never experience fatigue. They can close their eyes for a few minutes even while standing, and so prepare themselves for further work. Energy flows in their nerves when they relax, just as water flows when the tap is opened. Those who do not possess a knowledge of this science of external and internal relaxation waste their physical and mental energy considerably.

When you wish to contract a muscle in order to perform an action, an impulse is transmitted from the brain through the nerve to the muscle. Energy or prana travels through the motor nerves, reaches the muscle and causes it to draw its ends together. When the muscle contracts it pulls up the limb you wish to move. Suppose you wish to lift up a chair. The desire creates an impulse in the brain. The impulse is transmitted from the brain through the motor nerves to the muscles of the arms. A current of prana or energy is transmitted along the nerves from the brain. The muscles contract and you perform the action of lifting up the chair. All other actions — conscious or unconscious — are similarly performed by you. If the muscles are overworked, more energy is spent and you feel fatigue. There is much wear and tear in the muscles through overwork, strain and tension, on account of heavy expenditure of prana or energy.

An unconscious act is done instinctively or mechanically. The mind does not wait for orders. When the scorpion stings your finger, the finger is at once withdrawn. You do not argue here. This is an instinctive or mechanical movement.

The action of one set of muscles can be checked by the action of another set of muscles. One impulse may try to put one set of muscles in motion, and by sending another repressive impulse through another set of muscles you can counteract the action of the first set of muscles. For instance, if a man abuses you, you may jump at once to beat him. An impulse has already put one set of muscles in motion. You may check the impulse through discrimination and reflection — "I do not gain anything by beating him. He is an ignorant man. He does not know how to behave. Let me forgive him now." A repressive impulse will check at once the operation of the first set of muscles. Raising of impulses and counter-impulses or repressing impulses, cause high tension in nerves, muscles and brain. A large number of people are slaves of impulses; hence they do not enjoy peace of mind. They are tossed hither and thither.

The woman who can never relax, who never takes a real rest, will not retain her beauty. Her face will show signs of the fatigue her body is undergoing. Her body will lack poise. By being in a continual state of nervous tension (as many women are), she will grow old before her time, lose her looks and find that the tension has sapped all her strength away.

The science of relaxation is an exact science. It can be learnt very easily. Relaxation of the muscles is as important as contraction of the muscles. I lay great emphasis on the relaxation of the mind, the nerves *and* the muscles.

Relaxation is of two kinds, viz. mental relaxation and physical relaxation. There is another classification. If you relax certain muscles of certain parts only, it is partial relaxation. If you relax all the muscles of the whole body, it is complete relaxation.

If you can relax all the muscles, brain and nerves you will get sound sleep the moment you lie down on the bed. Mahatma Gandhiji knew this science well. Napoleon also had a full knowledge of it. They could get sleep at any part of the day or night, at any time, and could get up at the very second they wished to.

Even while at work you can relax if you are conversant with this science. You can take a nap even while sitting in a chair when several people are talking and laughing, or when there is beating of drums. There are many jobs which can be done in a sitting position — darning, mending, sewing and machine work. Be careful to sit correctly in order to avoid fatigue. Only a few women are aware of the fact that a faulty position may enlarge the hips.

He who has perfect mental poise can relax and sleep at any time. He who can relax well can turn out much work. Change of work or pose is rest or relaxation. Meditation gives perfect rest.

Relaxation for a few minutes will serve as a great restorer. Once in the morning and once in the afternoon relax completely for ten minutes at least. No matter how urgent the task, stick to this rule. Sit on a very comfortable chair or lie flat on a mattress; prop up the legs about eighteen inches from the ground with a stiff cushion under the knees and let every muscle go 'flop'. If lying on the mattress, a cushion under the head will relax the neck muscles. Close the eyes. Make the mind blank.

The idea of propping up the legs is to make the spine lie flat and to cool the feet by letting the blood run away from them. When resting in a chair, prop up the legs and relax every muscle. It will not come easily at first but it can be turned into a habit.

Never sit on the edge of a chair. Place the body well back and have a firm cushion to support the lower part of the back. Another thing to remember is to choose a chair of the correct height. Do not cross the legs. Sit with the knees and feet close together and firmly planted on the floor or on a stool.

Fatigue can be avoided at other tasks by adopting a correct standing posture. When a job necessitates your being on the feet for a long time, keep the knees and heels close together. This makes a pillar on which the body can rest. The weight of the body is not thrown on one leg or the other, but is distributed evenly on both.

Mental Relaxation

Just as you relax your muscles after having finished your asanas and physical exercises, so also you will have to relax the mind and rest it after concentration and meditation, after the practice of memory training and will culture. Relaxation of the muscles brings repose to the mind, while relaxation of the mind brings rest to the body as well. The body is a mould prepared by the mind for its enjoyment.

The mind gathers experiences through the body and works in conjunction with the prana, senses and body. The mind has influence over the body — for instance, if you are cheerful the body also will be healthy and strong, and when you are feeling depressed the body cannot work. Conversely the body has some influence over the mind. If the body is healthy and strong the mind will also be happy, cheerful and strong. If there is a stomach ache the mind cannot work. Thought takes form in action and action reacts on the mind. The mind acts on the body and the body reacts on the mind. Removal of tension in the muscles brings repose and calmness to the mind.

A man of easily irritable nature cannot enjoy peace of mind. His brain, nerves and muscles are always under high tension. Every minute he is wasting abundant muscular and nerve energy and brain power.

He is a very weak man though he may be endowed with physical strength, because he loses his balance of mind very easily. If you really want to enjoy unruffled peace and abiding joy, you must try to possess a calm, controlled and balanced mind by eradicating worry, anxiety, fear and anger, and by repressing impulses.

You do not gain anything by worrying yourself unnecessarily and manifesting anger for nothing at all. Fear, anger and worry are the products of ignorance. The muscles and nerves of a victim of anger and worry are always under contraction and high tension. Anger belongs to the brutal nature. Anger does positive injury to the brain, the blood and the nerves. You are not profited a bit by exhibiting anger. By repeating an action, a habit is formed in the mind. If you worry yourself frequently, a worrying habit is developed. Your vitality and energy are simply drained by worry, anger and fear. Why should you be afraid of anything at all, when everything is nothing but your own self?

Mental poise and calmness may be brought about by the eradication of worry and anger. Be careful and thoughtful. All unnecessary worries should be avoided. Expel all worry, fear and anger. Think of courage, joy, bliss, peace and cheerfulness.

By relaxation you give rest to the mind, tired nerves and overworked muscles. You will get immense peace of mind, strength and vigour. When you practise relaxation of either body or mind, the brain should not be occupied with various sorts of loose extraneous thoughts.

The practice of relaxation of mind will remove internal mental strain, will fill the mind with new mental energy and will make you cheerful and happy.

---

* For relaxation asanas, see page 172

EXERCISE

The Necessity for Exercise

Exercise is necessary at all periods of life and particularly during childhood and early manhood. It is very essential for keeping up good health, vim, vigour and vitality. It preserves the healthy tone of the body. Exercise bestows a general efficiency of body and mind, with a better social spirit and co-operation with your fellows. You learn to control the weak side of your nature and give fuller freedom to the best spirit that is in you. It checks overgrowth and develops the weak person. It quickly restores convalescent persons to better health. During growth it corrects various deformities. It removes debility and obesity.

Exercise is essential for the different organs of the body to function easily and effectively. It is necessary to promote the repair and formation of tissues, and excite the demand for oxygen needed for utilisation of food. Without exercise there will be no health. The whole system will refuse to function. The stomach will refuse to digest the food properly and the intestines will decline to function efficiently. The blood will be loaded with poisonous matter.

The heart cannot work efficiently without definite exercise. If you do exercise regularly it will drive the blood more vigorously. The lungs will take in the air with deep breaths. The chest will expand. More waste and used air will be driven out. When the action of the heart is improved by exercise, local congestions vanish. The blood is equally distributed and the circulation of blood in the lungs is improved. The amount of oxygen inspired and of carbon dioxide expired is greatly increased. It supplies more oxygen. The increased output demands increased supply of food and fresh air. It is best to take exercise in the open air, because you get much oxygen to purify the blood.

Exercise gives a healthy glow all over the body. Because it gives a rapid supply of blood, the kidneys, the lungs and the skin which remove the waste materials are stimulated. They do the function of cleansing more energetically and more efficiently. Muscular exercise has a beneficial effect on the body as a whole. It removes constipation and produces a regular action of the bowels. It leads to better mental efficiency and better performance of mental work. It promotes the action of the skin. There is increased perspiration. It reduces and regulates the temperature. After exercising, the body should be covered and protected from undue loss of heat.

All the movements of the body are done by muscles. Exercise increases the nutrition of the muscles. This contributes to their growth and energy. If you have well-developed muscles you can turn out more efficient work. If you do not exercise, the muscles will waste. You will be lazy and weak. You will have no power of endurance. If any organ or part of the body is not used, it gradually becomes smaller and less liable to work. For instance, if a broken limb is fixed with splints the limb will be found to be much smaller than the other when the splints are removed at the end of two or three weeks, because the muscles have wasted for want of use. But if the muscles are much used, they increase in size. A gymnast, an athlete, a blacksmith and a labourer in the field have strong, well-developed muscles in the arm, chest, etc. They have a wonderful and beautiful physique.

Well-developed biceps and chest are a source of great joy to a student. When he wants to show his general fitness he pulls up his sleeve and says, "Feel my biceps, O Ram. It is as hard as a stone." A football player says, "Look at the muscles of my calf. They are like big iron balls. I can walk thirty miles a day without any exertion." The gymnast shows his developed deltoid muscles and says, "Come along, Krishna, break a coconut on my deltoid muscle. I have a very strong deltoid muscle." However, strength and size are not always the same. Either a thin, a wiry or a heavy-built man may be strong.

A sick person after a prolonged illness is not able to walk or even stand by himself. As he has been in bed for a long time without using the muscles they have lost their strength. By doing mild exercises they gradually regain their lost tone and strength.

You should have a well-built body without adiposity. Fat hinders work by its extra weight, by giving rise to additional heat during work and by greater fatigue due to the accumulation of waste. Reduce the fat through regular and systematic exercise.

Exercise should be regulated and adjusted to the needs and capacity of the body. Violent exercises should be avoided. It is better to have recourse to graduated exercise.

Exercise should be systematic. Every muscle of the body should share in the exercise. Be regular in your exercise. Do not fatigue yourself or go beyond your capacity. If there is fatigue you have gone beyond your capacity. Reduce the number of exercises and the period of exercise. There should be perfect exhilaration of spirit after exercise. Infrequent, severe exercise is not very beneficial. It may do more harm than good.

(Some young persons become too fond of games. They neglect their studies and grow up with big bodies but little mental culture. Mental culture and spiritual culture should not be neglected. It is the mind that makes the man. It is the soul that makes the superman.)

Forms of Exercise

The forms of exercise are numerous. You should select that form which suits you best — whether it be riding, gymnastics, walking, running, swimming, rowing and boating, cycling, cricket, tennis, badminton, football, hockey and golf; the use of dumb-bells, bar-bells and Indian clubs; boxing and wrestling; or asanas, pranayama and suryanamaskara.

In cycling every muscle and nerve is used. The bowels are massaged by the muscles which form the abdominal wall and are thus made to act naturally.

Gymnastics develops and strengthens the muscles symmetrically. It increases the flexibility of the body and develops greater capacity for balance. Trapeze has a most excellent effect in shaping arms and shoulders.

No other exercise has so good an effect on the respiration and circulation as running. The outside air is pure and beneficial.

Nearly every muscle is called into play in rowing. The muscles of the back are particularly strengthened.

Swimming exercises all the limbs. It is a pleasant and invigorating form of exercise. It trains the respiratory muscles and it has a marked influence in straightening the back.

Cricket is very interesting. It keeps the players out in the open for hours. It provides the most varied movements and educates the hand and the eye to act in union.

Football is a good muscle-forming game. It promotes strength and develops the muscles of the leg and thighs, though it does not fully develop the arms and the chest.

Hockey necessitates much turning about and is beneficial to the trunk muscles.

The following rules for exercise should be observed:

1. Exercise should be taken in the open air. It should be repeated daily about the same hour. It should never be taken just after or just before meals.
2. The amount of exercise should be regulated according to the age, physical development or capacity of the individual.
3. Chills should be avoided after exercise.
4. Exercise should be regular and systematic.
5. Every part of the body should take part in the exercise.
6. After exercise the body should be washed or sponged.

SLEEP

If you want to enjoy good health you must take enough rest. There is always a cycle in nature. A period of activity is always followed by a period of inactivity. Even the heart has a period of rest, as there is a short pause between heart-beats. Sleep is the most perfect form of rest, because it is shared by every tissue in the body. The muscles are completely relaxed, the heart beats a little more quietly and the brain also takes rest.

As the day and night alternate, so there should be an alternating proportion of work and rest. Man works hard in daytime so that he may get what he desires most. He is tossed hither and thither by the two currents of likes and dislikes, so he gets tired. During work, and even when the limbs are resting, the nerves have to work. They also need relaxation. Relaxation is necessary for health. During rest the repair and renewal of the tissues takes place. Perfect relaxation is obtained in sleep. Nature takes him to her bosom at night to soothe his tired nerves and brain, to refresh him and to supply him with fresh energy and vigour so that he may continue his activities the next day. She makes him go to sleep. Sleep is a physiological phenomenon by which the mind, the brain and all the organs get rest for some hours. During sleep the mind goes back to its source. There is temporary absorption of the mind into its cause — avidya (ignorance).

Even when you are asleep some eternal principle is ever awake. He is the silent witness of the three states: waking, dream and deep sleep. He is the source, cause, substratum and support for everything. He is the Lord of Lords. He is the soul of all. The mind rests in Him during sleep and derives power, fresh energy and peace.

Vedantins make a deep study of sleep and draw conclusions about the all-blissful Atman, the silent witness of the state of deep sleep. The mind assumes a seed-like state in deep sleep. The tendencies and subtle desires become latent. All thoughts subside. The mind that was working in the brain during the waking state moves through susumna nadi into the heart and rests in Atman. The jiva (individual soul) is very near to Atman. A thin veil of ignorance separates him from Atman, just as the thin veil separates the husband from his wife. The husband rejoices as soon as his wife removes the veil; even so the individual soul rejoices as soon as the veil of ignorance is removed and he comes face to face with God. Mind, prana, senses and the body derive their power from the one silent witness of all minds. It is the soul that really moves the senses, mind and body, and nature works. So Atman is the all-doer and also the non-doer, all-enjoyer and also non-enjoyer.

Sleep is nature's tonic for a healthy life. The more sound sleep one has, the more healthy he will be. The hours of sleep necessary depend upon your physical and mental capacity for resisting fatigue. Without sufficient sleep you will not be efficient. The amount of sleep required varies with age, temperament and amount of work done. As age advances people require less sleep. Ten hours sleep is necessary for a child. For an old man over sixty years, six hours of sleep may be sufficient. Adults who work hard may sleep for eight hours. (Medical men and psychologists are paying great attention these days to the question of sleep.)

Too much sleep makes a man dull and lethargic. What is required is quality of sleep. Even if you have a sound, dreamless sleep for one or two hours, you will be perfectly refreshed. There is no benefit from rolling in the bed for hours. Too much sleep causes premature decay and weakens brain power.

There have been several instances of famous men who kept fit and active with less sleep than that enjoyed by most people. Scaliger, the French scholar and contemporary of Shakespeare, slept only for three hours. Wellington and Sir Henry Thomson, the famous physician who attained the age of 80, both considered that four hours of sleep was sufficient. So did Edison, who for thirty years limited his sleep to the same number of hours. Persons who do brain work are in need of more sleep and rest than those who do physical labour. Weak, debilitated and sick persons require more sleep and repose than healthy persons.

Avoid going late to bed. When you sleep keep all the windows and doors of your bedroom open. The more oxygen you inhale during your sleep the more refreshed you will feel throughout the next day. Do not take drugs to make your sleep. If you cannot sleep naturally take a brisk walk in the open air for fifteen minutes and then go to bed. You are sure to have refreshing sleep.

Sleep on your side, especially on the left side. This helps to empty the stomach. Keep the same time daily for sleep. Wear loose clothing. Do not cover yourself with heavy blankets or clothing.

Sleep with your head towards the east. Do not sleep with your head towards the north. You can sleep with your head towards the west or south.

Sleeping in the day time should be avoided, especially after a meal, as it tends to induce dyspepsia or indigestion and possibly diseases of the liver. However, a short nap, particularly in the summer in the afternoon, is refreshing and invigorating for those who do very active work in the morning.

Do not cover your head during sleep. It is quite unhygienic. You will inhale again the foul air exhaled by the lungs. Two persons should not sleep together for this reason. Lamps, candles and charcoal fires vitiate the air and should not be kept burning in the bedroom. Cooking should not be done in the bedroom. You will get sound sleep if you sleep in a quiet, dark, well-ventilated room.

Do not take any food late at night. Late supper makes the brain work and disturbs sleep. The brain is called upon to work the digestive organs vigorously while it should be sleeping restfully. If you wish to get sound sleep you must regulate the hour of your last meal of the day. If 9 or 10 p.m. is the usual hour for sleep, do not take food after 6 p.m. You will have sound sleep. If you suffer from constipation, if the bowels are loaded, take a douche one hour before sleep. You will have sound sleep. (Do not develop a douche or enema habit, however.) Massage also induces sleep. Massage diverts blood from the brain to the exercised parts and this induces sleep.

Review your actions of the day before going to bed. Write down your spiritual diary. Make fresh resolves for the next day — such as 'I will not use vulgar or harsh words, I will control anger. I will observe celibacy. I will control passion, etc.' Repeat some prayer or sublime slokas of the *Bhagavad Gita* or *Upanishads*. Roll the beads of your mala for ten minutes and meditate on the form of the Lord and His divine attributes. Do not build castles in the air. Give up scheming and planning. If you have ill-feeling against anyone, forget it. Have pleasant thoughts only. Good spiritual ideas will sink down deep into the subconscious mind. You will enjoy sound sleep, free from evil dreams.

In going to sleep your eye-lids close first. The brain does not receive any message or impression from the eyes. The sense of taste and smell then go and then your ears fall asleep. Last of all the skin ceases to feel touch. The whole body is asleep.

Keeping wide awake throughout the night is called vigil. You will derive incalculable benefits if you practise vigil on holy days. You can practise vigil on every Ekadasi also. Complete fasting helps in the control of sleep. Control of sleep by taking recourse to tea is not desirable. You will not gain spiritual strength thus, as you have to depend upon an extraneous drug.

Half of your lifetime is wasted in sleep. Those spiritual aspirants who want to do rigorous sadhana should reduce their period of sleep gradually. They can get real rest from meditation. For three months reduce the sleeping period by half an hour. Go to bed at 10.30 p.m. and get up at 4 a.m. During the next three months go to bed at 11 p.m. and get up at 4 a.m. Four hours sleep will amply suffice. You should not sleep in the daytime. In course of time you should become a conqueror of sleep like Arjuna and Lakshmana, and rest in the all-blissful, sleepless sleep, the nirvikalpa samadhi of yogis.

Sleep as a condition of rest cannot be governed by hard and fast rules. Much depends on a person's physical and mental capacity for resisting fatigue. Everything depends upon the constitution and on the amount of work as well as the kind of work which has been done during that day. Those who have reached the years of discretion should decide for themselves the amount of sleep they require.

THE BEST THERAPY

Natural Treatment

The natural form of treatment is the best form of treatment. Nature's cure is the best cure. Natural living is the best living. Natural food is the best form of food. Be natural in all ways of living. You will enjoy good health, long life and happiness. In truth, nature does everything in the cure of all diseases. Medicines help nature in the recuperative work and the regenerative or constructive process in the bodily mechanism. That doctor who tries to help nature is a judicious doctor. By injudicious treatment a doctor may do much harm to the patient. Nature's healing may be interfered with or retarded by drugs. He who says "I have cured such and such a disease," is also an ignorant man.

Avoid drugs. Give up high and loose living. Eat simple, natural foods. Live in the open air. Take cold baths. Be moderate in food, drink and everything else. Wear simple dress. Bask in the sunshine. Enjoy the ultra violet rays in the morning. Take exercises regularly. Do not go to doctors frequently. Eat simple, natural foods. Eat to live. Give rest to the organs by occasional fasting. Take raw things as much as possible. Do not throw away the water from rice and boiled vegetables. Use just enough water to cook them properly. You will be healthy, strong and vigorous. You will be endowed with a high standard of vim, vigour and vitality.

If you become ill, nip the malady in the bud. Do not allow it to strike deep roots. Your body is a mysterious machine. You are its driver. Learn how to take care of it properly, how to run it smoothly and efficiently and how to repair it when it gets out of order. Become a master-driver of this wonderful machine. Endeavour to qualify yourself as an expert nature-healer. Obey nature's laws. You cannot find health in bottles with beautiful labels, so do not be carried away by pompous advertisements. Health is nature's reward for obedience to her laws. If you obey the laws of nature the curative and reconstructive forces within your body will rebuild and renew your cells and tissues, heal them, and remove the deleterious effects caused by disobedience of nature's laws.

The man who does not care for his health, who leads a happy-go-lucky life and who is a glutton, is a sinner and a criminal. He must be rigorously punished. He has no business to be sickly when he can have abundant life, vitality, energy and health by natural ways of living and by observing the simple rules and laws of health and hygiene.

Shun all sweetmeats ruthlessly. In Bengal one out of five is suffering from diabetes. Horrible and pitiable! This is due to taking too many sweetmeats. After all, man needs very little food on this earth. The palate and the tongue kill him. Man should pay the penalty when he transgresses nature's laws. He will suffer. He must learn lessons.

(The juice of a small lemon, spinach, one or two tomatoes, a little fresh coconut, bananas, gram soaked in water, green gram sprouts, half a pint of milk and two teaspoons of honey can give you wonderful health, vigour, vitality and longevity.)

O man! Why are you lingering with disease and poor health. Why are you dragging a cheerless existence? Enjoy the joys of supreme health by treading the path of nature. Swim in nature's sweet stream. Take a plunge bath in it. Float in it and rejoice. Be always healthy, wealthy, strong and wise.

As a wise gardener acts in obedience to the law of nature, so it is laid down for us that we should treat our bodies as instruments of an infinite power, and not as opponents of its purpose. Nature requires but slight attention on our part in the task of maintaining good health.

Pure food, cleanliness, rest and reasonable exercise represent the easy service expected of us for our health, comfort and repair, and in return we may derive a thousandfold blessing.

Cheerfulness is a healthy tonic. Be cheerful always. Mind can cure all the physical diseases of the body by harmonious, healthy and divine thoughts, because all physical diseases have taken their origin in mental ill-health. Lack of cheerfulness contributes to physical ill-health. If one is always cheerful and entertains good, divine thoughts he will not suffer from any disease and will have perfect health at all times. It is in your power to continue to be well and youthful as long as you like.

Firm faith in God and reliance upon your eternal immortal inner Atman will keep the mind in a vigorous and positive state. Know that He is manifest as the pure air, as the energising sun, as the vitalising elixir in the mellow fruits. Feel His healing power working through every pore of your body, through every cell, blood corpuscle and nerve fibre. Try to actually feel how your entire system is responding to the recuperative action of the various methods of treatment employed.

Allow the body to freely respond to the action of the natural agents. Put yourself in tune with the source of all health, power and strength. The cosmic force for well-being will then fill you. This is the ultimate factor behind all therapeutics, the secret to bear in mind. The doctor cannot impart this vital secret to you. Now you know it. Use it as the background for the treatment of your bodily and mental ills.

With your being harmonised with the all-pervading cosmic Being, with a cheerful, optimistic mind and a body rejuvenated through sufficient rest, wise choice of diet, sunshine, exercise and bath, you will easily ward off all diseases, have wonderful strength and vitality and cross this ocean of earthly existence by vigorous spiritual practices. Through His abundant grace and blessing may you attain health and long life!

Important Factors

An important and prominent factor in keeping good health is the air. We must spend as much of our life as is possible in open air. This is difficult in the case of many persons who have to work indoors in offices, factories and business concerns, as they have to lead their life in congested areas. Those who can afford some time in the early morning should take a walk or run in the invigorating hours of the dawn or in the evening in the open air. The early morning air contains more ozone and hence is most pleasant and effective in giving us exuberant health.

In addition we should do some abdominal gymnastics, sun exercises (surya namaskar), yoga postures (asanas) and breathing exercises (pranayama). Those who cannot take a walk should certainly do some exercise. They should wear as little clothing as possible and should expose their bodies to the air as much as possible.

The second important element in the preservation of health is water. As soon as we get up from bed we should drink one or two glasses of water, which helps the evacuation of the bowels. A cup of hot water half an hour before meals helps much to keep up good health. A cold bath is also important, and that also should be taken in the morning. After the bath the body should be rubbed well with a towel.

The third most important element in the preservation of health is sunlight. Sunlight is most essential for the growth of both the plant and the animal kingdom. Those plants and trees which do not get enough sunlight become stunted in growth. If we expose our bodies to the rays of the morning sun we gain much vitality from the sunlight. There should be enough light in places of work. The doors and windows should be kept open to allow the sunlight to enter. Even in winter the doors and windows should be kept open and we should protect our bodies with enough clothes. The dress should always be light and loose.

The fourth important factor is food. Though we boast ourselves to be civilised men, when the question of food comes we make many imperceptible blunders. For instance, the English system of breakfast and taking food often is not compatible with the tropical climate of our country.

Food is a substance which builds up or repairs tissues and supplies material for the production of heat and energy. The right kind of food is most important. Half the illnesses of the nation are due to an ill-balanced diet. There is no mystery about diet. It can be learnt very easily. A correct diet is a fundamental factor in the maintenance of perfect health and a high standard of vitality. Good food is not expensive. A well balanced diet is not costly.

Unwholesome, stale food produces irritating poisons in the blood, which cause various kinds of disorders. The liver and the kidneys are taxed by high and luxurious living. Rich people who lead a life of dissipation suffer from organic diseases of the liver and kidneys. They have to pay a heavy penalty because they have violated the laws of nature and the laws of health. Drinking alcohol affects the liver. Eating meat, beef, etc. affects the kidneys. Nature puts a check on the man who violates her laws by inducing chronic structural diseases of the vital organs. This is the punishment by Mother Nature on her impertinent children who transgress her law.

Without food you cannot live, but you eat more than you need. You season the foodstuff with spices which harm the stomach and intestines. As all palatable food is tempting, man takes more food than is actually necessary for the upkeep of the body. He eats three times as much as is necessary to keep him well. He unduly overloads his stomach. He loses control over the tongue and the power of discrimination when he sits in front of tempting dishes. He says "I must eat to my heart's content today. It does not matter even if I load my stomach and suffer from dyspepsia. I will take a strong purgative and a dose of some carminative mixture in the morning." How powerful is the tongue! More people die of over-eating than of under-eating. You press your friends to eat some extra sweets even after a full sumptuous meal. Mothers overfeed their children. Women waste their time, energy and money in preparing different varieties of palatable dishes. They try to exhibit their utmost skill in presenting diverse tasty dishes. But, after all, man wants very little on this earth.

The most natural food of man is green vegetables, fruits, roots and milk, i.e. uncooked food. Fruits and vegetables which are sun-cooked are the elixir of life and are nature's remedies. Animals living on sun-cooked food have more strength and seldom fall sick. The animals that live on grass, green leaves, fruits and roots are stronger than man. The cooking of foods takes away many vital elements from the food and so we cannot get the needed vitality from the foods which are conventionally cooked.

Since ages men have been accustomed to cooked foods and it becomes difficult to change the old habits all of a sudden. So the golden mean is to take one meal as usual and the next meal should consist of milk and fruits only.

We should have no breakfast — only a cup of milk or juice of lemon, orange or tomato in a cup of hot or cold water, after bath. Instead of milk, buttermilk can be taken. If nothing is available, a cup of hot or cold water will suffice. We should not discard our usual meal in the morning, but avoid fried and spiced food and sweets as much as possible.

This alone is not sufficient. There is also the necessity of avoiding unwholesome foods. Tea, coffee and other stimulants should be avoided as far as possible. In the afternoon, instead of tea or coffee, we can take one or two fruits available in the season. Abstinence from alcohol, cold drinks and other beverages is also necessary.

On one day once a week we should have two meals of fruits, milk and vegetables only. Our evening meal should consist mainly of fruits and vegetables and milk. It should be finished before 7 or 8 p.m.

Occasional fasts to correct our errors against natural life are as essential as occasional feasts which are often inevitable. An occasional use of enema or castor oil or any vegetable laxative is necessary to clean the bowels when we feel constipated.

The practice of going to bed early and rising in the early morning is also most essential. Working till late hours at night should be avoided as far as practicable. We should go to bed between 10 and 11 p.m.

Celibacy is also necessary for maintaining radiant health. One who practices celibacy is free from diseases. He is healthy and attains longevity.

All excesses in enjoyment should be avoided. Too much cinema going is also a sin against health and nature.

It is the mind which controls the body, so we should try to keep cheerful under all circumstances. A strong mind helps much to ward off ill-health; not only this, but it aids us in preserving good health and effecting a speedy cure. It is the mind which creates heaven or hell, so we should always try to keep cheerful at all times.

An ordinary man cannot change the circumstances or effect a revolution. He must adapt himself to the circumstances. Knowing that they are not under our control, it is our duty to struggle hard against them with a hope of success, which is slow but sure if our attempts are in the right direction. We should not entertain pessimistic thoughts. God is always good. The apparent difficulties which we have to face in life are for our progress, and we must pray to God to find out means and measures to overcome them.

Before going to bed we must bring the image of our favourite deity before our mind's eye and pray to God fervently to give us health, wealth and power to fight the battle of life successfully.

The overproduction of luxuries and means of destruction has brought on a crisis. The current of the crisis is so strong that none can check it. Only an incarnation of God can give a right turn to the current of adverse circumstances which are drifting towards destruction.

The luxuries give a momentary enjoyment, but ultimately they have a very unsalutary effect upon our health. It has been found that with all the possible means of enjoyment man is losing his natural power of enjoyment. With natural methods of living the health of the past generation was very good. Now with all possible conveniences the health of the present generation is very delicate.

The present advance in modern civilisation has made the necessities of life expensive. The majority of people do not get nourishing food. The tendency towards self-appeasement and exorbitant profits has induced manufacturers to resort to unlawful and unjust means for their personal gain. Machinery has made a very few excessively rich, while the majority of people have become very poor and are not able to get even enough food for their maintenance. The only way out of this chaos is to turn towards plain living and high thinking. It will give us a healthy body and a sound mind.

Body building is the foundation of nation-building. Build the body through nature's aids. Avail yourself of the healing agencies of nature —sun, water, air, earth, fasting, herbs etc. Observe the laws of eating, drinking, sleeping, thinking and conducting oneself as laid down by the ancient sages. Live in tune with nature.

To sum up: good physical health can be achieved and maintained by observing rigidly the laws of health and the rules of hygiene; by taking wholesome, light, substantial, easily digestible, nutritious, bland food; by inhaling pure air; by regular physical exercise; by a daily cold bath and by observing moderation in eating and drinking. Good mental health can be attained and maintained by japa; meditation; celibacy; practice of *yama, *niyama and right conduct; right thinking, right feeling, right speaking and right action; enquiring into the nature of the Self; change of thought; relaxation of mind by dwelling on pleasant thoughts; mental recreation and the practice of cheerfulness, etc.

---

* See *Raja Yoga: The Yoga System of Patanjali*

FOOD

Man continually works, whether he sleeps or sits quietly. Breathing is work. When work is done, energy is spent. The body supplies this energy by combustion of food. Blood gets its supply from food-materials. The lamp burns oil as fuel and gives light as heat and energy. Even so the human body burns food as fuel and gives energy in the form of heat and motion. In an engine, oil or petrol is burnt; in this marvellous human engine, food serves the purpose of fuel. Engines are in need of different kinds of fuel — coal, oil or petrol according to their construction. All the fuels contain carbon. Carbon burns and supplies energy. In the human engine, which is very delicate and complex, carbohydrates, fats, etc., provide this carbon.

Proteins

Proteins are nitrogenous or flesh-forming substances. They supply material for growth and to replace wear and tear of tissues. They build and repair tissues.

In an engine, parts have to be renewed from time to time. So it is with the body. The working parts need continual overhauling and renewal. This necessitates the supply of protein. A piece of skin is torn off. The body promptly sets to work to renew it. New cells are manufactured rapidly. The part is reconstructed within a short time. Protein is necessary for this.

Proteins are formed by the linkage of twenty different 'building blocks' called amino-acids. The value of protein depends on its amino-acid content. The difference between proteins is due to the number, arrangement and proportion of the different amino-acids. They are essential for nutrition, and also provide energy. The daily requirement of the body for protein is approximately one gramme per kilo of body-weight.

Fats

Fats or hydrocarbons are great heat-producers. They are 'protein sparing foods', our main source of calories, and are more concentrated than carbohydrates. One gramme of fat when burnt in the body produces 9.5 calories, while one gramme of starch will yield only 4.8 calories and cane-sugar only 3.95 calories. Animal fats are carriers and sources of the fat soluble vitamins, vitamin A, D and E. Fat is not easily burnt in the body unless there are carbohydrates present. The fats delay the passage of food from the stomach and so give a feeling of lasting satisfaction. Fats yield about two and a quarter times as much energy as an equal amount of carbohydrates or protein and reduce the bulk of food intake.

Carbohydrates

Carbohydrates include substances like starch, rice, arrowroot, barley, wheat, sugar, etc. They are sources of heat and energy, and supply fuel for the human engine. Sugar is a concentrated and readily combustible form of carbohydrate. It supplies energy immediately when the body is exhausted. Other carbohydrates need a longer time for their conversion into sugar.

During digestion, rice and other kinds of starches, milk-sugar etc. are changed into glucose before they are absorbed. The excess sugar is stored up in the liver and muscles as glycogen. Prolonged muscular work during starvation may exhaust the entire store of glycogen in the body.

Carbohydrates are the most easily digested, absorbed and metabolised of the foods. If you take too much carbohydrate the islets of Langerhans in the pancreas are overworked. Diabetes is produced.

The body always needs carbohydrates to digest fats. The foods which give warmth and energy are fats and carbohydrates. They form 80 per cent of our diet. Protein forms only 20 per cent. Any protein is burnt and utilised for warmth and energy when the body has satisfied its needs for repair and growth.

Mineral Salts

Lime, iron, phosphorus, sodium, potassium, magnesium, copper, iodine, sulphur, common salt, etc. are found in the blood. These elements are lost each day by the body and must be replaced from the food. They are essential to the body. If we take any tissue of the body and completely burn it, we will find a small amount of incombustible material. This incombustible material is called ash. This ash contains the mineral salts.

Mineral salts form about one-twentieth of the body weight and are necessary for the maintenance of the body. They form part of every cell, and play a vital part in the regulation of the acid-alkali balance. There are fifteen different mineral elements. Each has its own special part to play.

Phosphorus, sulphur and chlorine are the acid-forming elements. Calcium, sodium, iron, manganese, copper and magnesium are found in the body in large amounts and are the alkali-forming elements. They are also the most important.

Every cell in the body contains phosphorus. It is necessary for the multiplication of cells and the growth of the body. The daily requirement in the diet is 1.5 gms., or more during pregnancy. Its deficiency is characterised by softening of the bones, stunted growth, rickets and caries of teeth. Foods rich in phosphorus are cheese, milk, oatmeal, almonds, nuts, peas, beans, whole wheat, spinach, potatoes and okra (lady's fingers).

Calcium phosphate is necessary for the development of bones. Milk is the best source. Green vegetables and certain of the millets are rich in calcium, but this calcium is not so easily absorbed as the calcium of milk. Calcium is essential for children, and during pregnancy and lactation. The minimum requirement of calcium in the body is O.45 gm.

Iron is the most important part of the red pigment of the blood (haemoglobin) and enables it to carry oxygen from the lungs to the tissues. Pulses, whole cereal grains, lettuce, dried fruits, spinach, dates, figs, raisins and tomatoes contain iron.

Iodine is an essential constituent of the thyroid gland. Goat's milk, fresh vegetables and sea vegetables contain iodine. Goitre is due to lack of iodine in the water.

Vitamins

In the last few decades a revolution has occurred in the history of dietetics. Scientists and doctors have found that although the required quantity of proteins, fats, carbohydrates and mineral salts are taken daily, the system can fail to discharge its functions. Growth is checked, loss of weight follows, leading eventually to death.

After repeated and continued research, they found out that in addition to the building, repairing and working materials, some other substances in minute amounts were needed to make the body function properly. These mysterious substances were named vitamins or life-giving substances.

Vitamins exist in food in minute quantities. A diet deficient in vitamins produces certain diseases, and may even cause death. Rickets, scurvy, pelagra, beri beri, xerophthalmia or keratomalnia and osteomalacia are some of the diseases produced by the lack of vitamins in food. Green vegetables and fresh fruits are rich in vitamins. Some vitamins are water-soluble, some are fat-soluble.

Vitamin 'A': It is a fat-soluble vitamin. It protects the body from infection. It is known as the anti-infective vitamin. Butter, milk, cheese, the green and yellow vegetables, fruits and tomatoes are rich in Vitamin 'A'. Carotene which is found in abundance in carrots can act as Vitamin 'A'. Deficiency in Vitamin 'A' leads to night blindness; ulceration of the eye; xerophthalmia; infection of respiratory and alimentary tracts, bladder and urethra; low resistance to bacterial infection and dryness of the skin.

Vitamin 'B': The substance removed while polishing rice is rich in vitamin 'B'. Vitamin 'B' is in the outer coating of rice and wheat. It is the most important vitamin for health and well-being. It is complex and consists of many factors. Vitamin 'B' protects one from skin trouble. Absence of Vitamin 'B1' causes beri beri. It is found in the outer layers of cereals and legumes, and in yeast, nuts, tomatoes, green leaves, oranges and milk. Marmite is a valuable source of this vitamin.

Vitamin 'C': Vitamin 'C' is present in the juices of a large number of fruit and vegetables. To ensure its presence in the diet some fresh fruit or salad is necessary. Apple has only a small amount of vitamin 'C'. Grapes are almost deficient in Vitamin 'C'. Oranges, lemons, cabbages, turnips, tomatoes, amla, citrus fruits, rose-hips and green vegetables are rich in Vitamin 'C'. The Vitamin 'C' is soluble in water, and suffers much destruction in cooking. (It is also called ascorbic acid.)

Scurvy is due to the prolonged absence of Vitamin 'C' from the diet. Sailors in sailing ships have invariably been troubled with scurvy when there is lack of fresh fruits and vegetables. The absence of this vitamin causes caries of the teeth, anaemia, etc.

Vitamin 'D': Vitamin 'D' is fat-soluble. It is an anti-rachitic vitamin. It is very necessary for the calcification of bones and prevention and cure of rickets. The human system can synthesise Vitamin 'D' from the sun's rays.

Vitamin 'D' is contained in milk, butter and ghee; vegetable oils develop Vitamin 'D' on exposure to the sun.

Even if calcium and phosphates are found in fair proportion, bones cannot be nicely developed without a proper supply of Vitamin 'D', the forming agency. The practice of smearing the body well with mustard oil and exposing it to the sun is a good method of imbibing Vitamin 'D'. The food one eats must contain the bone-forming materials calcium and phosphorous in the right proportion. If these are absent, exposure to the sun is not useful.

Vitamin 'E': This is an anti-sterility vitamin. It is fat-soluble, and is necessary for reproduction. It is found in abundance in the embryos of seeds, and in green leaves (chiefly lettuce), cotton seeds, maize, peas, oats, corn and wheat germ oil. If wheat germ oil is given to sterile women or women who have had repeated abortions, it helps them to conceive and give birth to normal children.

Vitamin 'K': This is a coagulation vitamin. It is fat-soluble. Deficiency of this vitamin causes prolongation of blood-clotting time. It is found in spinach, carrots, tomatoes and soyabean oil.

Water in the Human System

Water forms 64 per cent of the body weight. It helps the solution and dilution of solid foods, it compensates for the loss caused by the excretory organs and helps the free elimination of the products of metabolism. Thirst indicates the demand for water.

Vegetable Acids

These are not really foods, but they are essential for the preservation of health. Tartaric acid, citric acid, oxalic acid and malic acid are the important vegetable acids. They are derived from fresh fruits and vegetables, and form carbonates in the system, thus preserving the alkalinity of the blood and other fluids.

Calorie and Calorimeter

A calorie is the amount of heat needed to raise one gramme of water one degree centigrade at 15 degrees centigrade. A kilocalorie is the amount of heat needed to raise 1 kilogramme of water one degree centigrade. The kilocalorie is equal to 1000 calories. The heat value of 1 gm of protein and 1 gm of carbohydrate is 4.1 kilocalories each. The heat value of 1 gm of fat is 9.3 kilocalories.

The amount of heat and energy which each food can impart to the body, if it is completely digested and utilised, can be ascertained by a calorimeter.

A man of average weight doing a moderate amount of muscular work must take enough food to give 3000 calories per day. A man who does sedentary work needs 2170 calories. An agriculturist who does active work in the fields needs 3500 calories. In finding out the calories, age, sex, height, build and work etc. have to be taken into consideration.

The value of a certain food depends upon its digestibility and absorbability. A food that is easily digested is not necessarily one that is completely absorbed, and a food that is completely absorbed is not necessarily one that is easily digested.

The interval between two meals should be four or five hours. Regularity in the time for taking food is very important. The stomach should not be disappointed when it is eagerly hoping to get its food for digestion. If the food is not supplied at the proper times there will be griping pain and burning in the stomach owing to the action of gastric juice on the empty stomach and rubbing of the walls of the stomach against each other.

Philosophical Vitamins

The following philosophical vitamins excel the ordinary medical vitamins. They give wonderful health and pave the way for the attainment of God-realisation:

VITAMIN A: adaptability, abstinence, austerity.

VITAMIN B: brahmacharya (celibacy), bravery, balance of mind, Brahma-chintana (constant meditation on Brahman), bhakti (devotion).

VITAMIN C: compassion, consideration, charity, courage, co-operation, cleanliness, contemplation, contentment, constancy, concentration.
VITAMIN D: desirelesness, diligence, discipline, detachment.
VITAMIN E: equanimity, endurance.
VITAMIN F: faith, forgiveness, friendliness, firmness, fasting fortitude, fearlessness, forbearance, frankness.
VITAMIN G: generosity, good will, gentleness.
VITAMIN H: humility, honesty.
VITAMIN I: innocence, industriousness.
VITAMIN K: kindness, knowledge.
VITAMIN L: loyalty, love.
VITAMIN M: mauna (silence), magnanimity, mercy, moderation, modesty, meditation.
VITAMIN N: nobility, non-covetousness, non-violence.
VITAMIN O: obedience.
VITAMIN P: patience, perseverance, purity, politeness.
VITAMIN R: Renunciation, regularity, resourcefulness righteousness.
VITAMIN S: self-control, self-sacrifice, satisfaction, satsang, self-effacement, sympathy, serenity, simplicity, steadfastness, study of scriptures, self-realisation.
VITAMIN T: tolerance, tranquillity, truth.
VITAMIN U: understanding, uprightness.
VITAMIN V: vairagya (dispassion), vigour.
VITAMIN W: wisdom.

A WELL—BALANCED DIET

A well-balanced diet is very necessary for growth, development and maintenance of good health and a high standard of vigour, vim and vitality. This is particularly essential for growing children, pregnant women and nursing mothers.

The supply of the inorganic mineral salts such as calcium, phosphorous, iron and iodine; protein; fats and carbohydrates; vitamins etc. must be adequate. The diet should provide the same number of calories daily. The food-stuff must be readily digestible and assimilable. The different food-stuffs must be in proper proportion. The proteins should be of good quality and should contain the necessary amino-acids. Then alone will the diet be well-balanced.

If you have an unbalanced diet for a very long time you will develop deficiency diseases.

Vegetarian Food

Cereals, pulses, roots and tubers, green vegetables, fruits and nuts constitute vegetarian food. Cereals are rich in nitrogenous substances and starch, but poor in fat. The different cereals are wheat, maize or Indian corn, rice, millet, oats, bajra or cambu and barley.

Cereals contain phosphates of calcium, magnesium, potash and a small amount of iron, plus protein, carbohydrate and fat. Maize is relatively rich in fat and slightly deficient in salts. Rice is very rich in starch but poor in protein, fat and mineral matter. Millet is inferior to wheat in proteins but superior to it in fat. Oats are quite rich in fat and protein, and the most nutritive of all the cereals. As all cereals contain abundant carbohydrates they should be eaten with foods rich in protein and fat.

Pulses are abundant in nitrogenous substances. They contain the vegetable protein, legumine. Pulses should be taken with rice.

Potatoes, sweet-potato, arrowroot, tapioca, sago, carrots, beetroot and radish belong to the class of roots and tubers.

Fruits and milk form a very healthy, wholesome diet, and help concentration of mind. It is the diet of rishis and raja yogis. It is also the diet of hatha yogis who practise pranayama vigorously. Try to live on milk and fruits on Sundays. The value of milk as a tissue-building agent when taken alone or in combination with fresh fruits cannot be too strongly emphasised. Milk is a perfect food as it contains all the dietetic principles in well-balanced proportion.

Amongst the different foods, fruits stand foremost in importance in the yogi's menu or regimen. The curative effects of fresh juicy fruits are astonishing. These juices cleanse the tissues and throw out the morbid materials from the bodily system. They fill the body with vitalising or life-giving mineral salts, potassium, sodium, manganese, iron, calcium etc. They also supply Vitamin 'C' and roughage. They contain alkaline matter which helps to keep the blood pure and free from acidity. They keep the bowels open owing to roughage.

Fruits are very good for invalids, also for those suffering from acute diseases. Fruits freshly plucked from the tree are very good. Fruit juices are ideal beverages for children, the aged and convalescents.

The all-fruit diet is the finest eliminating medium. In the treatment of lumbago the patient is put on a diet of oranges alone. The uric acid that is accumulated in the system is eliminated quickly by this diet. The body becomes light when one lives on fruits alone. Tamas is destroyed. You can conquer sleep if you live on a fruit diet. Those who live on fruits alone experience a peculiar inexpressible ananda or bliss. They sometimes feel that they have no body. Some people when they change their diet and live on fruits, feel weakness in the beginning, because their stomachs were habituated to heavy starchy food. They used to load their stomachs to the brim. After sometime, through force of the new habit, the feeling of weakness will vanish. The all-fruit diet can be carried on for two weeks or more with ease by most people. When all other remedies fail in the treatment of chronic diseases, an all-fruit diet may work wonders.

Fruits are rich in acids and sugar but deficient in proteins and lime. Milk contains plenty of these two necessary principles. Hence a diet of fruits and milk combined is a proper diet. This is more suitable for aspirants who wish to do a lot of meditation, old persons and those with weak digestive power.

This diet keeps the urine alkaline and prevents the formation of stones in the bladder and acidosis. The best time for eating fruits is the morning or after breakfast. 'Fruit in the morning is gold, in afternoon silver, and in evening lead.' This is the popular proverb. Overripe and unripe fruits should be avoided.

If you remove fruits from this world, half of its attraction will vanish. If you remove fruits, milk, sugar and woman, the attraction of the world will totally disappear. They are all products of maya to make the passionate man cling to this world.

Friend, why do you take carnivorous foods and spoil your health? Carnivorous foods excite passion and make the mind restless. Fruits exercise a soothing influence on the mind and subdue passion. Man leads an artificial life in these days of modern civilization and scientific advancement. He lives on patent foods, drinks alcohol, puts on tight collars, attends theatres, eats all sorts of things in hotels and restaurants, forgets God and the goal of life, leads an unnatural life of dissipation and meets with various sorts of diseases and premature death. What a sad, lamentable state!

If you take pure food you will have a pure mind. Mind is formed out of the subtlest essence of food. If you have purity of mind you will remember Atman, and the knots of the heart — ignorance, desire and ignorant action — will be rent asunder. You will attain liberation.

If you would attain longevity and possess good health and vigour you must go back to nature. Lead a simple natural life with high sublime thinking. Develop ethical virtues, control the senses and the mind, practise meditation, realise the Self and be forever free.

He who dwells in the fruit-juice, who is within the juice, whom the juice does not know, who rules the juice from within, is your immortal Atman or inner Ruler.

Grapes

Grapes are one of the best blood-purifiers. They are a valuable general tonic. The functional activity of all the organs of the body is stimulated by eating grapes. They cause general improvement in the tone of the body.

Grapes contain citric and tartaric acids. These acids are converted into alkalis after digestion and increase the alkalinity of the blood. Citric acid helps the absorption of uric acid deposits. Grapes can be taken as a laxative in constipation. They are useful in treating swelling of the feet and abdomen, dysentery and diarrhoea.

Grape juice allays thirst and is a delicious, health-giving, refreshing beverage. It can be given in all fevers, influenza, pneumonia, malaria, typhoid fever etc. It gives nutrition in wasting diseases like consumption, chronic diarrhoea, etc. Of all the delicious fruits, one of the most nutritious and luscious is the grape. It produces a keen appetite and promotes digestion. It is highly beneficial for invalids and convalescents.

Grapes contain Vitamin B in abundance, which help physical growth and development and removes malnutrition. There is a small quantity of Vitamin A also, which can remove many kinds of eye-diseases like chronic sore-eyes, night-blindness, etc.

Grapes contain several mineral salts which help to build the tissues of the body. They contain plenty of iron. Hence they are useful in anaemia or poverty of the blood. They are highly beneficial to women who suffer from excessive menstruation. After delivery they can take grapes with much benefit.

Oranges

The orange is rich in Vitamin B and very rich in Vitamin C. It contains a small quantity of Vitamin A. It promotes growth and prevents rickets and helps the development of bone and teeth on account of the Vitamin A. The orange is a blood-purifier. It tones up the entire system of the body, and invigorates and energises. It is a good appetiser. It possesses anti-scorbutic properties and hence cures scurvy. It cures constipation also. It is useful in anaemia or poverty of blood, indigestion, constipation, loss of appetite, weakness and lack of vigour, on account of Vitamin B. It prevents scurvy, loss of vigour, on account of Vitamin C. The juice of the orange contains sugar, citric acid and mucillage and organic salts such as potassium citrate. It is refreshing and life-giving. It has a nice flavour, and contains predigested food in a most delicious and attractive form, ready for immediate assimilation and absorption. It is useful in typhoid fever, pneumonia and other acute diseases. It sustains life. The juice of one or two oranges first thing in the morning or the juice of half a lemon in a glass of hot water at night, will exercise the most beneficial effect on the kidneys and the eliminative functions generally.

The adding of fruit juices, preferably orange juice, to the diet in infant feeding is highly beneficial. It is the best preventative for infantile diarrhoea, scurvy and constipation.

Orange juice renders the blood alkaline. When in season it should form a regular part of your diet. It supplies nutrition to the body. It helps concentration and meditation. It is a sattvic article of diet. Live on orange juice for a week or fortnight and practise vigorous meditation.

Mango

In India the mango is regarded as a valuable medicine. A confection made of the juice of ripe mangoes, sugar and aromatics is recommended as a restorative tonic. The ripe fruit is invigorating, fattening, laxative and diuretic. It is endowed with excellent health-giving properties.

Mangoes contain sugar, iron and useful acids. Mango with milk is a wonderful combination. You can live on this diet for two or three months. Many people live on mangoes in the season.

The mango is a very potent source of Vitamins A and C. 'Alphonso' mango is one of the most potent known natural sources of Vitamin C. It contains comparatively greater amounts of Vitamin C than lemons, oranges, grapes and apples.

Pineapple

The pineapple has considerable food value. It is both a medicine and food for singers and speakers. The juice has a remarkable effect on the vocal organs. It is an old fashioned domestic remedy for quinsy and ordinary throat infections of an acute nature. A pineapple is very beneficial in cases of enlargement of the spleen. Take one fruit daily at bed time and you will have free movement of the bowels in the morning.

Apple

Apples supply food to the nerves and muscles. 'An apple a day keeps the doctor away,' is an English proverb. Apple and cream is a good combination for those who suffer from blood pressure. Do not throw away the skin.

Bananas

Bananas contain much starch and sugar. Banana or plantain fruit contains A, B, C and D vitamins. This is a very good soothing food. You can live on milk and bananas alone. They are very nutritious. They promote growth, augment vigour and add flesh to the body. The fully ripe fruits act as a laxative. Take one or two fruits at bed time. You will have free movement of the bowels in the morning.

Figs and Others

Prunes and figs are laxatives. They are useful in constipation. Green figs are an excellent food. Tomato may be called a fuit or a vegetable. It is an ideal article of diet. It is rich in Vitamin A, B, and C. Dates are rich in sugar. They are staple articles of the Arabs. They contribute very greatly to the caloric value. Tamarind is rich in mineral salts and contains Vitamin C.

Bael Fruit

Bael fruit is used as a drink. The pulp is mixed with water. Sugar is added to make it tasty. It is a cooling drink useful in chronic diarrhoea. It is a mild laxative. A sherbet can be formed out of this fruit and drunk in summer. It is useful in dysentery as it stops the passing of blood and heals the ulcers that may have formed in the lower bowels.

Lemon

Lemon possesses anti-scorbutic properties. It is useful in bleeding gums. It is a blood purifier and restorative. It is rich in Vitamin C. It contains citric acid in abundance.

Pomegranate

Pomegranates are highly delicious, refreshing and nutritious. The juice is useful in pneumonia, typhoid and acute diseases. It sustains life. Pomegranates are also very invigorating, cooling and strengthening. The juice is very refreshing and toning. Those who want to supply energy to their system quickly, should take this juice.

Papaya

Papaya contains the active principle of alkaloid papain. The latter digests food readily. Papaya fruit should be included in the daily diet. It is easily digested, and is very useful in dyspepsia.

Jambul and Others

Jambul fruits are useful in diabetes-mellitus. They remove excess sugar in the urine. The chikku or sapota is a blood purifier. It contains iron in abundance.

Cranberries are useful in malaria and erysipelas. Blackberries are useful in fevers. Jack fruit is tasty but is difficult to digest.

Value of Vegetables

Green vegetables contain a large quantity of water, a little starch and a very small amount of protein and fat. They contain a relatively large amount of mineral salts and cellulose. Their value in the diet is due to mineral salts and vitamins. They contain important mineral elements such as calcium, sodium etc. They maintain the proper alkalinity of the blood by balancing the acid producing tendencies of cereal grains. They contain vitamins A, B1, B2 and C.

Vegetables may be divided into three classes:

1. With seeds (or fruit vegetables)
2. Greens
3. Roots or tubers

Beans, peas, snake gourd, brinjal (egg fruit or aubergine), ladies' fingers, pumpkin, red cucumber, lauki (bottle gourd), white pumpkin, tori, tomato and gourd come under the first category.

Tori, lauki, snake gourd and white pumpkin are particularly useful for the diet as they are easily digestible. Spinach, purslane, fenugreek, cabbage, cauliflower and watercress are all green vegetables. Purslane and spinach are the best for sick patients.

Carrot, tapioca, potato, sweet potato, radish, yams, turnip, onions and garlic are all roots or tubers.

Carrot is a brain tonic. It is nutritious and is rich in vitamin A and mineral salts such as calcium. Carrot halva is very palatable and nutritious. Radish raw or cooked is useful in piles and jaundice. Celery is useful in rheumatism and dyspepsia. It is a nerve tonic. Onions are useful in cholera and sunstroke. They are an aphrodisiac. Garlic is useful in lumbago and tuberculosis. Onions and garlic are fairly rich in vitamin C and they contain a powerful antiseptic substance.

Leafy Vegetables

Mother Nature has demonstrated her marvellous skill and power in cultivating these wonderful eatables for her children in her cosmic garden. How kind and merciful She is; She has compounded and beautifully blended all the essentials of life in various kinds of fruit and vegetables to give proper strength, vitality, vigour and energy to her children.

Leafy vegetables are a blessing to humanity. They are the very basis of life. They help the growth and development of the body. They are protective foods. Alkaline mineral salts are abundant in leafy vegetables; hence they afford effective resistance against infection. They give protection to the body against invading infection and pathogenic or disease-causing germs. If you add a liberal supply of leafy vegetables to the pulses, then it becomes a perfect diet. The deficiencies of the pulses are made good by the leafy vegetables. The vitamins of the leafy vegetable stimulate the secretion of the bile and aid the digestion and perfect assimilation of the proteins of the pulses. The leafy vegetables contain all the mineral elements. These serve the purpose of milk for the poor.

Vegetables supply roughage for the proper functioning of the organs of evacuation. The leaves of green vegetables are the lungs and livers of plants. Hence they are storehouses of vitamins and mineral salts. Leafy vegetables should find a place in the diets of all. The Chinese use a large quantity of leafy vegetables, so rickets is unknown to them.

Cabbage is the most valuable of all leafy vegetables. Spinach, tops of radish and beetroot, watercress and other leafy vegetables are valuable supplements to food. They afford nutrition to a cereal diet, make up the deficiency and make it a perfect diet. Leafy vegetables are protective foods. They supply the mineral salts that are deficient in our staple food grains.

There is no fat in vegetables. Broad beans, fresh peas, apricot and butter beans, dried peas and lentils contain 4 to 8 percent protein.

Leguminous vegetables like peas, beans and lentils contain more protein than meat (25 per cent). They should be taken with juicy fruits or vegetables. Dried peas, beans and lentils are wholesome.

Leafy and juicy vegetables are useful in balancing the acid-generating sugars, fats, proteins and starches. They prevent the blood from becoming acid and they balance the acid-producing tendencies of meat and cereals.

Some vegetables are beneficial when eaten raw. Some others require cooking, singly or in combination with other food materials.

Fresh tomatoes, cucumber and various kinds of gourds contain a fair amount of vitamin C. Pumpkin supplies roughage which helps the evacuation of the bowels and prevents constipation.

Potato is the most important among roots or tubers. It supplies an excellent form of starch. It contains iron and vitamin C also. It retains a high percentage of vitamin C even after cooking.

Tomato is one of the best of all vegetables. It contains citric acid and a small quantity of oxalic acid. It contains large quantities of five of the six vitamins. (Cooking partially destroys the vitamin content, therefore it should be eaten raw.) Tomato contains potash, lime, magnesia and iron. It exercises a beneficial effect on the liver, kidneys and other organs. It also cures constipation. It gives sure protection against beri-beri and scurvy.

Lettuce, celery, cabbage, spinach and watercress rank highest in organic mineral salts. Tomatoes, cauliflower, onions, radish and cucumber come next. Eat a variety of vegetables. You will supply all the organic mineral salts to the body. Vegetarians keep up sound health till old age. Even in western hospitals doctors are now putting patients on a vegetable diet. They convalesce very quickly.

Water-melons and musk melons are cooling summer foods. They are abundant in organic salts which purify the blood.

Fruits or vegetables with nuts are the best food of all. Nuts are rich in proteins and fats but they are not easily digested. They are suitable for those who suffer from diabetes. They are a substitute for meat. They are rich in vitamin B.

Honey

Honey is a first-class food and tonic. It is very easily digested and assimilated and a most nutritious natural food. It will strengthen a weak heart, a weak brain and a weak stomach. Honey is the product of the nectar of flowers. It is a mistake to say that honey is gathered by bees from flowers. Bees are nature's sweet makers. They manufacture sweets better, finer and healthier than any sweetmeat maker — with all his skill, dexterity, ingenuity and many ingredients — can ever make.

Green plants manufacture sugar for their own use. This is carried with the cell sap to the different parts of the plant either for direct assimilation or future use. All the flowering plants concentrate a quick supply of food at the base or the bottom part of their flowers to help the proper growth of the ovaries. The excess solution is thrown out at the base of the flowers. This solution of the cell sap with sugar is known as 'nectar'. This nectar is changed into honey in their mouths by the honey bees. Every hive imparts a new flavour because in every hive the nectar is drawn from different flowers and plants.

Honey contains all the mineral elements found in the human body. It contains 80 per cent nutriment in a most assimilable form. It contains the sugars levulose and dextrose, formic acid, iron and various accessory components. Because it contains enzymes which disintegrate or break up complex foods into substances that can be easily digested and absorbed, honey does not require digestion at all. It is ready for absorption into the blood without any change, and goes into the blood stream directly. It should form part of your diet. A teaspoonful of honey per day will keep the stomach in order.

Honey is a heart stimulant. It is useful in cases of malnutrition, and should be given for general physical repair. Honey kills bacteria and thus enables the body to overcome diseases. Disease germs cannot grow in honey. Honey is useful in bronchial catarrh, sore throat, coughs and colds. It also acts as a laxative. As soon as a child is born its tongue is smeared with honey. This is the first food that the child takes.

Honey can be taken with milk, cream or butter. It is a restorative after serious illness. It invigorates, energises and vitalises the system and improves health. It is more stimulating than alcohol.

Honey is a diffusible stimulant. If you take a tablespoonful of honey in hot water when you are tired or exhausted by over-exertion it will brace you up immediately. You will become strong and active again. (If the honey is bitter do not take it.)

Soak 10 almonds in water at night. Remove the skin in the morning. Take them in the morning with one or two tablespoonfuls of honey. This is a potent brain tonic.

Milk and its Products

Milk is an ideal diet. It is a perfect and complete food in itself. It contains all the nutritive principles in a well-balanced proportion. You can live on milk alone. In India there is a sect among the sadhus known as 'Dudhalharis'. They take no other food but milk and they possess sound and perfect health. One man has lived on a strictly milk diet for more than fifty years. He has never been ill even for a day during that period. He is healthy and well-nourished. Charaka Rishi says: "Give no other medicine to your patients but milk and cure them one and all." Milk contains proteins (casein), fat, milk sugar and mineral salts. All infants grow properly on an exclusive milk diet. The sick recover their health and strength when put on milk alone. Take plenty of milk. Not only is it rich in proteins and minerals, but it also contains the four most important vitamins.

Curd, lassi, cheese, whey, butter, cream, ghee etc., are the products of milk. Lassi can be made out of milk or curd. Equal parts of milk and water with sugar, or one part of curd with four parts of water and some sugar, form lassi. Lassi is very cooling. If taken in the morning it opens the bowels.

The clear liquid left after curd or cheese have been separated is called whey. This is highly beneficial in constipation and diseases of the stomach and intestines. It is very good food for invalids and convalescents as it is easily digestible.

Buttermilk is very cooling to the system. It quenches thirst. It is useful in diseases of the stomach and intestines, and dysentery. The lactic acid contained in buttermilk kills the pathogenic germs that may be present in the stomach and bowels.

Dangers of Meat Eating

Meat is not at all necessary for the keeping up of health. Meat-eating is highly deleterious to health. It brings a host of ailments such as tapeworm, albuminuria and other diseases of the kidneys. Killing of animals for food is a great sin. Instead of killing egoism and the idea of 'mine-ness', ignorant people kill innocent animals under the pretext of sacrifice to a goddess; but it is really to satisfy their tongues and palates. Horrible! Most inhuman! Non-violence is the greatest of all virtues. It is the first virtue that a spiritual aspirant should possess. We should have reverence for life. Lord Jesus says: "Blessed are the merciful for they shall obtain mercy." Lord Jesus and Mahavira shouted at the top of their voice: "Regard every living being as thyself and harm no one." The law of karma is inexorable, unrelenting and immutable. The pain you inflict upon another will rebound upon you, and the happiness you radiate to another will come back to you, adding to your happiness.

Mark how the meat-eating tiger is ferocious, and the cow and the elephant, which live on grass, are mild and peaceful! Meat has a direct evil influence on the compartments of the brain. The first step in spiritual advancement is the giving up of a meat diet. The Divine Light will not descend if the stomach is loaded with meat. Meat decomposes readily, producing irritation of stomach and bowels, colic, diarrhoea, collapse, urticarial rashes, etc.

The flesh of animals suffering from anthrax, glanders, tuberculosis etc. is dangerous. Tape worm, taenia solium, taenia saginata, distomum hepaticum and tridhinella spiralis are communicated by eating contaminated meat. Meat-eating is unnatural and dangerous. Therefore meat-eating should be totally abandoned.

Pythagoras, the Grecian sage, preached: "Do not kill or injure any creature." He condemned a meat diet as sinful food. Just hear what he says: "Beware, O mortals, of defiling your bodies with sinful food! There are cereals, there are fruits bending their branches down by their weight, and luxurious grapes on the vines. There are sweet vegetables and herbs which the flame can render palatable and mellow. Nor are you denied milk, nor honey, nor fragrance of the aroma of the thyme flower. The beautiful earth offers you an abundance of pure food and provides for meals obtainable without slaughter or bloodshed."

If you want to stop taking mutton, fish etc, just see with your own eyes the pitiable, struggling condition of the sheep at the time of its killing. Now mercy and sympathy will arise in your heart. Then you will determine to give up flesh-eating. If you fail in this attempt, just change your environment and live in a vegetarian hotel where you cannot get mutton and fish, and move in that society where there is only a vegetarian diet. Always think of the evils of flesh-eating and the benefits of a vegetable diet. If this also cannot give you sufficient strength to stop this habit, go to the slaughter-house and the butcher's shop and personally see the disgusting rotten muscles, intestines, kidneys and other nasty parts of the animal which emit bad smell. This will induce dispassion in you and a strong disgust and hatred for meat-eating.

Yogic Diet

A yogic diet is that which helps the aspirant to keep the mind calm and to curb the restless senses. A yogic diet helps him to squeeze out the rajas from his mind and fill the mind with sattva, and to practise unceasing meditation. All the senses should be filled with pure material; then only will the mind attain one-pointedness; then only can you attain Self-realisation. The eyes should see the picture of your chosen deity or any other holy object; the ears should hear the *Upanishads*, the *Ramayana* or the *Bhagavatam*; the tongue should speak of matters that concern God. These are all pure materials or food for the senses.

The nature of food that is taken determines the character of individuals. Carnivorous food makes men callous and bestial. It excites the passion and renders the intellect gross. A meat-eater cannot become a philosopher and sage. His intellect is so dull that he cannot solve the problems of life here and hereafter.

The intellect is rendered keen, subtle and sharp by a vegetarian diet. A vegetable diet is highly conducive to sublime thinking and divine concentration. It gives greater vitality than animal foods.

The diet should be carefully chosen and arranged. Condiments, tea, coffee, alcohol, foods that are rich in starch, sugars and fats and all stimulating drinks should be avoided. Fresh fruits, salads and raw vegetables, cheese, nuts, cereals, wholemeal bread, soya beans, dried fruits, cream, milk, barley, honey, dates and almonds are highly beneficial. Raw foods are more vitalising, make better blood and build better bodies. They should therefore make up at least eighty per cent of the diet. Occasionally live on juicy fruits for a week. This will help greatly towards the elimination of impurities from the system.

Food should also contain some roughage to stimulate the peristaltic movements of the intestines. Raw foods contain more than cooked.

Indigestion or dyspepsia induced by an unnaturally heavy meal or unwholesome irritating food or unsuitable diet will cause all kinds of reflex effects on the nerve centres.

Masticate the food thoroughly. Eat only when you are hungry. Nowadays people mistake the cravings of the palate for hunger. Perhaps hunger is a joy they have never experienced. Real hunger is indescribable in its nature, even as God Himself is. To know this one has to experience it. One cannot be told by another.

Food does not need to be eaten with appetisers, which act as aeroplanes to carry the food to the stomach, since such food is not demanded by the life-fire within. This life-fire is God Himself. Man should wait for the appearance of this God within and only *then* offer Him some food.

Eat slowly. Drink plenty of water after finishing the food. Do not drink water before meals as it will dilute the gastric juice and will cause indigestion and other stomach complaints.

The mouth is the gate-keeper of the digestive system. It should always be kept sweet and clean by rinsing it with a solution of potassium permanganate several times, soon after taking food. Many germs breed in an unclean mouth. Cleansing of the teeth is of paramount importance. Chewing of a few neem leaves keeps the mouth sweet and clean. Neem leaves act as a powerful germicide.

We require a variety of foods with a variety of contents and properties. Variety in food is necessary; but too many different kinds at one time are not good. The fewer the kinds, the better. Mother Nature provides judiciously and amply for all our needs and varies the contents of foods in accordance with our needs.

A simple diet containing a minimum of unnecessary food or waste will throw less strain upon the kidneys than a rich diet. Proper diet ensures healthy tissues by preventing the accumulation of waste in the system. An eminent doctor says, "The perfect food consists of a mixture of honey, cream, hot water, oatmeal, lemon juice, grated apple and ground hazel nuts, which contains all the vitamins."

Appetizing food and mastication stimulate the flow of saliva. The increased production of saliva, in its turn, tends to increase the secretion of gastric juice. This again stimulates the mucous membrane of the duodenum — the first portion of the small intestine — and leads to the production of hormone secretion. Therefore mastication of food is most necessary and its neglect is fraught with danger. If you do not masticate the food well, the stomach will be overworked. It will have to do the work of grinding the food.

Starchy food is digested in the mouth by saliva which is alkaline. This cannot be done unless the food is throughly masticated. Hence, thorough mastication is very necessary. Food must never be taken in haste because it produces dyspepsia.

The secret of enjoying and ensuring good digestion of food is to masticate every morsel so thoroughly that it glides down the throat in a liquid state. Proper mastication of food prevents and cures dyspepsia. If you thoroughly chew every bit of food a much smaller quantity gives more nourishment, better digestion, more rest to the stomach and less amount of excreta than a large quantity of half-chewed food.

Eating For Health

Man eats too much. This is admitted by all. Even when you are not hungry you try to stuff your stomach by taking recourse to spices, chutneys and pickles. It is the tongue that deludes you and does so much havoc. It goads you to eat this thing and that thing. The stomach really wants only a little. If you overload the stomach it throws out the extra food through vomiting and makes you give up the next meal by producing a bad sensation in your throat.

Simple natural foods are quite sufficient to keep up good health and a high standard of vigour and vitality. You will have to create a good appetite by fasting and not by taking recourse to highly seasoned dishes, pickles and chutneys.

You eat even when you are not hungry. This is a sad mistake. If you are not really hungry, fast. You will have a good appetite for the next meal. Thousands of educated people load their stomachs even when they have no appetite, even when they suffer from dyspepsia, on the strength of some digestive mixture. They do this act of folly daily and suffer afterwards, and still they call themselves highly educated, cultured and civilized. Do not over-load the stomach. Such is the law. You will have wonderful health if you follow this simple law.

Nature herself does rationing. If you eat too much sweet-meats and take too much sugar, the pancreas is overworked, you get diabetes and nature forces you to give up sugar. If you eat too much meat and proteins, the kidneys are overworked and you get albuminuria. Nature forces you to give up protein substances.

Some persons are sensitive to certain kinds of food on account of inherent or acquired idiosyncrasy. They exhibit some inconvenient symptoms when they take certain foods. The symptoms may be gastro-intestinal. They may get colic or diarrhoea. They may have certain urticarial eruptions on the body. They may exhibit symptoms of an asthma attack.

Food should be protected from contamination, from dust, flies and other insects. Ptomaine poisoning takes place on account of taking foodstuffs which are undergoing putrefaction. The symptoms are vomiting, purging, colic, headache, great muscular weakness and severe collapse. (It is generally mistaken for cholera.) The collapse should always be guarded against by keeping the heart stimulated by coffee and a stimulant mixture. Hands and legs should be kept warm by hot water bottles and by rubbing turpentine liniment.

Botulism is a form of food poisoning. There are no symptoms of gastro-enteritis in this form. Poisoning results from absorption of a specific toxin from the digestive canal. Canned, preserved and pickled foods are generally the sources of danger.

Fasting

Nowadays many have recognised and realised the value of fasting. They resort to fasting whenever any form of ill-health manifests itself, and save doctor's bills. Fasting is nature's greatest curative agent. The fast gives an opportunity for nature to cleanse the system and remove the materials that clog certain organs or parts. It is a very efficacious therapeutic agent. Many kinds of poisonous materials and toxins are eliminated by fasting. In numberless cases it has restored health when everything else has failed. If you fast as soon as a disease is manifested it will soon disappear and many serious complications will be avoided. If you feel feverish, if you suffer from dyspepsia, fast for a day and you will be cured immediately. Nature is your reliable guide, doctor, friend and nurse. Seek her help always.

Some people are unnecessarily alarmed when they hear the word 'fasting'. Fasting does not impair vitality, nor does it produce weakness and loss of weight. Strength and vitality are usually increased by fasting, the mind becomes clear and the body becomes very light.

During fasting the internal digestive organs — such as stomach, liver, pancreas, etc. — take rest. Epicureans, gluttons and those who are tireless eaters do not allow rest for the organs even for a few minutes. Hence these organs soon get diseased. After all, man needs very little on this earth. Ninety per cent of the people in this world take more food than is really necessary for the body. Over-eating has become their habit. Many diseases arise from over-eating. Hence, a fast is a great desideratum for all to keep up good health, relieve the internal organs and maintain celibacy. It overhauls the respiratory, circulatory, digestive and urinary systems. It destroys all the impurities of the body and all sorts of poisons, eliminates uric acid deposits and reduces fat. Diseases that are pronounced incurable by allopaths and homeopaths are cured by fasting.

Give rest to the internal digestive organs by fasting. You can have a healthy long life. May you grow wise from today at least and lead a healthy life by taking simple natural foods and giving up over-eating.

Fasting develops will-power. It increases the power of endurance.

Mahatma Gandhi had developed his will-power considerably through fasting. He was a great votary of fasting. If anything went wrong in the Ashram, if any one conducted himself in a wrong manner, he would fast for some days. He took the burden and sins of others on himself by fasting. He fasted for effecting Hindu-Muslim unity. He had a long fast of forty-five days for the political and economic good or freedom of the country.

Fasting is the message of the heart. By fasting you can melt the heart of even a hard-hearted man. By fasting you can influence anybody.

Fasting is a form of austerity to destroy the effects of evil tendencies and purify oneself quickly. Fasting is a sacred resolution or vow amongst the Hindus. They observe a complete fast on Sivaratri and Gokulasthami days. They do not take even a drop of water during these days. Some religious-minded persons fast every Ekadashi day (the eleventh day of the Hindu lunar fortnight). Christians observe Lent: forty days (from Ash Wednesday to Easter Eve) are devoted to fasting and penitence in commemoration of the fast of their Saviour in the wilderness. Mohammedans fast during Ramadan. Fasting helps in controlling the mind and makes the mind sattvic. It subdues passion.

If the mind does a wrong action, if it hurts others' feelings, seriously punish it by observing a fast. It will come under your control gradually. Just as impure gold is rendered pure by melting it in the crucible again and again, so also this impure mind is rendered purer and purer by fasting again and again.

The practice of fasting may be distasteful in the beginning for some, but later they will take great delight in it. You will be troubled by hunger on the first day and second day, but from the third day you will have no appetite. If you find it difficult to observe complete fast even for a day, at least observe partial fast. Do not take anything in the daytime. Take milk and fruits at night. Continue for two or three days.

Those who fast for two or three days should not break their fast with any solid food, but should slowly sip fruit juice, either orange or pomegranate. You can take an enema during fasting. You should drink water copiously for four or five days when you observe a fast, to flush out the system. What do the municipal people do when the sewers are clogged? Do they not flush them with plenty of water? You should do the same thing when your system is clogged. The water drunk may be flavoured slightly with a little of the juice of an orange, a lemon or grapes. Take an enema of soapy water in the early morning to cleanse the bowels thoroughly. Just as a car after thorough overhauling looks like a new car and runs smoothly, so also our body which is clogged by overeating and stuffing of all sorts of food, gets thoroughly overhauled by fasting and becomes like a new machine.

Avoid excessive fasting. It will produce weakness. Use your common sense. Practise fasting for a day to start with and gradually increase the period to a week. Slowly increase the number of days according to your strength and capacity. The first day may be very tiring. You will experience bliss on the second or third day. The body will be very very light.

You can turn out more mental work while fasting. Those who are in the habit of fasting will rejoice. On the first day the mind will tempt you in a variety of ways to eat something or the other. Stand firm. Be bold. Do more japa during fasting. Do not allow the mind to think of various articles of food. The chief object of fasting is to practise meditation rigorously, as during that period the mind and all the senses are calm. You will have to withdraw all the senses and fix the mind on God. Pray to God to guide you and throw a flood of light on the path. You will get purity and light, strength and knowledge.

Fasting is more a spiritual cleansing exercise than a physical one from the view-point of health. You will have to utilise the fasting days for higher spiritual purpose and in the contemplation of God. Always entertain thoughts of God. Dive deep into the problems of life such as the why and wherefore of the universe. Enquire: "Who am I?", "What is the purpose of life?", "What is this Brahman or Atman?", "What are the ways and means to attain knowledge of God?", "How to approach Him?". Then realise your own blissful state and rest in purity for ever and ever.

Fast and calm your emotions and passion. Fast and be healthy. Fast and control the tongue and other sense-organs. Fast and destroy your sins. Fast and eliminate the poison from your system. Fast and control your sleep. Fast and pray. Fast, purify and meditate, realise the Self and be free. Fast and shine with divine splendour and glory.

The Yogi's Secret

You can give up food for some days, but you cannot do without water for some days; you can give up even water for some time, but you cannot give up air even for a short time. Yogis suspend their breath, get themselves buried for some months and yet there is life in them. Their life is kept up by some mysterious vital fluid, the nectar that flows from the sahasrara (the thousand-petalled lotus on the crown of the head). Modern physiologists cannot explain how life is kept up in yogis even when food, water and air are entirely withdrawn, and how their bodies derive their nutrition when they are buried. Earth, water, fire and air are all products or modifications of the space element. If you know through yoga how to tap space, it will provide you all the things supplied by food, water and air, because space is the mother substance.

Yogis tap the source which is in the brain, drink the nectar and maintain life in their bodies. This is a secret known to yogis only.

Dietetic Rules

1. Take a moderate diet. Get up when three-quarters of the stomach is full. Do not overload the stomach.
2. Eat only when you are really hungry. Beware of false hunger.
3. Do not eat anything between meals. Do not drink between meals.
4. Eat wholesome food, in proper quantity, at fixed times.
5. Do not take food too cold or too hot, because it will derange the stomach and produce indigestion.
6. Do not eat anything which you do not like, but do not eat everything that you like most.
7. Reduce cooked food to a minimum. Take always some raw vegetables like radish with your food.
8. Eat only four or five kinds of food at one meal. Abandon too many mixtures or combinations. It is difficult for the digestive juice to digest complex diverse combinations.
9. Eat combinations that are compatible. If you take incompatible mixtures, there will be fermentation in the stomach and intestines. All cereals can be taken with milk, fruits and vegetables. Do not take milk with milk-products, such as milk-based sweetmeats. Nuts, breads, apples, lemons, whey and butter can be taken with everything. Proteins and starches, fruits and cereals or other carbohydrates, are compatible combinations. Experience and instinct will guide you in making compatible mixtures.
10. A little lemon juice or buttermilk may be added to give flavour to food. Buttermilk can be taken after meals or an hour or two before meals. These rules are for persons whose digestion is not

good, and the number of such persons is numerous. Only very few persons of robust health can digest any kind of food and can overcome any irregularity in food.

11. Do not take tinned foods and old butter. Vegetables and rice should be steamed. Overcooking will rob the vegetables of their value and flavour. Do not throw away the water in which rice and vegetables are boiled. They contain valuable minerals. Drink it also.

12. Do not remove the skins of apples and carrots, because the skin has valuable minerals and vitamins.

13. Take only two meals at fixed hours. Never heat the food again over the fire.

14. Protect all food from flies. Keep the milk in a cool place.

15. Take food when the breath is passing through the right nostril.

16. Sit on vajrasana for ten minutes after meals. This will help the digestion.

17. Observe silence when you take your food.

18. Make a change in your diet gradually. If any article of diet disagrees, reduce the quantity. It will be agreeable to you.

19. Do not do any strenuous work, physical or mental, after taking food. Take rest for half an hour. Do not run immediately after food to catch the train.

20. Avoid late dinner.

21. Do not eat when you are angry. Rest for a while till the mind becomes calm, and then take your food. Poisons are secreted by the glands when you are angry, and thrown into the blood stream.

22. Take food as medicine. Give up gluttony.

23. Fast one day in a week. Fasting eliminates the poisons, overhauls the internal mechanism and gives rest to the organs.

24. Remember God, the Indweller in all foods, fruits and vegetables and the bestower of bounties, during meals and at all times. Pray to Him just before and after meals.

HEALTH AND HYGIENE

Life here is a continual battle. It is never-ending adventure. There are dragons to be destroyed. You will have to wage war with the enemies of health — impure water; bad ventilation; overwork; unwholesome food; disease-germs; domestic pests such as mosquitoes, flies, rats and so on. You are surrounded on all sides by invisible foes, the pathogenic or disease-causing microbes or bacteria. You should certainly learn all you can about your enemies, their ways, habits and strength. In some cases you will have to attack them directly. In some other cases you will have to starve them out. You must adopt the most up-to-date weapons which modern sanitary science and preventive medicine have given you. You must husband your resources in every way possible.

Every citizen, every individual is directly and intimately concerned in the preservation of the health and welfare, not only of himself, but of the community as a whole.

Most of the diseases which are preventable are produced by some specific germs which are carried by air, water, food, clothing or insects. A study of the life story of these disease-causing germs and the methods to exterminate them will be extremely helpful for the health and welfare of the community. Impure air, impure water, infected food, uncleanliness of houses and their surroundings, and improper or bad disposal of excreta play a vital part in the dissemination of disease.

Every individual must be educated in the science of hygiene and sanitation so that he may be able to appreciate the value of sanitation not only for his own health but also for the community at large.

The child must be protected before birth by ante-natal precautions. The health and well-being of the child is the primary foundation of its education. Pregnant and nursing mothers must also be well protected. Maternity and child welfare centres must be established in each district. People must be protected from diseases like small-pox, plague, cholera and typhoid, by taking recourse to artificial immunity through injection of vaccines. For the sake of our fellow creatures, as well as for ourselves, it is our duty to use all proper means for preserving health.

May you all possess good health and vitality by observing the rules of health and hygiene and study of the science of sanitation and preventive medicine.

Personal Hygiene

Man is a criminal if he suffers from any disease by violating the rules and laws of health and hygiene. The responsibility of maintaining good health rests with every individual. Personal hygiene deals with matters that pertain to the health of the individual. Only a healthy man can turn out good and useful work, only a healthy man can serve humanity, only a healthy man can meditate well, only a healthy man can earn money. Therefore good health is a great blessing indeed. He who observes the laws of health and hygiene will be endowed with good health.

Cleanliness is next to godliness. Cleanliness bestows good health. You must observe cleanliness with regard to the food you eat, the air you breathe and the water you drink.

You must take a daily bath in the early morning. A cold bath is invigorating and highly beneficial. Old people, convalescents and invalids can take a hot water bath. Daily cleaning of the skin is of paramount importance. If this is not done, the pores of the skin will be blocked by dirt and various skin diseases will develop. The parts where hair grows must be kept scrupulously clean. The armpits give out an offensive smell and so require cleaning.

A plunge bath in the running water of rivers is very exhilarating and strengthening. A shower bath is also very enjoyable. Baths in sulphur springs cure diseases of the skin. A cold hip-bath prevents wet-dreams. A tepid hip bath stops renal colic and helps the flow of menstrual fluid and urine. A steam bath is useful in rheumatism. Tepid sponging is useful in fevers for bringing down the temperature.

Do not take a cold bath immediately after performing asanas or any kind of physical exercises. Allow the body to cool down first. Wait for an hour. Never bathe soon after meals as it will interfere with the digestion.

The application of soap in a tropical climate is injurious. It keeps the skin dry. Nature supplies a little oil to the body for keeping it smooth and soft through the secretion of the sebaceous glands of the skin. Ignorant, fashionable man removes this natural secretion by application of soap, and wastes his money. If soaps are not manufactured properly they corrode the skin. Rub the body vigorously with a rough towel. This will open all the pores of the skin and cleanse the latter properly. Resort always to easy natural methods that cost nothing. If you like you can use a mixture of soap-nut powder and green-gram powder for cleaning the skin. This is cheap and very cooling also.

Cleanliness of the mouth is very important. The mouth is the gateway for the entry of micro-organisms, hence the teeth should be thoroughly cleaned twice a day. The tongue should be cleaned daily in the morning with a tongue cleaner.

The nails should be cut short and kept clean, otherwise dirt will accumulate under them and may carry infection. Wash the hands before taking meals. This will prevent the introduction of infection.

Do not use the brushes, combs, bed-clothes etc. of other persons. Ask the barber to wash his hands, razors, etc. before you take a shave. It is better to have your own razor, soap, and brush. Dhobi's itch and other kinds of skin diseases are communicated through dirty hands of a barber, his brushes and razor. Do not use another man's pillows, bed, clothing, etc. Diseases may be communicated through these articles.

Clothing

You must protect yourself against the extremes of heat and cold; then alone can you maintain good health and general well-being. Excessive cold and heat are unpleasant and injurious to your health. You must wear suitable clothing. Children in particular should be guarded against the dangers of extremes of climate. Clothing should keep you warm in winter and cool in summer. This is the main object in wearing clothes.

The most important function or use of clothes is non-conduction. In temperate and cold climates they prevent heat flowing away from the body too rapidly. In tropical climates they prevent the heat flowing to the body from the sun. Without clothes you will lose so much heat from the body in cold weather, that even if you eat enormously you will not be able to generate enough heat to keep you going. In the tropics and in very hot weather the skin may get badly burnt from the heat of the sun's rays if it is not protected by clothing. Clothing affords protection to the body against heat and cold and external injuries. It assists in the maintenance of body-heat. It is used for decency and personal decoration or ornamentation, although this is of lesser importance.

The protection given to the skin by clothing is an acquired habit of comfort. Had it not been for this acquired habit, man may very largely do without clothing. Agriculturists use very little clothing. Their skin has become more resistant to the influences of the weather in maintaining the body temperature. There are naked and part-naked sannyasins even in the icy regions of the Himalayas. No-one covers the face even in cold weather. If the sensitive skin of the face can withstand cold, the skin of other parts of the body ought to be able to bear cold if called upon to do so.

The animal kingdom supplies two of the best materials for clothes — wool and silk. To these may be added fur for special clothing. The plant kingdom furnishes cotton, linen and artificial silk.

Cotton and linen sheets always feel much colder than the blankets, because cotton and linen conduct the heat away more rapidly than wool does. Silk does not prevent the loss of heat as well as wool does, but it does better than linen or cotton. The greatest amount of heat will be retained by wool and the least by linen.

The same material will absorb different amounts of heat when dyed with different colours. Black absorbs the solar heat rays and white reflects them.

Cotton can be boiled without injury and is therefore easily sterilized and may be said to be more hygienic than wool from the point of view of infection, but it quickly conducts away the warmth of the body and fails badly as an absorbent. It simply becomes wet and cold when we perspire.

Wool does not absorb moisture so readily as cotton. This is the reason why chills occur more quickly with linen or cotton than flannel clothing. When you perspire the woollen material absorbs and retains this moisture. The fabric remains quite warm to the touch and thus prevents a chill.

Silk is a bad conductor of heat and so it gives warmth but it does not absorb moisture nearly so well as wool. It is less liable to shrink than wool and does not irritate the skin as some wools do.

If a cloth is loosely woven there are many tiny air spaces in the meshes. As air is not a good heat-conductor its presence in the meshes of the cloth makes the latter warmer than if it were very closely woven. For the same reason loose clothing is warmer than tight clothing.

Air in between two folds of cloth is more efficient than two thicknesses of cloth. Where protection is the object it will be comfortable and less costly if clothing is arranged in layers. One coat or shirt over another, or one wrapper over another would be more non-conducting and lighter than a coat or wrapper made of thicker cloth.

The dress should not interfere with healthy action of the skin. For this purpose materials which absorb moisture readily should be preferred.

All tight clothes should be avoided as they interfere with circulation, respiration, digestion and the action of muscles.

Garters should be condemned as they compress the superficial veins, produce a feeling of heaviness, and they cause varicose veins.

Clothing should be of good quality, strong, durable and light. It should be capable of being easily washed or cleaned. The material should be of an attractive appearance. Such clothing is ideal.

Hygiene of the Eyes

The eye is a very important organ. It is one of the five organs of perception. It is a window in this body for the soul, the proprietor of the body. The 'will to see' or the 'desire to see' has become the eye, the organ of sight or perception. The presiding deity of the eye is the sun.

The external eyeball is only an instrument to catch the vibrations of colour and light and to send them to the centre in the brain

The eye consists of a cornea, a transparent, curved window which receives the rays of light. The white part is the sclerotic coat. The space behind is filled with a transparent watery fluid. There is a coloured curtain next to the cornea, called the iris. It has a hole in the middle which can automatically become large or small to receive more or less light. The hole is called the pupil. In the bright light the pupil becomes small; in the dim light it becomes large. The lens is behind the pupil. Behind the lens is the hollow of the eye which is filled with a vitreous body, called the vitreous humour. Light passes through this vitreous humour and strikes the screen or retina behind the eye. Then the optic nerve takes the impression of the object seen from the retina to the brain. If the optic nerve were to be cut, sight would be totally lost.

The muscles of the eye move the eyeball up, down and sideways.

A little tear gland (lachrymal gland) is placed in each socket in the outer corner of the eye. A continuous secretion of tears keeps the surface of the eye moist. A little duct opens at the inner edge of each eyelid and carries away tears into the nose. When dust enters the eyes they water involuntarily. This bathing of the eyes with tears helps to wash the particles of dust into the corner of the eye.

The eyeballs are very safely placed in the boney eye sockets. They are well protected on all sides by the boney walls. The eyebrows act as little drains to keep perspiration out of the eye, and they act as brushes to prevent dust from falling into the eyes. The eyelids also prevent foreign bodies or dust from getting into the eyes. Mark how the all-merciful, all wise Mother Nature has given all sorts of protection from external injuries and foreign bodies.

Behind the eyeball there is a soft pad of fat which serves as a cushion and lessens the chance of injury to the eye when it gets a blow. The disappearance of this pad of fat causes the shrunken eyes in very old and sick people.

The eye is like a camera. It photographs the outside world on the retina. It perceives the light rays from the sun. Just as images are printed on the plate of the camera, so also images of external objects are printed on the retinal plate of the eye.

If you are taking a photograph of something near at hand you have to focus your camera differently from the position for a distand landscape view. So also there is the adjustment of the eye for seeing near objects. The shape of the lens is altered, and the pupil also adjusts in size. When you look at near objects the pupil is smaller than when you are looking at distant objects.

Good eyesight is very necessary for success in life. The eye should always be examined by a doctor in cases of headache or where there is any difficulty in reading the blackboard at school. Squint is caused by straining the eye. Do not read in a bad light or in a light that flickers. This is a great strain on the eyes and will produce eye trouble. The light should come from the left side, behind and above. Do not read in a kerosene light. It will spoil your eyesight. If you are forced to work in that light, place it behind your head and have a green shade. Too much reading and close work such as fine sewing are not good for the eyes.

The eye is the most sensitive organ. Do not apply anything and everything which laymen suggest for diseases of the eye. The eye will be spoiled. Always consult an eye specialist. (Do not neglect early treatment in granular lids. The granules should be frequently touched with copper sulphate. Do not remain in smoke.)

The common causes of diseases of the eyes and defective eyesight are: over use and straining of the eyes by reading in bad light, by reading books printed in too small type on glazed paper, by glare, foreign bodies getting into the eye, draughts of cold air, lack of proper food and fresh air, and general bad health. Do not read a book lying down in bed.

Use brahmi amla oil. It will cool and refresh tired eyes. If there is a foreign body under the eyelids, use boric eyewash. Open and shut the eyes within the eye-cup or open them under clean water. Put a drop of castor oil in each eye at night. The foreign body will come out by itself in the early morning. If these methods fail, consult a doctor.

The knowledge of this sense universe is obtained chiefly through the avenues of the eye and the ear. All colours and forms are centered in the eye, in the mind and Atman. It is really the brain that sees and interprets the impressions conveyed to the eye from the external universe. To be more correct, it is the mind that really sees the objects.

The eye is ever wandering and restless. It makes the mind also ever restless. Steadiness of the eye is steadiness of the mind. Tratak, concentration, devout meditation and worship, etc. make the mind steady. Practise these three times a day — morning, evening and night.

The following simple eye exercises have improved eyesight to the extent of allowing some people to again read without glasses, depending of course on the nature of the eye weakness:

Exercise i: Focus intently on a distant object — for a normal-sighted man on the horizon, but for a weak-sighted man on the farthest object you can see clearly — day by day coaxing the eyes to see further. Then without moving the eyes, straighten out an arm in front of you and lift the forefinger to cover the distant object. You will see the original object plus two fingers, because the finger is out of focus.

Stare at the finger, then at the distant object. Repeat five times. Focussing on the finger-tip, slowly move the finger towards the eyes until it rests on the forehead between the eyebrows. Now the eyes are closed. Hold them thus until you feel a slight strain, then slowly straighten the arm, returning the finger to its original position before the distant object. As soon as the finger leaves the forehead, concentrate again on the finger-tip. When the arm straightens, focus on the distant object, then on the finger-tip and repeat several times.

Exercise ii: Repeat the above exercise, but bring the finger, eyes focussed on its tip, slowly to the end of the nose.

(While doing these eye-movements, try to remain unblinking, eyes open continuously, thus practising a form of tratak and improving your concentration and one-pointedness of mind.)

Exercise iii: Without moving the head, turn the eyes to look as far as possible first to the left, then slowly to the right, up to the sky, down to the ground; then along the diagonals, starting with the left top corner, slowly down to the bottom right corner, to the bottom left corner and finishing at the top right corner.

Exercise iv: (This exercise will help concentration because you must think simultaneously of both your breathing and movement of the eyes.) Look down to the ground then slowly make a big circle to the left, above, to the right and down again with the eyes, breathing in deeply and trying to have capacity breath when the eye-circle is completed. Repeat the slow circling to the left, this time breathing out to empty the lungs as the circle is completed. Repeat both sequences to the right. The circles must be as large as possible.

Exercise v: There are endless shapes — letters of the alphabet, the square, the diamond, the figure eight firstly upright and then lying on its side — which can be drawn with the eyes.

Practise these exercises conscientiously in the open air, but not in direct sunlight. Each time as you finish, cover the eyes with the palms of the hands, open them in the dark and breathe deeply, concentrating intently on the open eyes, especially as you breathe out, thus sending plenty of pranic energy along with fresh blood supply to the eyes. Close the eyes again before removing the hands, to avoid sudden glare. You can do the breathing three times.

Hygiene of the Skin

The whole body is covered, protected from injury, kept warm and made beautiful by the skin which covers its surface. This garment never grows old because Mother Nature in constantly renewing it. New cells are continually being formed in the deepest layers of the skin. When they grow they push off the old cells on the surface of the body.

The skin is a most wonderful and intricate piece of bodily mechanism designed by nature for various purposes. It protects all the internal organs of the body. As it is elastic it allows free play to the muscles which are below it. It keeps the body clean by throwing out impurities from it as sweat. It regulates the temperature of the body. It keeps it from getting too hot or too cold. When the perspiration evaporates it cools the body.

The skin is an organ of touch. You get the sense of touch from the nerve endings arranged in it, though it is the mind that really feels. It is not only the organ of touch, but the organ for sensation of temperature and pressure also. Some carbon dioxide also passes through the skin. We breathe through the skin and lungs.

The skin consists of two parts — an outer layer called the epidermis and an inner layer called the dermis, or true skin. The sweat glands, sebaceous glands and hair are in the true skin or dermis.

The epidermis consists of pavement cells, tiny cells which are seen only under a microscope. They are flat and very tightly packed together. The upper layer cells are dry and peel off if you rub them well. The under cells then take their place and the same thing happens again.

The dermis or the true skin is full of blood-vessels and nerves. If you prick it with a pin, blood comes out. The nerves send the news or telegraphic message to the brain and you feel pain.

There are three million pores in the skin. There are pores with hair and pores with fine body-hair into which oil glands open. (There is a small muscle at the side of these body-hairs. It is these muscles which contract and make the hairs stand on end — goose pimples or horripilation.)

The sebaceous glands secrete an oily substance which lubricates the skin and serves the purpose of a natural pomade. It makes the skin shining and smooth and preserves the delicately sensitive sense of touch. It keeps the skin from getting dry and cracked.

The sweat glands open through pores in the dermis. Sweat (or perspiration) is saltish acid water which contains organic dead matter. The sweat glands are simple tubes which open on the surface of the skin and relieve the body of a portion of the effete material. The amount of sweat given off by a full-grown man in twenty four hours is about two pounds in weight, or two pints. The sweat increases in hot weather and during exercise and running. It decreases in winter. The sweat glands are numerous in the neck and back.

In hot countries much of the work of the kidneys and lungs is done by the skin. The amount of sweat and excretion of solids is very great. Hence the cleansing of the skin is very important in hot countries. If the pores of the skin are blocked by dirt, the function of the skin is interfered with. The lungs and the kidneys will have to overwork.

The skin, the kidneys and the large intestines represent the sewers of the body. If the kidneys are in a diseased condition, the skin works more vigorously and tries to throw out the poison as quickly as possible. From each of its pores a stream laden with poisonous products of disintegration constantly flows. When the perspiration evaporates it leaves behind it waste products which are deposited as a thin film over the whole surface of the skin. If the dirt of the skin is not removed the accumulation continues to increase. It undergoes decomposition, it putrifies and emits a stinking odour. The unclean accumulation chokes the millions of pores on the skin and stands in the way of its proper functioning. Various diseases of the skin develop and the functioning of the whole system seriously suffers. The waste matter that accumulates in sickness is more abundant than in health, and is more poisonous. Hence it is very necessary to keep the openings of these glands free, by daily baths and gentle rubbing of the skin. Bathing in cold water followed by friction with a towel cleans the skin and invigorates the body.

The skin is the great gateway through which nature tries to throw off the waste materials and poisons collected in the system through errors in diet, unhygienic living, etc. Good food, exercise, fresh air and daily baths are essential if you wish to have a beautiful complexion. Remain in the sun and apply mustard oil to the body. Massage the body well. The circulation of the blood is quickened, the muscles are exercised well. You will experience an exhilaration and refreshing feeling. It keeps the body cool and makes the skin soft and supple. It entangles the dirt of the body and makes its removal easy during bathing when soap is used.

Care of the Teeth

Teeth are hard organs developed in connection with the mucous membrane of the mouth and implanted in the jaw bones. They serve for biting and grinding the food as well as aiding in speech.

The teeth are really intended by nature to serve the purpose of a mill for crushing the food. The tongue acts the part of a millhand by bringing the food under the mill.

Each tooth is composed of four substances: dentine, enamel, cement and pulp. Dentine makes up the greater part of each tooth both in the crown, where it is covered by a layer of enamel, and in the fang, where it is surrounded by cement. This coating protects the soft dentine. If it is broken or worn away, it does not grow again.

Each tooth consists of three parts: the root, neck and crown. The crown projects into the cavity of the mouth and the root or fang is embedded in a socket in the jaw-bone. At the point where the crown and the fang join there is a constriction known as the neck.

The centre of the tooth is hollowed out to lodge the pulp. The dentine is composed of animal matter and earthly matter, chiefly lime salts. Enamel is a brilliant white layer forming a sort of cap to the tooth. Cement or tooth-bone is a thin layer of bone covering the dentine in the fang. Pulp is one of the most important parts of the tooth. It contains the blood vessels and the nerve fibres derived from the fifth cranial nerve. It consists of connective tissue.

There are a few different shapes of teeth, viz. incisors, canines, premolars or bicuspids, and molars or grinders.

The teeth appear in a definite order and at definite periods. In childhood there are teeth called the 'milk teeth'. They begin to appear from the sixth month, are twenty in number and are temporary teeth. The whole set is out by the second year. The permanent teeth are thirty-two in number. They begin to appear gradually from the sixth year when the milk-teeth begin to fall out. There are sixteen in each row, and the set is completed between the seventeenth and the twenty-fifth year.

The order of the milk teeth is as follows:

Middle incisors — about the sixth month.
Lateral incisors — about the ninth month.
Canines — about the eighteenth month.
Second molars — about the twenty-fourth month.

As regards the permanent teeth, the first molar appears when the child is six years old, the incisors about seven or eight, the bicuspids about nine or ten, the canines about twelve, the second molars about thirteen and the wisdom teeth frequently do not cut the gum until the age of twenty or twenty-five.

Vitamin A is necessary for the growth of the jaw bone and vitamin C for the health of the gums. Vitamin D helps the calcification and hardening of the teeth. The teeth are composed of calcium and phosphates.

You should have a perfect set of teeth so that you can masticate your food in an efficient manner. If every particle of food that enters your mouth is not thoroughly masticated, you put an unnecessary amount of work on the digestive organs. In the long run they get diseased. The gums also should be healthy in order to keep the rest of the body healthy.

In your search for health and strength you may undertake a series of beneficial exercises that have been expressly designed to improve your breathing organs, to tone up and strengthen the various muscles of the body, strengthen your nerves and put your digestive system in a very healthy condition. These exercises will certainly go a long way in this direction, but if your mouth and teeth are not in a healthy condition you will find that the body will not respond to these exercises in anything like the way it will when your mouth and teeth are perfect.

The mouth is the first line of defence in the system. Chemical and mechanical irritants, poisons and gritty particles are detected here and thrown out. Every particle of food that you eat and the liquid you drink goes through your mouth to your stomach. If your mouth and teeth are not in good order then germs that are always in the diseased tissues will become mixed with your food and drink and find their way into your intestinal organs. For this reason, decayed teeth are one of the great causes of intestinal trouble such as gastritis, dyspepsia or indigestion, constipation, intestinal ulcers, flatulence, etc.

Tartar collects at the root of the teeth. This tartar is composed of secretions from glands and from food particles left over. This helps the accumulation of germs and bacteria. These germs are swallowed with food. They cause many disturbing conditions in the stomach and affect the system generally. The gums recede and waste on account of irritation set up by tartar on the teeth. The teeth get loosened. Have the tartar removed by a dentist.

If particles of food are allowed to remain in the teeth, they irritate and injure the teeth. They decompose and produce fermentation, the gums get swollen and pus forms there. The enamel is eaten away and the dentine exposed. This causes the teeth to decay, and dental caries occurs.

When pus is formed in the gums, it is called pyorrhoea. Most of the pus is swallowed into the stomach. The throat, the larynx (wind-box) and tonsils get diseased. The stomach and the intestines are affected by the pus. Then all sorts of diseases, disorders of the stomach and general poisoning of the system from the toxins generated in the pus, occur. Many complications also take place. There is general debility.

Avoid too cold or too hot food and drink. This is injurious to the whole system and produces caries in teeth, and pyorrhoea.

The mouth should be kept scrupulously clean. Cleaning with salt water daily is very beneficial, and at the end of each meal the mouth should be rinsed twice with salt water, especially after eating sweets. Potassium permanganate gargle is highly effective in the treatment of pyorrhoea. Chewing a few neem leaves and keeping the juice in the mouth for a few minutes is also very efficacious and beneficial.

From this it is quite obvious that every seeker after health should keep his teeth in a very clean and healthy condition. Remove the particles of food that stick to the teeth with a toothpick or fingers. Clean the teeth twice daily with a nice toothpowder composed of alum, black pepper and ochre. Do not use tooth sticks or brushes. Violent rubbing with these sticks removes the enamel quickly. Use your finger only. This is the most readily available and cheap tooth brush. Do not use any tooth powder or paste that is sold in the market. Do not be carried away by pompous advertisements. Salt mixed with mustard oil is a valuable dental paste. It is used in inflammation of the gums and pyorrhoea. Do not use carbolic tooth powder. Carbolic acid corrodes the enamel quickly.

Daily massage of the gums with the fingers improves the circulation of blood in the gums and their nutrition. Massage your gums with mustard oil mixed with a pinch of common salt. Always massage and brush your teeth and gums either in a circular way or from the gums towards the teeth. Brushing horizontally harms. Finish by rinsing with common salt and water.

Fresh milk, whole grains, cereals, fresh vegetables and fruits are highly beneficial in preserving the teeth in a healthy condition. Take some sour fruit at the end of a meal. The acid helps to keep the teeth clean. Cleanse the mouth several times with water and force the water through the teeth.

Constipation is the mother of many diseases which the human flesh is heir to. Inactive or sluggish liver is the cause of constipation. The liver becomes inactive because of indigestion, improper function of the stomach being the cause. The function of the stomach is to digest food which is forwarded to it in crushed ground form from the mouth, wherein Providence has provided a mill of sixteen stones in each of the upper and lower jaws. So, ultimately the cause of constipation, the mother of almost all troubles, is to be found in the teeth. Hence the desirablility, rather necessity, of keeping this mill — the teeth — in perfect order.

Toothache is a symptom of several affections of the teeth and neighbouring parts. The commonest cause of toothache is caries or decay affecting one or more teeth, particularly when the cavity in a tooth exposes the pulp.

Gum boil, consisting of an inflammatory condition connected with the root of the tooth, which often precedes the formation of an abcess, is another cause of dull, throbbing pain.

The want of effective cleansing of the mouth, leading to the presence of acid secretion on the gums and between the teeth, which eats gradually into the enamel, is another cause of very annoying toothache.

An attack of toothache is started by exposure to cold, a hot drink or some sweet or acid article of food.

The mouth is essentially the gateway of health. By observing the following rules the teeth can be maintained in perfect order:

1. Never take too cold water or icy water after hot meals. If you do so, there will be congestion in throat and gums.
2. Never develop the habit of eating with only one side of the jaw. If you do not heed this, the other side will suffer from poor blood circulation, tartar will cover your teeth, and thereafter spongy gums will lead to pyorrhoea.
3. Avoid taking sloppy foods. The harder the food, the better for teeth and gums. Sloppy foods give no exercise to teeth. Every

organ of the body needs exercise for maintenance of health; otherwise it degenerates and dies.

4. Rinse your mouth thoroughly after each meal, especially after sweets. Sweets, if they cling to the teeth, are converted into an acid which makes holes in the teeth.

The Benefits of a Sunbath

The sun is the source of all energy and power. You derive energy and power from the sun. If the sun does not shine for a day or two on account of clouds, your vitality falls to a low level and you are not in good spirits. Flowers, plants, animals and men rejoice as soon as the sun rises above the horizon. The sun supplies energy to all plants and living beings, and yet its energy is never exhausted. Its energy is inexhaustible because it derives its energy from the inexhaustible source — the Atman.

The rays of the sun bestow on us wonderful health. The *Vedas* have glorified the rising sun. Ayurveda has extolled its efficacy. The sages have sung its praise in a variety of ways.

Build your house on the western side of a river, lake or tank. Then you will daily enjoy the reflected light, which is more beneficial and potent than the direct rays. The rays of the rising sun are a blessing from God for the preservation of health as well as for the cure of diseases. The rays of the sun possess antiseptic and germicidal properties. Expose your blankets, bedsheet, pillows and mattress to the sun once in fifteen days. In the rays of the sun you will find a cheap and easily available tonic, a disinfectant, an antiseptic and potent germicide.

Sunlight is a food. You can make Vitamin 'D' by exposing your naked body to the sun. The skin and the nerves will absorb the energies of the sunlight. The sunlight provides the heat needed to sustain life.

Sunlight as a healer of leprosy and various other skin diseases was known to the ancients. They built temples dedicated to the sun. The temple of Konarak was built upon a tradition that Samba, the son of Sri Krishna, was striken with leprosy because he saw his father in the act of connubial pleasure. When entreated to be forgiven, Krishna asked Samba to worship the sun in order to be freed of the loathsome disease. Accordingly he did so and was cured. In Egypt, the sun god is Ra; in Greece, Apollo; in Phoenicia, the sun. In Syria also the sun and moon are worshipped. In France and Germany the peasants even now take off their hats to the rays of the sun. The sun is looked at and worshipped by Hindus when they take a bath in the morning.

The morning sun gives out ultra-violet rays, as does also the evening sun. If persons suffering from leprosy and other skin diseases strip themselves of all clothing and remain in the sun naked till their body is properly tanned, then the sun's rays will penetrate their body and work wonders there. Only the head must be protected from the sun. Besides leprosy, tuberculosis, rheumatism, obesity, anaemia, neurasthenia, eczema, colds, coughs, rickets, diseases of the teeth, etc. can also be treated with the sun's rays.

Wear a thin light garment and walk on the western bank of a river, on the west side of the sea, a lake or tank early in the morning at sunrise. Run also. You will doubtless enjoy a sunbath. Practise asanas and physical exercises in the sun. Expose your mouth to the rays of the rising sun. Open it wide. Let the rays penetrate your nostrils also. Close your eyes when you expose your mouth. Practise deep-breathing exercise and pranayama in the sun.

The various parts of the body should receive a regulated sun-bath. Turn the body round frequently. Bask in the sun. Expose your body to the rays of the sun for a short time. Lie down on the ground on a blanket or lie on a cot. (If the rays are very hot, cover your back with a green plantain leaf.) This will prove useful in lumbago and rheumatism and diseases of the skin.

Have sunlight treatment for the eyes. You will have clear vision. You need not take recourse to spectacles. First, sit in the sun. Close your eyes. Slowly move your head from side to side. Let the sun shine directly on the closed eyelids for ten or thirty minutes. Let the eyeballs also move with the movement of the head, and not against. Now, turn your back to the sun or come into the shade. Do not open your eyes. Cover the eyes with the palms of the hands for five or ten minutes. This is palming. Have the sun treatment in the morning and evening, 7 a.m. and 5 p.m. Let the exposure of the eyes to the sun be gradual. When the eyes get accustomed to the light, you can gradually have stronger light.

The sages of yore who had knowledge of the curative power of the rays of the sun revealed the mysteries of the sun and its beneficial rays, and the uses of this radiant energy.

Even in the West, doctors are using the rays of the sun as a powerful therapeutic agent in the treatment of diseases. They call this heliotherapy. In the sanatoriums in the Alps the consumptive patients are directly exposed to the mild rays of the sun. In olden days in India babies were put in the cradle and their bare bodies exposed to the rising sun. In California and other parts of the West boys and girls now take sun-baths.

Whence comes the mysterious power in the sun which causes the seeds to germinate and flowers to turn into fruits? Whence comes this radiant energy in the sun which bestows wonderful health, power and vigour to living beings? Whence comes this power to heal? Whence comes the vital energy in the sun that invigorates and galvanises the young and rejuvenates and vitalises the old? Whence comes this vegetative vigour which enables the plants to synthesise the vitamins? The sun derives its power and energy from Atman or the Eternal, the Absolute, the Sun of suns, the Light of lights, the Source of everything, the first of all causes, the store-house of all energies. Brahman willed; the sun came into being to bestow health and happiness to all beings.

Repeat the twelve names of the sun at sunrise:

Mitraya namah, ravaye namah, suryaya namah, bhanave namah, khagaya namah, pushne namah, hiranyagarbhaya namah, maricaye namah, adityaya namah, savitre namah, arkaya namah, bhaskaraya namah.

He who repeats this at sunrise will possess wonderful health, vigour and vitality. He will be free from any kind of disease of the eye. He will have powerful eyesight. Pray in the sun in the early morning before sunrise:

O Lord, Suryanarayana, the Eye of the world, the Eye of God, give me health and strength, vigour and vitality.

Repeat the prayer of the *Isavasya Upanishad*, slokas 15 and 16:

The face of Truth is covered by a golden vessel. Remove, O Sun, the covering, so that I, who am devoted to truth, may behold it. O Pushan (nourisher of all), the only seer (sole traveller of the heavens), controller of all, Surya, son of Prajapati, disperse thy rays and gather up thy burning light; I behold thy glorious form, I am He, the purusha within Thee.

In the words of the *Yajur Veda:*

O Sun of suns! You are all-energy, give me energy; you are all-strength, give me strength; you are all-powerful, give me power.

MENTAL THERAPEUTICS

We are accustomed in this age of scientific advancement to hear of marvels. Many people all over the world are expecting that nuclear physics will be utilised by experts for providing amenities of life to the common man, in a manner hitherto unimagined. Very probably it may also happen that the advancing practical philosopher may show the world how, by a purely mental process, physical ills can be cured. If any such thing happens, one need not wonder at it; because it is said that such things happened in our country in the remote ages past.

Our sacred scriptures tell us that the whole world comes out of the mere thought of the Creator. They also say that everybody himself, in real essence, is identical with God. The great sentence of the *Upanishads* is *Aham Brahmasmi — I am Brahman*. If that is the truth, if even the entire universe is only the external manifestation of the potency of a single thought, it must be very simple for an individual to project a thought which has got the potency to destroy the evil effects of a malady and create a curative process by which a disease is removed.

But who knows this trick? Sacred books say that the yogi knows it, that the yogi can cure himself of all diseases and also can cure others of their diseases. Is it possible in the present day for anyone to learn this secret? It seems to be so. At any rate, one can well think about the rationale behind such treatment of physical ills.

At the outset, let it be clearly stated that such a treatment is not of the nature of the widely advertised hypnotic cures. Spiritual treatment is the sending out or projection of vibrant, forcible, harmonising thought waves which will take control of the patient's mind — not for the purpose of subordinating it, but for the purpose of charging it with those energies which alone will make that apparatus (the mind) function effectively to do away with the discord-creating tendencies and impulses which are the root cause of the disease that the patient has been suffering from.

Disease is only the consequence of the absence of peace. If peace is infused into the patient, it will automatically get into his subconscious mind which will make the necessary changes in his mental make-up, so that the activity of aggression and anxiety will be suitably counter-balanced by the extra charge of purity and peace. The result will be that the conscious mind will begin to perceive that change in the form of diseaselessness.

If the spiritual healer is to be competent to give peace vibrations to the patient, he must have them himself. In other words, he must have stored up within himself a sufficient stock of peace. That is possible only if he has gone through the regular practice of raja yoga, which is control of the mental modifications.

The question now is: will there be in the world of the future a sufficiently large number of raja yogis who will be qualified to straightaway get at the root cause of all diseases — the absence of peace in the mind of the sufferer — and administer spiritual treatment in the form of successive potent doses of peace? If such a thing happens, most of the work of the medical practitioners will be taken away and they will thereby be able to devote their energies in some other constructive manner. If marvels can be achieved in the field of science, as is being done today, nothing stands in the way of the achievement of marvels in the field of spirituality.

This body is the moving temple of God, the sacred shrine for the Supreme Soul. It should be kept ever clean, healthy and strong. The individual soul is a reflection of the Supreme Soul in the mind. The mind is like a mirror. Selfishness, lust, hatred, anger and egoism are the dirt which spoils the transparency and purity of the mind.

The Supreme Soul is the source for all life and all intelligence animating the universe. It is a mass of pure consciousness and bliss. It is spirit. The physical body is dominated and guided by the mind, which is a higher power than the physical body. The mind draws its power and light from the Supreme Soul.

For many the body is all in all, it is everything for them. They worship this body; they have become abject slaves of this body — a mass of flesh and bone, a combination of the five elements. They have no idea of the soul; the body has become their Lord. They have no self-control at all. They neither practise any asana or regular exercise nor lead a well-regulated and disciplined life. They fill their stomach with sweets, pastries, etc., giving no rest to their digestive and eliminative organs. They ever suffer from physical weakness and disease. The atoms, molecules and cells in their body produce discordant and inharmonious vibrations. They have neither hope, confidence, faith, serenity nor cheerfulness. They are unhappy. The life force is not operating properly and their vitality is at a low ebb. Their mind is filled with fear, despair, worry and anxiety.

The physical body should be kept under your perfect control. It is only your instrument. It should be your willing servant ever ready to obey your commands. You are always the master and proprietor of this body. You are in essence the soul.

The influence of mind over the body is now well understood by the vast majority of educated persons. Every thought and every emotion exercises a direct influence over the body. Cheerfulness, faith, serenity, joy, happiness and love produce good, harmonious vibrations in the physical body. Hatred, doubt and depression generate disharmonious and discordant vibrations in the physical body. The influence of the mind upon the body excels all other agencies which can be brought to bear upon it. Mental therapeutics in the treatment of disease is exceedingly beneficial. Particularly in the treatment of nervous diseases, it surpasses all other kinds of treatment.

Health and Psychology

You must have a healthy state of mind if you want to lead a happy and healthy life and if you want to progress in the spiritual path. Most of the physical ailments spring from a diseased state of mind. Kindly bear this fact in mind. Emotional imbalance leads to all sorts of nervous troubles and physical illness also. That is why a real sannyasin, even if he is starved, homeless and friendless, is happy and full of vigour. He has inner strength.

You should lead a well-regulated life. Proper hours of work and rest are necessary. Then alone can you be healthy and peaceful, and have ample time for sadhana (spiritual practices). Then alone can you achieve success in all your undertakings. Go to bed at 10 p.m. and get up at 4 a.m. You will have strong nerves.

One reason why people suffer from nervous breakdown is that they do not know how to utilise their holidays. They are more busy on holidays than they are on working days! They waste more energy on holidays, in the name of recreation. There is in fact no re-creation but a re-doubled destruction. Observe the vow of silence on all holidays. Devote all your time to spiritual practices. Do this for six months from now; you will yourself experience the truth of what I say.

Cheerfulness, harmony, serenity, faith, love and compassion co-operate with the constructive principles in nature. They harmonise the physical vibrations, relax the tissues and muscles and open them wide to the inflow of the vital force and purity.

Develop the power of will through elimination of desires, cravings and low corroding emotions and thoughts. You can dominate and regulate the activities and the life-currents in your body through the power of strong, pure and resolute will. The organs and the nervous system, etc. will perform their work intelligently, harmoniously and serenely even under the stress of disease and other unfavourable conditions.

Through the power of will you can harmonise the blood circulation, you can direct the currents of prana to those parts or organs which need them most, you can remove congestion from certain areas or organs, you can charge certain diseased parts with vigorous prana and abundant nerve force, you can recharge your battery with new vigour and force and you can fill the vital sheath with abundant energy.

The more you are endowed with faith, serenity, love, courage, tolerance, devotion and sympathy, the more you open yourself to the inflow of divine energy or the vital forces.

Constant thinking of a disease intensifies the disease. Divert the mind. Keep it always occupied on some interesting work or other. You can minimise the force of a disease. If the mind constantly thinks of the heart as being in a diseased condition the mental pictures of disease, weakness and fear vibrations are telegraphed to the cells of the heart through the efferent nerves. The cells of the heart become more weakened and diseased through the discordant vibrations sent to them from the mind. Affirmations of health remove disease. Auto-suggestion is another form of psycho-therapy. This is beneficial in the treatment of diseases. By auto-suggestion one can turn his thoughts away from the idea of disease. He can break away from the habit of thinking he is ill and can create the habit of thinking he is well. The subconscious mind responds to constant and repeated phrases such as, "Through the grace of God, I am getting better every day, in every way."

You can cure diseases in others by giving healthy suggestions. A higher mind has influence over a lower mind. Diseases are produced by the sickly excited imagination. Bodily functions are influenced by ideas and imagination. The sickness is in the brain. The diseased imaginations must be combated in a proper manner through healthy, harmonious, powerful thoughts and good suggestions. Suggestions have powerful influence. In the mind of a sick person put the idea, "You will quickly become alright". He will become better.

He who has great magnetic force or animal magnetism can help others in the treatment of disease. He can impart his magnetic power to weak, diseased persons. You can increase the healing power through exercising right thinking, concentration and meditation. Magnetism is a nerve force. It radiates or flows from the operator when an affinity exists between the mind of the healer and the one to be healed. He who is pure in mind, who has sympathy, goodwill, fellow-feeling, mercy and fear of God, can really magnetise others.

Selfishness, egoism, fear and worry contract the blood vessels and the nerve fibres and obstruct and dominate the inflow of the vital force or life-current, and lower the vitality and the power of resistance to external, immoral influences or forces.

Mental Health

Mental health is more important than physical health. If the mind is healthy the body will necessarily be healthy.

Mental hygiene deals with the condition and laws of mental health. It aims at conserving and improving the mental health of the individual and of the community. It touches many aspects of practical human life. It represents a systematised mass of knowledge which it derives from researches in psychology, psychiatry, medicine, sociology, biology, child-study and education.

An understanding of the principles of mental hygiene is highly desirable. A careful practice of these principles will lead to great happiness, strength and joy. Everybody should acquire a general knowledge of psychology, psychological medicine or psychiatry and some idea about the principles of education.

Man is a composite of three parts. He has a body, a mind and a soul. In dealing with the health of a complete human being you must remember: (1) the body which is visible and tangible, and which is the organ of expression of your invisible and intangible (2) mind and (3) soul.

This body is the mould prepared by the mind for its enjoyment. It is another form of the subtle, invisible mind. The unseen mind has become the visible body.

The body is a counterpart of the mind. If there is pain in the tooth or the stomach or ear, the mind is at once affected. It cannot think properly. It is agitated and disturbed. If there is depression in the mind, the body also cannot function properly. For instance, if a man receives a telegram that his only son has died of pneumonia, at once his face becomes pale, his mind is agitated, he becomes nervous, he has no appetite and his red corpuscles are destroyed. The mind is affected at first. He receives a shock. Afterwards the whole body reacts. Mark here the influence of the mind over the body!

As physical health is an important condition of mental health, strain of any organ, excessive fatigue and mental strain should be avoided. Your life must be well-regulated and disciplined, and excess of any kind should be avoided. You must stick to the happy, golden medium. Rest is necessary.

Tobacco, alcohol and intoxicating drugs affect the brain, nerves and the mind also. He who is addicted to these drugs cannot enjoy mental health or physical health. Give up these intoxicants at once.

Mind is a mysterious subtle force. It is the power of the Atman. It is a product of nature. It is a non-entity that appears as an entity. It is a bundle of desires, thoughts and imaginations. It creates and destroys this world. It is manifestation of para shakti (supreme energy). It is an offspring of illusion or ignorance. It is composed of three qualities: sattva (purity, harmony, light, goodness), rajas (passion, motion) and tamas (inertia, darkness, ignorance). If sattva prevails you will enjoy wonderful health and peace. If rajas predominates, the mind will be restless, perturbed, agitated and distracted. If inertia or tamas predominates, the mind will be heedless, indolent and lazy.

Fill the mind with sattva. Have satsang or association with the wise. Cultivate faith, serenity, truthfulness, courage, mercy, devotion, love, cheerfulness, confidence, divine thoughts and divine virtues. Change worldly thoughts. Allow the mind to run in the spiritual direction, in divine grooves. Your mind will be peaceful, harmonious.

You will have excellent mental health. You will have no physical disease.

Practice of ahimsa (non-violence), satyam (truthfulness) and brahmacharya (celibacy) is necessary in maintaining good mental health. Truth is an honest endeavour to convey a real expression of what has occurred or what is intending, to those around you. The truth, the whole truth and nothing but the truth can satisfy God and your own heart. Truth cannot be measured by rods and furlongs, minims and ounces. Thought must totally agree with the speech and the speech with the action. This is truth.

Himsa (violence), falsehood and impurity fill the mind with restlessness, cares, worries and anxieties. You cannot have peace of mind even for a second. How then can there be good mental health where there is no peace of mind?

If you wish to have a successful and useful life and good mental health it is absolutely necessary for you to acquire the virtue of self-control. Life will be a long series of futilities, a succession of follies if the quality of self-control is absent.

Psychologists are of the opinion that disease is not primarily of body or flesh, but of mind. They say that disease is caused by poisons generated in the blood by anger, revenge, hatred, lust, etc.

The root cause of all diseases is ignorance. Ignorance leads to desire, greed and anger. These torture the heart. From these spring 'mine'ness, jealousy, attachment, envy, malice, egoism, pride, hypocrisy and hatred.

The pains which afflict the body are called the secondary diseases, while the desires that afflict the mind are called mental or primary disease.

In the *Yoga Vasishtha* Sri Vasishtha says:

> Now listen, O Rama, as to the manner in which the two forms of disease, primary and secondary, perish in two days. The wise say that primary disease has two sub-divisions — ordinary and essential. The former includes the diseases incidental to the body, while the latter includes the rebirth men are subject to. If the diseases which afflict the body return to their primal source, then they are destroyed. Their primary causes being (bad) thoughts, if these thoughts are destroyed, all bodily diseases will vanish. But the disease of rebirth will never perish except through Atmajnana (direct knowledge of the Self). Is it possible to suppose that the

> misconception of a serpent in a rope will be removed except through the discovery of real rope? But those grievous diseases of the body which do not arise through the original cause, can be extirpated through mantras, medicine and the many means proposed by men well-versed in medical lore. I need not expatiate upon this subject any further here.

Then Rama asked Vasishtha how mental diseases arise and how they are destroyed. Vasishtha proceeded thus:

> When the mind is agitated, then this body also follows in its wake. And when the body is agitated then there is no proper perception of things that are in one's way, and prana flies from its proper road like an animal hit by, and reeling under, the impact of an arrow. Through such agitation prana, instead of pervading the whole body steadily and equally, will vibrate everywhere at an unequal rate. Thereby the nadis will not maintain a steady position (like electric wires), but will quiver. The food which settles itself down in this body amidst such a commotion is transformed into incurable diseases. Thus through the primary cause (of the mind) is the disease of the body generated. If this primary cause can be annihilated at its root, then all diseases will be destroyed.
>
> Now hear the path by which diseases may be removed by the uttering of mantras. Like base gold which, when placed in the crucible, is transmuted through alchemical process into pure gold, the mind is unfailingly rendered pure through true, virtuous and pure actions and through dependence upon the wise. In the mind thus purified there will arise unalloyed bliss. Is not the whole world exhilarated with joy when the soft moon begins to shed its silvery light on it?
>
> If the mind becomes purified with the true sattva guna, then prana will begin to circulate freely throughout the body, the food taken will be digested properly, and hence no diseases will arise. I have thus described to you the path through which the two kinds of diseases can be destroyed.

If your mind is pure, if your thoughts are pure, you will be free from all diseases, primary and secondary.

If you want to possess good mental health, you must be always cheerful. You must cultivate this virtue again and again. Cheerfulness acts as the best mental tonic. Depression, gloom and cheerlessness corrode the mind. If there is depression you do not have a good appetite, you feel very weak, you cannot talk briskly, you cannot do any work with intense attention and application. If there is pain in the physical body, you cannot think properly, you cannot meditate. This is the common experience of all.

Removal of hatred through cosmic love, service, friendship, mercy, sympathy and compassion, removal of greed through disinterested service, generous acts and charity and removal of pride through humility will help you a great deal in the achievement of good health.

Fortitude, forebearance, patience, endurance and balance of mind keep the mind in a good healthy state. Therefore endeavour to possess these divine virtues.

If you are sulky, irritable, greedy and selfish, these bad traits will produce a deleterious effect on your own physical and mental health and will have a definite influence on others. They are positively harmful to others.

In many cases both mental and physical troubles are due, not to inexorable fate or inevitable misfortune, but they arise for want of knowledge and as a consequence of a weak and wrong management of the circumstances of life.

Eliminate fear, care, worry and anxiety by relying on God. God is the source of power, wisdom and bliss. Fear, worry and anxiety corrode the mind. They paralyse the mind and fill it with despair, depression and despondency.

Avoid all mental conflicts. Do not interfere in the affairs of others. Have perfect tolerance and broad adaptability. Allow individuals to grow in their own ways. Every man has his own way, his own predilection, his own natural capacity, temperament and outlook. No two men are alike. Endeavour to remove any undesirable and unsocial trait in yourself.

The real supreme healer is God. His grace alone can make you hale, hearty, cheerful, joyful, blissful and healthy. Take refuge in Him alone with all your being. Be righteous. Lead a well regulated, disciplined life. Observe the rules of health and hygiene and be happy forever.

Japa, chanting, study of sacred scriptures, meditation, enquiry, reflection and pranayama all pave a long way to the attainment of mental health. Therefore practise japa and meditation. The flow of divine grace, the flow of purity from the Lord towards the pious student of yoga, heals the mind. When the mind is healthy the body is also healthy. Purity and divine grace are mighty spiritual forces.

Do not become a faddist or slave to some fad. A faddist is intensely, hopelessly and terribly attached to his own weak pet theories or beliefs. A yoga student, an allopath, a naturopath, an ayurvedic vaid, a scientist and a philosopher have their own fads. They never listen to other people's arguments, however cogent, convincing, sound and strong they may be. A faddist develops intolerance and bigotry, which make his mind hard and thus prevent his intellect from vibrating harmoniously to receive others' views.

Brahman or the Eternal is infinite. His expressions are also infinite. Allopathy, homeopathy, hydropathy, chromopathy, electropathy, naturopathy, ayurveda, etc. are all His expressions. All these systems are very essential. Temperaments are different: therefore different systems of treatment to suit men of different temperaments are also necessary.

Auto-Suggestion

Every one of you should practise auto-suggestion, as it has marvellous benefits. Whatever medicine cannot do, this psychic method powerfully accomplishes. It gets rid of disease and establishes admirable health, power, energy and vitality. It consists of powerful assertions: e.g. 'I am becoming better and better, every day in every way.' Constantly repeat this mentally. Constantly dwell on these thoughts. As you think, so you become. Think you are strong, strong you become. Think you are weak, weak you become. Think you are a sinner, a sinner you become. Think you are Brahman, Brahman you become.

Mind makes a hell of heaven and a heaven of hell. Mind is the cause for bondage and for liberation. Never give-in to dark negative thoughts. Drive them out. Kill them on the spot.

Even if you are the poorest of the poor, the dullest of the dull, never move a fraction of an inch from your real position. *Tat tvam asi — 'Thou are That'* — Thou art Brahman. You are the sun. The whole world moves around you. There is nobody superior to you in the whole world. Assert strongly. Affirm. You will feel tremendous strength and power.

If you want to get rid of constipation (or any other disease) do any of the following:

1. Personify the disease. Assert. Command: "O disease constipation, get out!" The disease will die. The vital force inside will bring about repair and renewed energy. This method demands strong will-power.
2. Ignore and do not think of the disease. Divert the mind when thoughts of the body arise. Do this several times. The disease will disappear. Children do not feel cold while at play. Sleep vanishes when you are attending a cinema show. Hunger passes when you are interested in a music party. Why? Because the mind is diverted and kept occupied in something else. This is an easy method. Combine no. 1 with no. 2. This is a healthy combination.
3. Deny the existence of disease.
4. Truce method. Make alliance and friendship with the disease constipation. Praise the disease, "O disease constipation. You are a great power of Brahman. You have troubled me enough. I know your potency. Kindly get out of my system!" The disease will die out. The vital force inside will attend to the wear and tear and induce renewed energy and vitality. This is an easy method also. In the treatment of cobra poisoning, those who use a mantra praise Garuda, the vehicle of Lord Vishnu (Garuda mantra). This corresponds to the above method.

You can derive the beneficial results in a couple of days. You must calmly wait for some time. Have constant practice till you establish a mental habit. Then the subconscious mind will do the work for you.

Auto-suggestion is a powerful cheap agent to develop your will-power. You can get over any difficulty. You can tide over despairing situations. You can smile in any adverse situations. Have the word-image POWER—STRENGTH—VITALITY before the mind always.

Twenty-Four Precepts

1. Yoga brings a message of hope to the forlorn, joy to the depressed, strength to the weak and knowledge to the ignorant.
2. Fear is the deadliest disease. It is the cause of worldly cares and

anxieties. Remove this by cultivating courage and meditation on the fearless Atman or Immortal Self.

3. Temperance, exercise, pure air, wholesome food, rest, refreshing sleep and God's name are the best of all physicians.

4. Mere wholesome diet, fresh air and exercise alone cannot give you lasting health and happiness. Spiritual life alone can bestow real health and happiness.

5. The mind vibrates discordantly and the five sheaths vibrate inharmoniously on account of the force of passion and inertia, likes and dislikes, lust, greed, hatred, fear and jealousy. How can you expect real happiness and health when such a state of affairs prevails in the system?

6. Mental health is more vital than bodily health. Diseases take their origin in the mind first and then manifest in the physical body.

7. Do not think of a disease too much. Too much thinking of the disease intensifies and strengthens the disease. Forget the body and the disease. Keep the mind fully occupied on useful works.

8. Abandon imaginary fears, unnecessary worries, cares and anxieties. Have perfect faith in God and do what is right.

9. When you were small children you had tummy aches and bilious attacks. When you were young you got egoistic-fever, lust-fever, anger-fever, jealousy-fever. When you are old you get headaches. Remove inertia, lust, egoism, likes and dislikes. Get knowledge of the Self and attain eternal health and happiness.

10. The practice of pranayama has a wonderful influence over the body, the mind, the intellect and the senses.

11. Pranayama regulates the breath and the mind also, and brings about harmonious vibrations. You will enjoy good health and happiness. Therefore be regular in your daily practice of pranayama.

12. The practice of asanas develops the body, and the practitioner is agile and nimble. He has a very elastic spine and a supple body.

13. Practise celibacy (brahmacharya). Entertain pure divine thoughts. Study sacred books. Have satsang. Dwell in the company of saints.

14. He who boasts, "I have never had any disease in this life," has lost the greatest lesson of life, the most beautiful lecture room in the great school of humanity — the sick chamber.

15. Disease is indeed a blessing. It opens your eyes to the realities of life. It instils mercy and sympathy in your heart and turns your mind towards God.
16. When a man is suffering from an acute unbearable pain he abandons his vanity and recollects that there is God. He becomes humble and penitent.
17. If you visit a patient, do not talk about his disease but cheer him up. Tell him some stories of saints or great mahatmas and their great deeds. Make him laugh through educative humour. Chant with him. This is a potent and unfailing tonic.
18. Cultivate divine virtues such as purity, magnanimity, humility, cosmic love, courage and forgiveness. Then there will be harmony and peace in the mind, and consequently you will enjoy real good health and happiness.
19. Enquire 'Who am I?' There cannot be any disease in the ever-pure all-pervading immortal diseaseless soul. Disease belongs to the material body and not to the resplendent spirit or soul.
20. The ingredients of health and long life are prayer, japa, chanting, meditation, serenity, cosmic love, temperance, regulated life, fresh open air, regular exercise, regulated breathing exercises or pranayama, sunbath and good wholesome food.
21. Do unconditional and unreserved self-surrender to the Lord. He will take care of you. Be at ease. You will be free from fear and worries. You will enjoy health and happiness.
22. Practise the presence of God. Behold Him in all faces, in all beings, in all forms. See Him everywhere.
23. Prayer, chanting, japa and meditation fill the mind with purity. Divine energy flows from the Lord to the devotee.
24. Meditate ceaselessly on the desireless, ever-blissful Atman. Chant OM. Sing OM. Do japa of OM. You will be blessed with health and happiness.

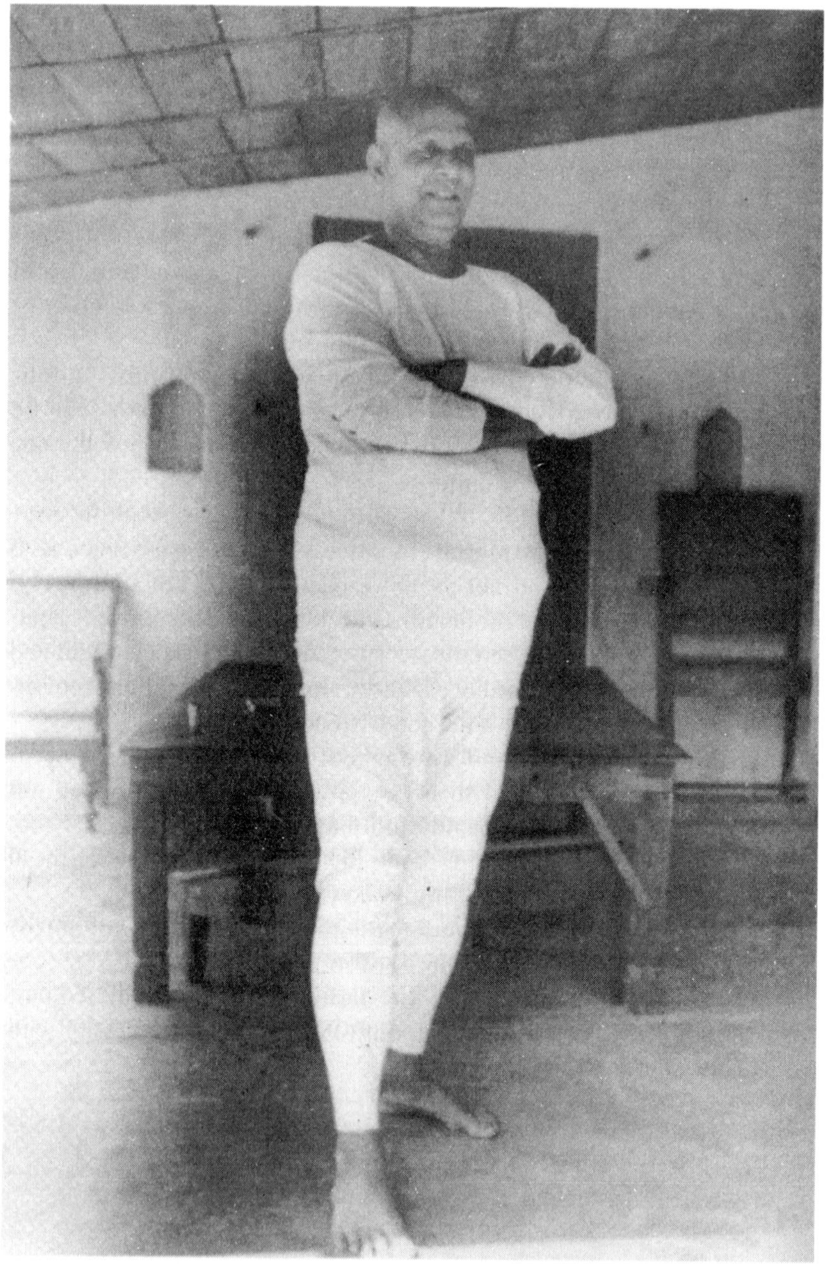

Though Swami Sivananda's body was not always well, he radiated health and energy.

Section II

HATHA YOGA

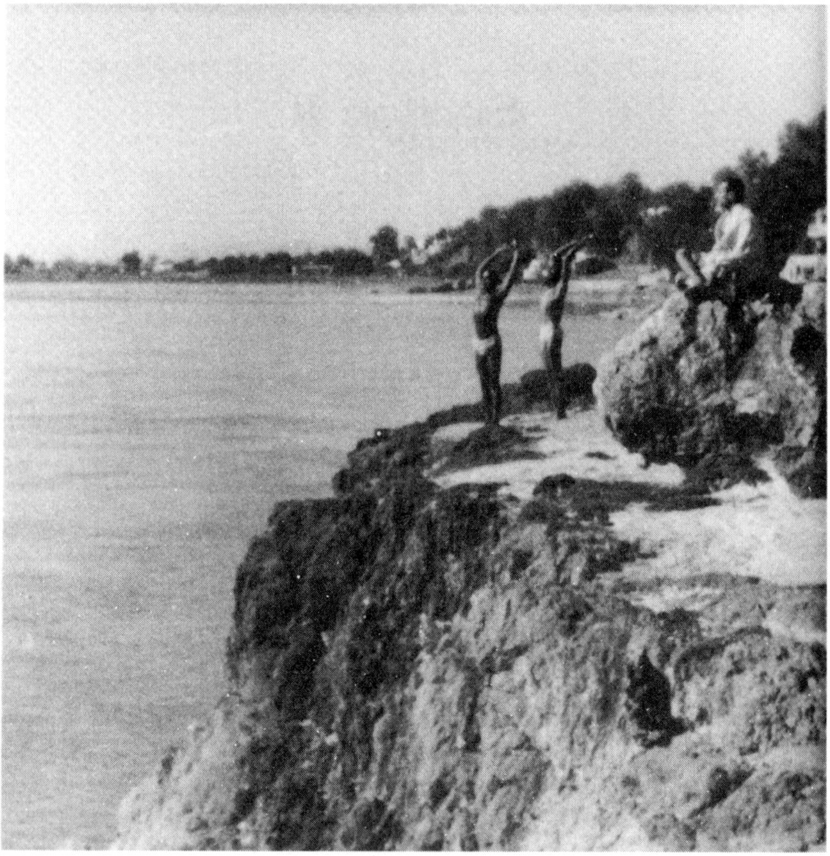

Surya namaskara on the Ganges bank

HATHA YOGA

Physical and Mental Efficiency Through Yoga

Every human being has within himself various potentialities and capacities of which he may never really have any conception. He is a magazine of power and knowledge. As he evolves he unfolds new powers, new faculties, new qualities. He can change his environment. He can influence others. He can subdue other minds. He can heal others. He can get plenty of material things. He can conquer internal and external nature. He must awaken these dormant powers and faculties through the practice of yoga. He must purify himself, develop his will, control the senses and the mind and and practise regular concentration. Then he will become a superman or Godman.

Yoga is a perfectly practical system of self-culture. You attain harmonious development of your body, mind, intellect and soul by the practice of yoga. It is an exact science. It is a system of yogic exercises of the Indian rishis and yogis of yore, based on exact principles. Yoga exercises are adapted for both men and women, for people of the East and West. It imparts to every practitioner definite practical knowledge of the means to enjoy fine health, longevity, strength, vim and vitality. You can acquire absolute control over the whole of nature by the practice of yoga. It will help you to attain ethical perfection and perfect concentration of the mind, and to unfold various psychic powers. Yoga brings a message of hope to the forlorn, joy to the depressed, strength to the weak and knowledge to the ignorant. Yoga is the secret master-key that unlocks the realm of Elysian bliss and deep abiding peace.

A yogi or a sage always keeps a balanced mind in all conditions of life and at all moments. A yogi's vision is deeply penetrating because he has gathered all the dissipated rays of the mind by discipline through patient sadhana. He can get full knowledge of either a distant or an internal object in no time. His mind is like a searchlight. Just as the diver in the pearl fishery dives down deep and brings up the pearl, so also the mind of a yogi dives deep into an object and brings out its truth in a moment. If the magnet is very powerful it will influence iron filings even when they are placed at a long distance; even so, if the yogi is an advanced person he will have great influence over the people with whom he comes in contact. He can even exert his influence on persons living in a distant place.

The yogi has the ability to laugh heartily and he radiates joy, strength and vigour. He always accomplishes his aims, getting success in all his attempts. He looks very young even at the age of sixty. He is endowed with a peculiar glow in his face and eyes and possesses a peculiar charm in his smile.

Now that you understand that you can attain physical and mental efficiency through yoga, destroy all weakness by regular and systematic practice of it. Attain harmonious development of your body, mind, intellect and soul by a regular practice of yoga. Health is thy birthright, not disease; strength is thy heritage, not weakness; efficiency, not inefficiency; courage, not fear; bliss, not sorrow; peace, not restlessness; knowledge, not ignorance; immortality, not mortality.

Attain this birthright or divine heritage and shine as a fully developed yogi radiating joy, peace, bliss and knowledge everywhere.

Hatha Yoga

Hatha yoga relates to pranayama, asanas, bandhas and mudras. 'Ha-tha' means the union of the sun and the moon, union of prana and apana. 'Hatha' means any tenacious practice till the object or end is achieved. Hatha yoga is inseparable from raja yoga. They are interdependent, and are the necessary counterparts of each other. No one can become a perfect yogi without a knowledge and practice of both. Hatha yoga prepares the student to take up raja yoga.

A hatha yogi starts his sadhana (spiritual practices) with body and prana; a raja yogi starts his sadhana with his mind; a jnana yogi starts his sadhana with intellect or will.

A hatha yogi gets siddhis (psychic powers) by uniting prana and apana and by taking the united prana-apana through the six chakras (centres of spiritual energy) to sahasrara at the crown of the head. A raja yogi gets siddhis by samyama — combined practice of dharana (concentration), dhyana (meditation) and samadhi at one time. A jnana yogi exhibits siddhis through pure will. A bhakta gets siddhis through self-surrender and the consequent descent of grace.

Kriyas, asanas, pranayama, mudras, bandhas and exercises in concentration and meditation constitute hatha yoga, which leads to the awakening of the kundalini shakti and ultimate union with God in samadhi.

Kriyas or preliminary purificatory processes — neti, dhauti, nauli, basti, tratak and kapalabhati — belong to hatha yoga. All need not practise these kriyas. However, those who have got too much phlegm in the body should practise them. Learn them under an expert hatha yogi.

Asanas pertain to the physical body and the nerve-centres. They render the body firm and steady and eradicate physical ailments and inertia. Pranayama aims at the control of the vital breath. Bandhas pertain to the prana. (That which binds prana is a bandha.) They do not allow the prana to move upwards and the apana to move downwards. They bind and unite the prana with the apana and send the united prana-apana along the sushumna nadi. Mudras concern the mind. They represent seals. (Mudra means a seal.) They seal the mind with the soul or Atman. They do not allow the mind to wander outside towards objects. They direct the externalising mind towards Atman in the chambers of the heart and fix it there. A combination of these is essential.

Hatha yoga is not the goal. It is only a means to an end. Take to raja yoga after possessing good health.

Brother! Attain good health. Without health how can you live? Without health how can you earn? Without health how can you get success in yoga or any undertaking? Possess wonderful health through the practice of hatha yoga. Drink the nectar in sahasrara and live in the immortal abode of Siva.

The Benefits of Yoga Asanas

This body is the moving temple of God. It is an instrument for crossing the ocean of samsara (or the round of births and deaths) and attaining the supreme abode of immortality, eternal bliss and perennial joy. It is a horse that can take you to the destination or the goal of life.

Therefore it must be kept quite healthy and strong. Proper training and care of the body on an intelligent basis are necessary.

These yogic exercises are preventive and curative. That is the beauty of this system. Some exercises twist the body forward and backward. Others help the lateral movement of the spine. Thus the body as a whole is developed, toned up and strengthened. The whole course can be finished in fifteen minutes. Within this short period you can realise the maximum benefits. All the organs of the body are toned up and exercised. This system is simple, exact, efficacious, economical of time and capable of being self-practised.

The practitioner of hatha yoga is agile and nimble. He has a very elastic spine, supple body and a keen vigorous appetite. Any trouble is removed from its starting point by the practice of asanas.

There should be a harmonious development of all the muscles of the body, the organs, nerves and frame. Some people try to develop the chest and the arms only; some try to develop only the lower limbs and the chest. To develop certain parts of the body at the expense of the rest of the body is irrational and unscientific. The general health must be maintained. There must be symmetrical development of all the parts of the body. The muscles of the extremities or limbs, chest, back, neck, abdomen, etc., should be developed equally. Then only will there be grace, elegance and beauty. Another important point is, there must be no violent exertion.

You should have a comprehensive understanding of the laws of health, hygiene and dietetics; of the causes of ill-health, how they arise and how they may be prevented or removed. An elementary knowledge of physiology (the functions of the human body) and anatomy (the structure of the body) will be of immense help to you.

The three important organs — heart, lungs and brain — and the cerebro-spinal system are kept in a healthy condition by a regular practice of asanas. The heart and the lungs are under the control of the brain. The heart and the lungs and the other organs are stimulated or retarded through nerves that proceed from the brain and the spinal cord. The vital forces are also preserved and increased. The circulation of blood in the arteries and veins is kept in proper order by the practice of asanas. There is no stagnation of blood in any part of the body. The spinal cord is toned up. The practice of asanas prevents the development of arterio-sclerosis or hardening of the arteries. The practice of asanas, in fact, lubricates the whole bodily system.

The endocrine glands play an important part in the economy of nature. The practice of sarvangasana keeps the thyroid in a healthy condition. A healthy thyroid means healthy functioning of all the organs and systems of the body. The suprarenals (or adrenals) and the pituitary glands are also toned up and maintained in a healthy condition.

Abundant blood is supplied to the brain by the practice of sirshasana (head stand). Hence the memory and intellectual powers are increased. The practitioner regains his memory-power that may have been lost owing to overwork or some other causes. It transmutes the sex-energy into spiritual power or ojas shakti. The nerves of the body are energised and galvanised. The spinal nerve-roots and the spinal cord receive an abundant supply of blood. Eyesight improves by the practice of sirshasana. Grey hairs also disappear. Many incurable diseases are cured by the regular practice of this asana. Wet-dreams are checked.

The diaphragm — the muscular partition between the chest and the abdomen — is also developed by certain exercises such as dhanurasana, mayurasana and paschimottanasana. The movement of the diaphragm massages the abdominal viscera or organs. There will be evacuation of the bowels daily in the morning. Constipation, dyspepsia and a host of other ailments of the stomach and the intestines will be eradicated.

For those who have a poorly-developed chest, respiratory exercises are necessary. For those who have excess of fat in the abdomen, abdominal exercises are essential. They should pay special attention to them. Exercises that are best calculated to improve the function of the vital inner organs of the body and tone them up to counteract their tendency to disease, are also indispensable. Then only will a high standard of health, vigour and vitality be maintained.

The lungs can be developed through the practice of deep breathing exercises. By pranayama the apices of the lungs will get proper supply of oxygen. There will be an improvement in quality and quantity of the blood. All the tissues and cells will be nourished with plenty of pure blood and lymph. The process of metabolism will be carried out in an efficient manner.

If the joints move freely the ligaments and the surrounding tissues will be in a healthy condition. Free movement of the spine will prevent stiffening and contraction of the spine. Ossification and degeneration of the bones of the spinal column will be checked. A thickened and immovable joint with consequent lack of free movement gives a great deal of discomfort and uneasiness. By the practise of asanas, free movement is given to the elbow, wrist, ankle, shoulder and spinal joints. Muscles of the cervical, dorsal and lumbar regions are stretched and relaxed. The body is kept in a fit condition.

If the muscles are not properly exercised, they will contract. The blood circulation and nerve force will consequently be impeded. Then functional disturbances of the organs and of the general nerve-tone will result. The muscles will get atrophied. Practice of asanas keeps the muscles, organs and nerves in a very healthy condition. Sound functioning of the organs depends upon good healthy nerves. Therefore yoga is the perfect system of physical culture. This is the king of all systems of exercises. Practise these yogic exercises and have a strong healthy body. There is no use in theorising. What is wanted is regular, systematic, sustained practice. An ounce of practice is better than tons of theory. Many people practise these exercises by fits and starts and give up the practice after some months, and hence they do not derive the maximum benefit of this system of exercises. Regularity in the practice is very necessary.

The Accessories for a Yogi's Gymnasium

You do not need barbells, springs, weights and parallel bars for constructing the yogi's gymnasium. At the most what you need is a simple soft blanket to practise asanas on.

You are not practising asanas and pranayama in order to gain big muscles. Muscles do not mean health. The healthy and harmonious functioning of the endocrine glands and the internal viscera, and more so of the nervous system and the mind, is what you need and what the regular practice of yoga asanas and pranayama will bestow on you.

For this purpose it is good to possess a few internal accessories to the practice of these wonderful exercises:

1. An abiding faith in God and a great love for the repetition of His name. Contemplation on God and mentally uttering His name while you are practising the asanas, and particularly pranayama, will greatly enhance their value and utility.
2. Punctuality and regularity. Nothing is ever achieved by the unpunctual and irregular man. What he gains when he practises he loses when he does not; and he loses, moreover, the very

tendency to practise! Practise for five minutes a day, but never miss a day's practice. In due time you will realise that these five minutes have greatly enriched the rest of the day's activity. You will then want to increase the period of practice.

3. Brahmacharya (celibacy). A bachelor should not even entertain lustful thoughts. A householder should exercise as much control as possible over sex-relations. Then you will derive the maximum benefit from these asanas and pranayama. These practices will themselves help you in maintaining brahmacharya.

4. Sincerity, earnestness and zeal are the three great equipments that would soon transform you into a great yogi. Even if you take up these practices for the sake of health and long life, you will soon aspire to realise God through them if you are sincere, earnest and zealous.

The ideal for the sadhak (or yogi) is to secure a place where he will not be disturbed by too many people, animals or insects, and where nature would favour his practice. There he should build his hut. It should give no cause for anxiety and therefore be free from destruction by landslides, flood and fire. Damp, marshy ground would only breed mosquitoes and other disease-producing agents; so the hut should be far away from them. It would be excellent if the place chosen enjoys an equable climate.

The yogi's hut should be small and elegant. It should have good ventilation without too many windows. There should be no room for the eyes to wander about; and there should not be too many things in the room lest they should distract his attention. The room should be kept scrupulously clean. It may be surrounded by a garden of sweet-smelling and beautiful flowers. A good well within the outer compound is a useful addition.

It is not always possible to have such an ideal place for practising yoga. The basic principles should be borne in mind. Peaceful atmosphere, solitude, freedom from distraction — if these are ensured you can convert your own room into an ideal hut for the practice of yoga.

EXERCISES FOR FLEXIBILITY

To increase your mastery over asanas, start daily with some flexibility exercises, mostly based on the largest possible circular movement at the main joints of the body, beginning with:

1. *Neck* (Can be done seated or standing).
(a). With neck relaxed drop head back as far as possible. Hold for a few seconds, then slowly lift head. Let it drop forward till chin touches chest at the hollow at base of throat. Hold for a few seconds.
(b). With head upright and shoulders steady, turn head slowly to look as far as possible over left shoulder. Hold for a few seconds, then slowly turn head to look as far as possible over right shoulder. Hold for a few seconds then slowly face front.
(c). With head facing front and neck relaxed, drop head towards left shoulder as far as possible. Hold for a few seconds then slowly lift head. Let it drop towards right shoulder as far as possible. Hold for a few seconds.
(d). Begin slowly to circle head on completely relaxed neck, three times in each direction.

2. *Shoulder circling* (Can be done seated or standing).
(a). Circle as large as possible with left shoulder only, forward, down, back and up, three times. Repeat with right shoulder. Then moving both shoulders together.
(b). As (a) above but circle in reverse, back, down, forward and up.
(c). Raise left shoulder as far as possible. Hold for a few seconds, then

drop. Repeat with right shoulder. Then repeat with both shoulders together.
(All the following exercises are done standing).

3. *Arm circling* (With concentration on shoulder joint).
Here the arm is straight but relaxed.
(a). Make a smooth circle as large as possible with left arm three times — back and up, breathing in, forward and down breathing out. Repeat with right arm.
(b). As (a) but forward and up breathing in, back and down breathing out.
(c). Make a smooth circle as large as possible with both arms moving to the sides and crossing above the head, breathing in. Then continue circling of arms across body on the way down, breathing out. Repeat three times.
(d). As (c) but begin crossing arms in front of body on way up, breathing in deeply till arms part above head, then breathe out as arms come down to sides of body.

4. *Lower arm circling* (With concentration on elbow joint).
Here the upper arm is steady. Begin with arms stretched to sides, then bend at elbows, moving lower arms up, down and stretch three times. Reverse.

5. *Hand circling* (With concentration on wrist).
Here the arms are stretched to the sides:
(a). Forward, down, back and up three times, then
(b). Reverse.
(c). Lift hand as far as possible, not moving the rest of arm. Let hand drop. Repeat three times.

6. *Flexibility of knuckles.*
(a). Stretch arms fully to sides then relax at knuckles, letting fingers drop. Stretch first and drop, three times.
(b). With arms stretched to sides clench fists tightly, then stretch fingers. Repeat three times.

7. *Flexibility of elbows.*
Stretch arms to sides, then relax at elbows and wrist, letting arms bend. Stretch and relax as far as possible. Hold for a few seconds, then let arm drop.

8. *For muscles of arms, shoulders, chest and back.*
(a). Raise arms to side as you breathe in deeply, then clench hooked fingers together in front of body with arms parallel to ground. Hold breath and pull hard as though to pull fingers apart. Hold for a few seconds, then let arms drop and relax. Once only.
(b). Hands pressed together as in Indian salutation but with arms stretched above the head. Breathe deeply and hold breath. Press hands hard then slowly bring arms down, keeping fingers pointing upwards, until at about waist level hands start to part. Flick them apart suddenly breathing out. Once only.

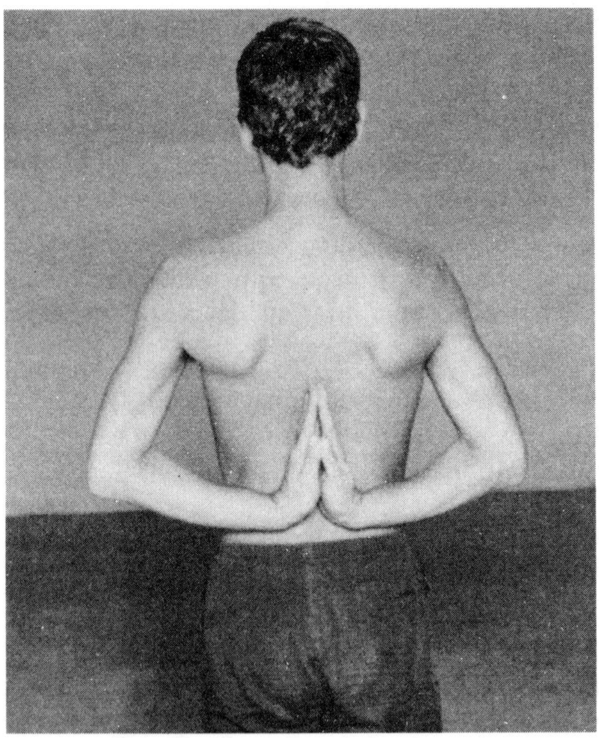

(c). Hands pressed together as in Indian salutation but with arms behind the back. Slowly work the hands as far as possible up the spine. Then press them together hard and pull them down the spine, keeping fingers pointing upwards, until at about waist level hands start to part. Flick them apart suddenly, breathing out. Once only.

(d). Bring left arm up the back as far as possible. At the same time bring right arm over right shoulder till you can clench fingers of both hands behind back. Breathe deeply, hold breath and pull. Hold for a few seconds, then relax. Once only. Repeat over left shoulder.

9. *For flexibility of hips and lower spine.*
(a). Stand erect, heels together. Relax by bending left leg and putting weight of body on straight leg. Keep heels flat on ground. Pelvis slopes down from right to left. Reverse position of legs. Pelvis slopes down from left to right. Repeat five or six times, gradually increasing speed. Concentrate on movement of pelvis.
(b). Stand erect, heels together. Bend slightly at knees. Keeping rest of body steady, tip pelvis backward and forward as far as possible. Due to stiffness of lower spine at first little or no movement may be possible.
(c). Bend slightly at knees as in (b). Make small, smooth circle of hips, connecting movements of (a) and (b). Three times clockwise and anticlockwise.
(d). Stand erect, heels together. Push lower spine and pelvis over to left as far as possible, retaining balance with head directly above feet, i.e. body arched to left. Outside leg straight, inner leg bent. Bend both legs, pushing lower spine and pelvis across to right as far as possible. Repeat to left and right three times.
(e). Stand erect, heels together. Push belly forward as far as possible, so that the whole of the body is arched to front with head remaining directly above feet. Bending legs, push lower spine and pelvis back as far as possible till legs are straight and upper body bent forward, with arms hanging vertically. Again bend legs and push lower spine and pelvis forward through the hanging arms till the body is again arched forward. Repeat three times.
(f). Make circle as large as possible connecting movement of (d) and (e), pushing hard in each direction. Three times clockwise and anti-clockwise.
(g). Stand erect, heels together. Without moving legs, push trunk as far as possible to left, feeling stretch at right side of waist, contraction at left. Reverse. Repeat three times.
(h). Arching body forward bend back as far as possible, letting head drop back relaxed and arms hang to sides, legs bent. Hold for a few seconds then slowly straighten up and bend forward with straight legs, trying to place palms of hands on ground. Slowly straighten up. Repeat three times.

10. *Combination exercise* (for concentration and flexibility). Stand erect, heels together. Keep left arm hanging straight down at side of left leg, with fingers touching leg and sliding up and down leg during movements of rest of body. Start to make a large circle sideways, raising right arm and keeping eyes fixed on right hand. Breathe in as arm is raised. As arm reaches above head start to bend body to left. When body cannot move further to left side, drop forward, breathing out, completing circle with right arm, hand touching ground in front of body. Immediately start lifting right arm and the body to right side, breathing in. Continue till body is straight, then let arm continue upwards on second circle. Repeat three times then with right arm, practise four times with left arm. Concentrate on breathing and movement at waist.

11. *Exercises to twist spine.*
These stretch the muscles behind the legs and increase flexibility at waist:
(a). Feet well apart, legs straight, arms stretched out at sides for whole exercise. Breathe in. Keeping head and body erect, turn as far as possible to left at waist (till you can see behind you) then breathe out as you bend to left without changing arms, touching ground with right fingers behind left foot and with vertical line through arms. Breathing in, straighten till arms are again parallel with ground. Hold breath as you turn as far as possible to right at waist (till you can see behind you). Then repeat as above to right. Do three times to both sides, then return to front and lower arms.
(b). Feet well apart and legs straight for whole exercise. Breathe in. Keeping head and body erect, turn to left at waist till head is over left leg. Bend body over left leg breathing out, keeping legs straight, and sliding hands down left leg till they touch ground. Straighten up, breathing in and still facing over left. Hold breath and turn to right at waist till head is over right leg. Then repeat as above to right. Do three times to both sides.

12. *For inner sides of thighs and behind legs.*
(This also gives flexibility of spine).
Slide feet apart as far as possible to sides, with body upright. Legs are straight throughout exercise. Bend forward to place palms of hands on ground in front of and close to body. Bend arms and put whole forearm on ground. Put top of head on ground. Hold for a few seconds. Lift

head. Straighten arms, leaving palms of hands on ground. Gradually work feet closer till heels touch with legs straight, arms straight and hands on ground. Hold for a few seconds. Straighten. Breathing normal. Concentrate on back of legs and inner side of thighs. Once only.

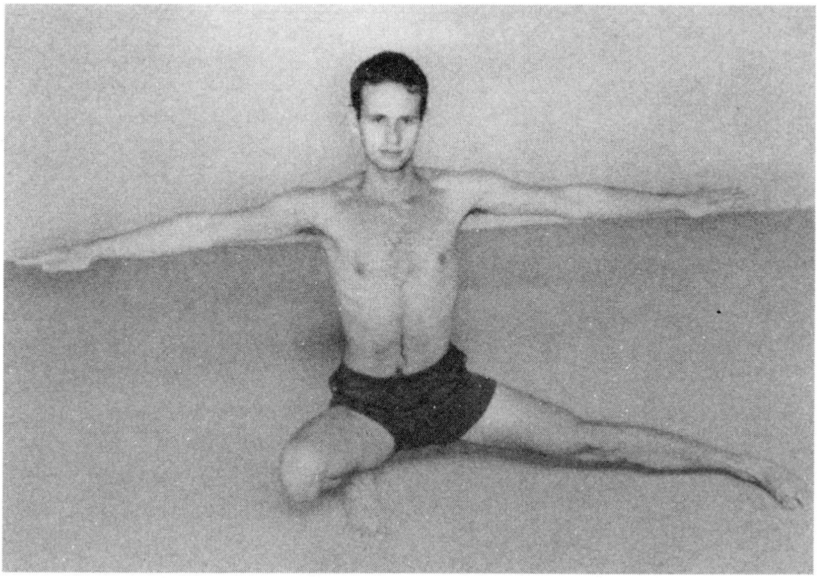

13. *For balance and to increase flexibility at hip joints*:
(a). Feet well apart and arms raised to sides for whole exercise. Straighten legs, then lunge to left, bending left knee and raising heel from ground, right leg stretched to side, with body as upright as possible. Keeping body low and upright, move slowly over to right side, bending right knee and raising heel from ground, left leg stretched to side. Repeat three times to both sides, then return to first position. Breathing normal. Concentrate on hip joints.
(b). Stand erect, heels together. Keeping rest of body still, swing left leg back and forward, completely relaxed and gradually getting higher. Height is not as important as stillness of rest of body. Four or five times each leg.
(c). As (a) but swing left leg out to left side and let it fall again. Repeat with right. Four or five times each leg.

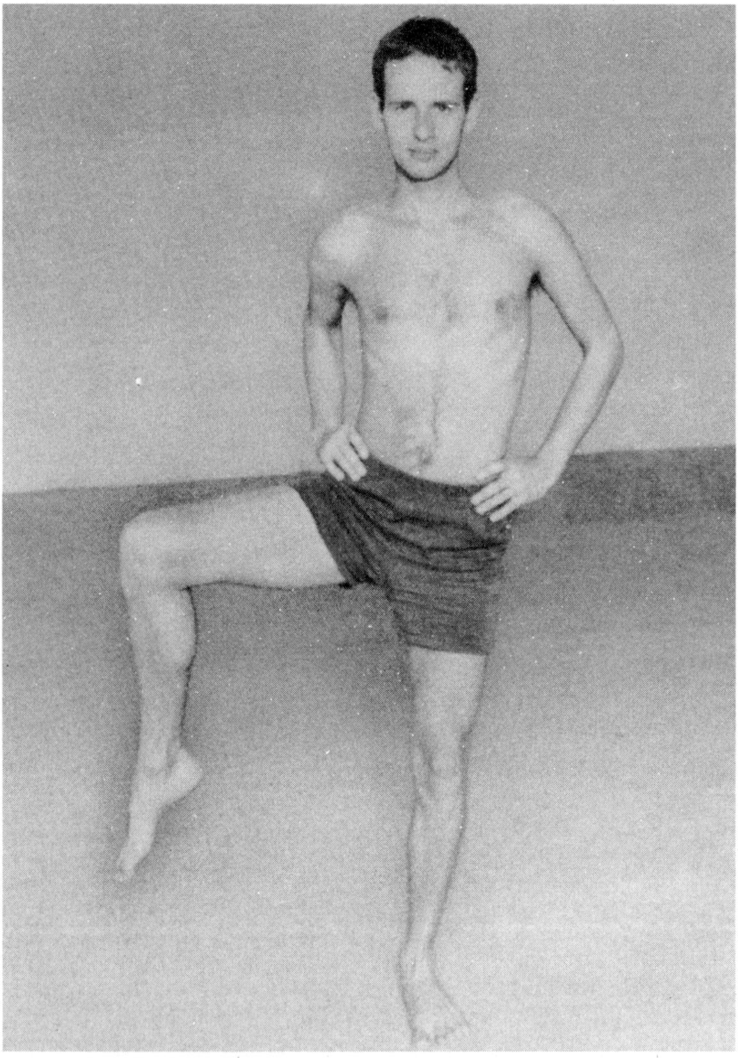

14. *For maximum flexibility at hip-joint.*
(a). Stand erect, feet together. Lift left leg to front, knee bent, till thigh is horizontal. Open leg out to left as far as possible, concentrating on hip-joint. Lower leg. Repeat three times. Then repeat with right leg.
(b). Reverse of (a). Begin by lifting left leg as far as possible to side till thigh is horizontal. Then bring leg to front, concentrating on hip-joint. Lower leg to front. Repeat as (a).

15. *Lower leg circling.*

Here the concentration is on the knee.

Have the left leg stretched to the front. With the upper leg kept still, circle in, out and stretch, three times; then reverse. Repeat with right leg.

(Exercises 16, 17, and 18 are to be completed first with left foot, then repeated three times with right foot.)

16. *Foot circling.*

Concentration on the ankle, left leg stretched to front. Movement at ankle only. Circling in, out and stretch, three times; then reverse.

17. *Up and down movement of foot.*

The foot should be moved as far as possible. Concentration on the ankle, left leg stretched to front. Movement at ankle only, three times.

18. *Toe clenching and stretching.*

Alternate with big toe on top, big toe underneath. Repeat three times.

Thus the joints have been loosened and the whole body put into a flexible condition for your yoga asana practice. When the sequence has been learned, all these exercises can be done within twenty to thirty minutes. Most can be done easily by the householder and will suffice with a little pranayama, till such time as he can slowly add some asanas.

Surya Namaskara

A few surya namaskaras before the actual practice of yoga asanas will not only confer their own benefits, but will also 'loosen' the rigid muscles and joints and make the asana-practice easier.

These surya namaskaras combine the benefits of several yoga postures, breathing, vigorous body movement, sun-bathing (for the exercises are generally done facing the sun in the morning) and prayer to the God manifest in the sun. The sun as a deity is adored with the following twelve 'names' which are mantras:

Om Mitraya namah
Om Ravaye namah
Om Suryaya namah
Om Bhanave namah
Om Khagaya namah
Om Pushne namah
Om Hiranyagarbhaya namah
Om Marichaye namah
Om Adityaya namah
Om Savitre namah
Om Arkaya namah
Om Bhaskaraya namah

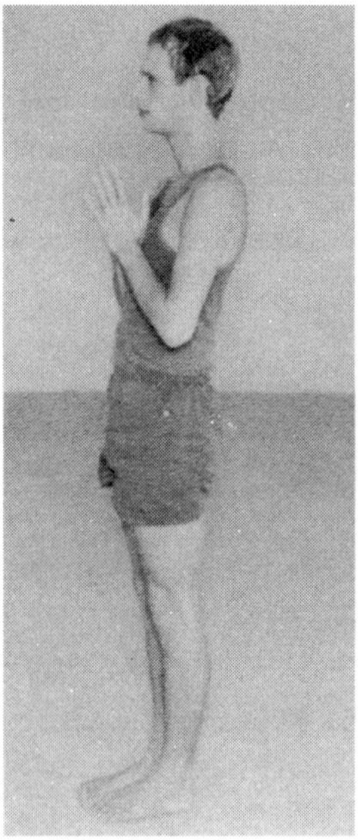

1 & 12

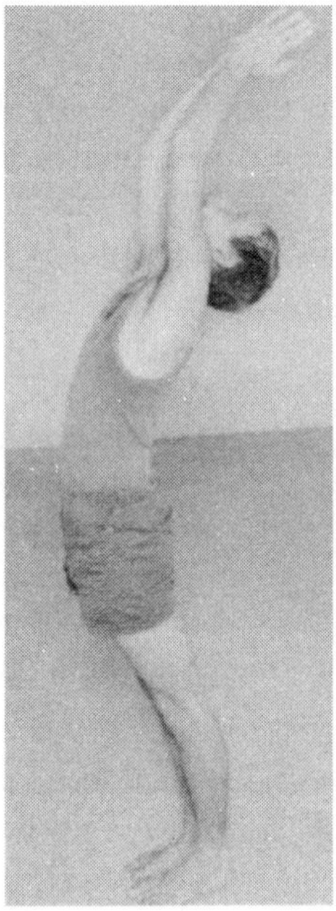

2 & 11

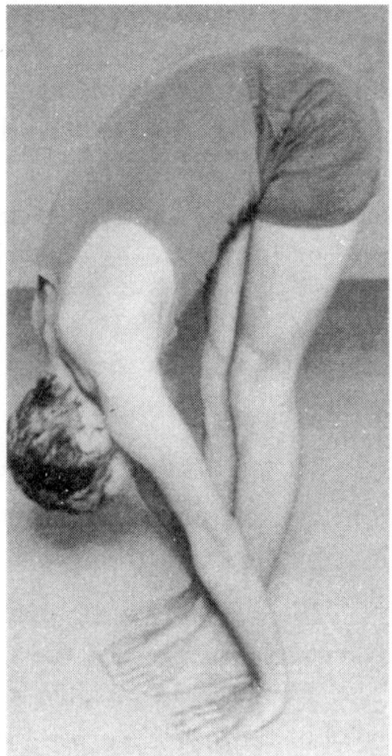

3 & 10

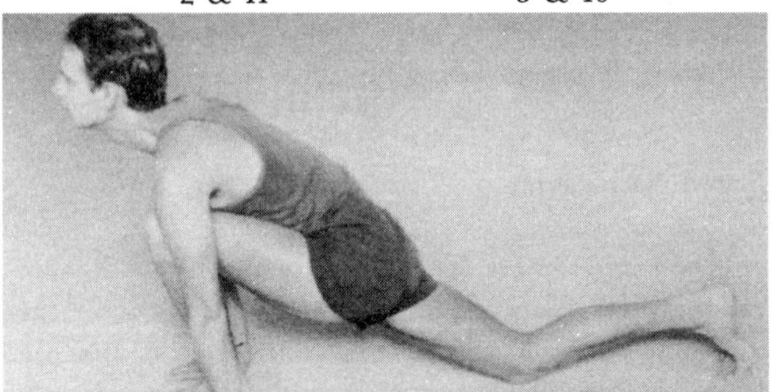

4

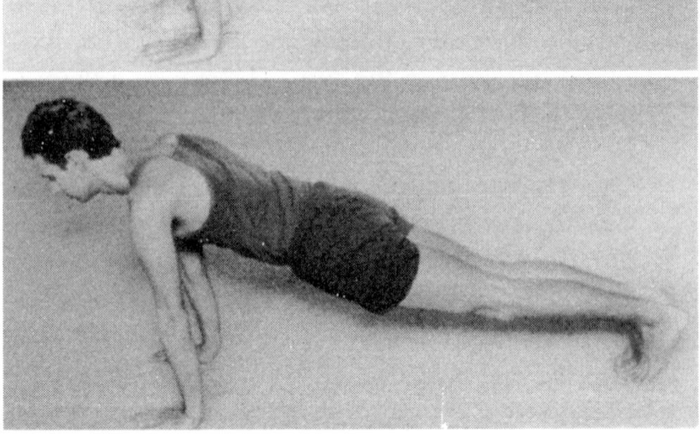

5

6

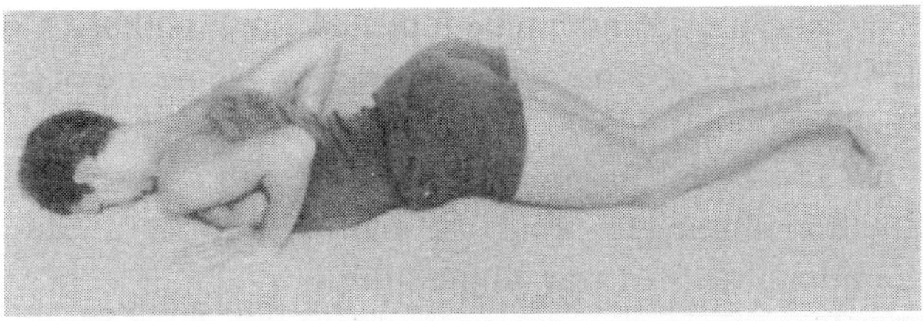

7

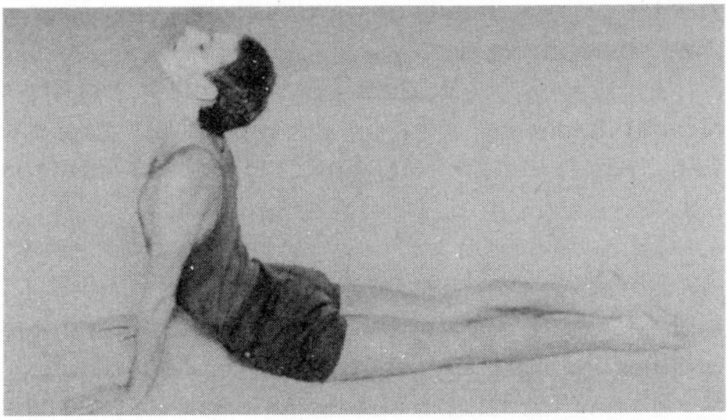

8

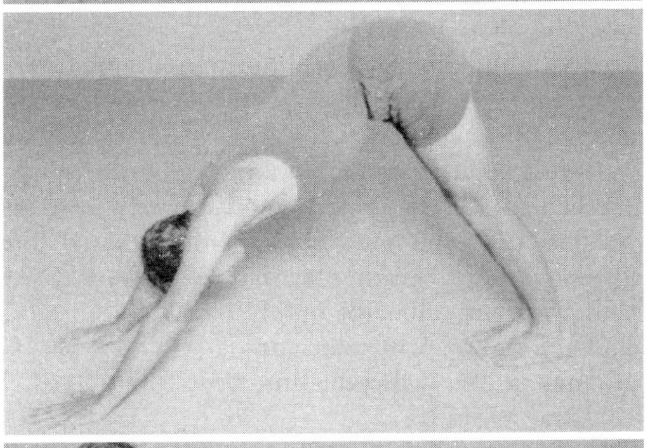

9

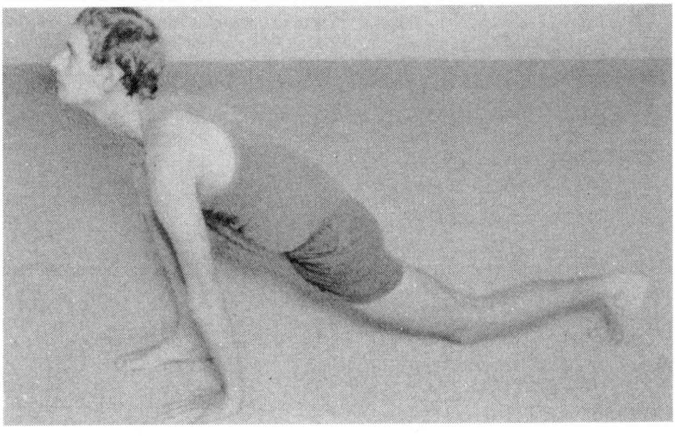

These mantras can be repeated along with each posture (12 for the 12 postures), or after each mantra a whole round of the 12 postures can be done.

The following are the twelve postures of surya namaskara:

1. Stand upright. Fold the palms in front of the chest, as in the traditional Indian way of greeting.
2. Throw your hands up, stretch them above your head, at the same time breathing in deeply.
3. Swing forward. Without bending your knees, try to place the palms of your hands squarely on the ground, fingers pointing straight in front, parallel to the feet. Bury the face between your knees. Breathe out.
4. Throw the right leg back, touching the ground with the knee. Flex the left leg at the knee, and bring the thigh in close contact with the body. Look up. Breathe in. (For the next round throw the left leg back, and flex the right leg. Alternate the legs with each round.)
5. Throw the left leg also back. Straighten the back. Straighten the arms too. Hold the breath.
6. Flex at the elbows. Touch the ground with forehead, chest, palms, knees and toes. The other parts of the body should not touch the ground. Breathe out.
7. Swing the head up and backwards, like the cobra pose. Breathe in.
8. Swing the body upwards and backwards, to assume the inverted V position, heels and palms resting on the ground. Breathe out.
9. Same as No. 4. Bring the right leg forward. (Next round bring the left leg forward.) Breathe in.
10. Same as No. 3. Breathe out.
11. Same as No. 2. Breathe in.
12. Same as No. 1.

Then normal standing position, with hands at the sides.

ASANAS FOR MEDITATION

Four asanas (postures) are prescribed for the purposes of japa and meditation. They are padma, siddha, svastika and sukha asanas.

You must be able to sit in any one of these four asanas for full three hours at a stretch without shaking the body. Then only will you get mastery over the asana (asana jaya); then only can you take to the practice of pranayama (control of breath) and dhyana (meditation). Without securing a steady posture you cannot get on well in meditation. The more steady you are in your posture the more you will be able to concentrate and make your mind one-pointed. If you can be steady in the posture even for one hour you will be able to acquire one-pointedness of mind and feel thereby infinite peace and bliss of the Atman.

When you sit in the posture, think: "I am as firm as a rock. Nothing can shake me." Give these suggestions to the mind a dozen times. Then the posture will soon become steady. You must become a living statue when you sit for meditation, then only will there be real steadiness in your posture. In one year, by regular practice, you will have success and will be able to sit for three hours at a stretch. Start with half an hour and gradually increase the period.

If there is severe pain in the legs after some time, unlock the legs and then massage them for five minutes and sit again in the posture. When you advance you will not experience any pain; on the other hand you will experience immense joy. Practise both morning and evening.

After sitting, close the eyes and concentrate on the space between the two eyebrows (ajna *chakra) or in the lotus of the heart. As the ajna

* See Kundalini section

chakra is the seat of the mind, the mind can be quite easily controlled if you concentrate gently on this spot. One-pointedness of the mind supervenes quite readily. Concentration at the tip of the nose (nasikagra drishti) also has the same advantage, but it takes more time for the focussing of the mind. Those who cannot concentrate either at the space between the eyebrows or the tip of the nose, may concentrate at any other outer point or inner chakra of heart, head, neck, etc.

Keep the head, neck and trunk in one straight line. Stick to one posture — either padma, siddha, svastika or sukha — and make it quite steady and perfect by repeated attempts. Never change it. Adhere to one tenaciously. Cling to it like a leech. Realise the full benefits of one posture for meditation.

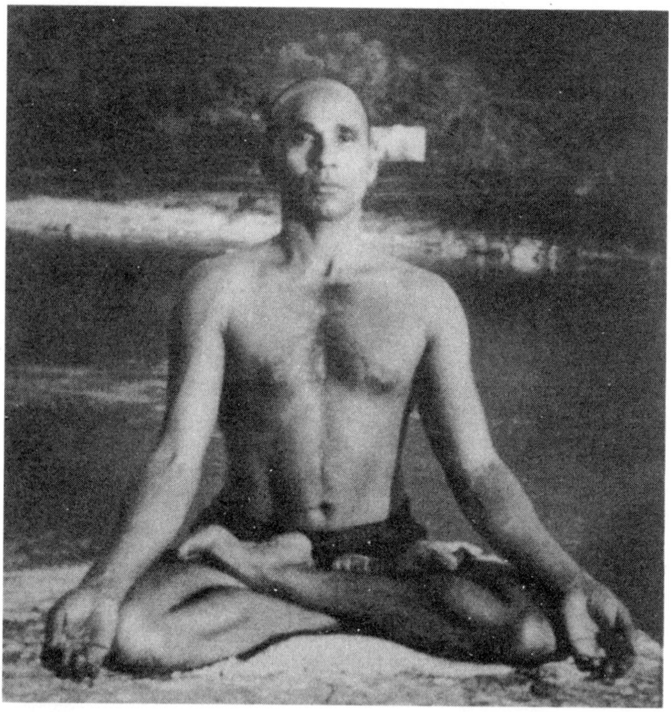

Padmasana

Padma means lotus. When the asana is demonstrated, it presents the appearance of a lotus, in a way. Hence the name padmasana. This is also known by the name kamalasana.

Amongst the four poses prescribed for japa and dhyana, padmasana comes foremost. It is the best asana for contemplation.

Rishis like Gheranda, Sandilya and others, speak very highly of this vital asana. This is highly agreeable for householders. Ladies can sit in this asana. Padmasana is suitable for lean persons and for youths as well.

Technique: Sit on the ground by spreading the legs forward. Then place the right foot on the left thigh and the left foot on the right thigh. Place the hands on the knee-joints.

You can make a finger-lock and keep the locked hands over the left ankle. This is very convenient for some persons. Or you can place the left hand over the left knee and the right hand over the right knee with the palms facing upwards and the index fingers touching the middle portion of the thumb (chinmudra).

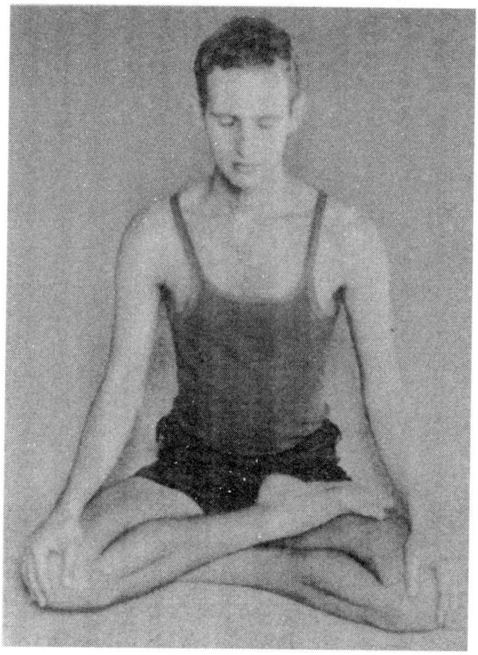

Varieties

i. *Ardha-padmasana*:

If you cannot place both the feet on the thighs at the very start, just keep one foot on one thigh for some time and the other foot on the other thigh for some time. After a few days' practice you will be able to keep both the feet on the thighs. This is half pose of padmasana, or ardha-padmasana.

ii. *Virasana*:

Sit at ease. Place the right foot on the left thigh and the left foot underneath the right thigh. Lord Gauranga used to sit in this asana for his meditation. This is a comfortable posture. Virasana means hero posture.

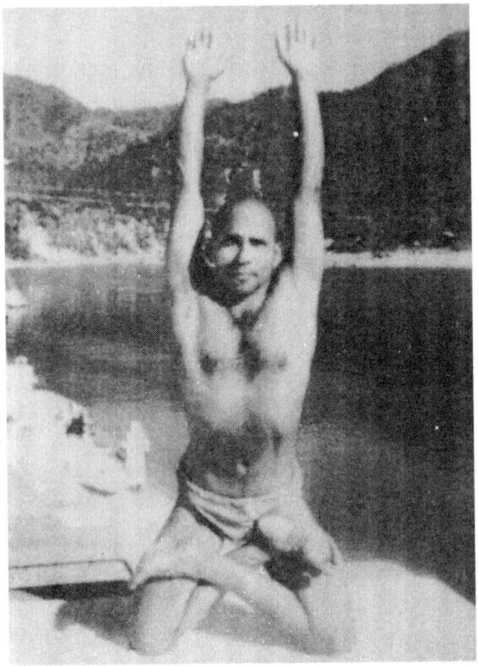

iii. *Parvatasana (Mountain Pose)*:

Do ordinary padmasana. Stand on the knees and raise your hands above. This is parvatasana. Keep a thick blanket on the ground and then do this asana so that you will not injure your knees. In the beginning, for a few days, catch hold of a stool or bench till you get the balance. Afterwards you can raise the hands above.

Sit in virasana and then raise the hands above and be steady. Some persons also call this parvatasana.

iv. *Samasana (Equal Pose)*:

Place the left heel at the beginning of the right thigh and the right heel at the beginning of the left thigh. Sit at ease. Do not bend either on the left or right. This is called samasana.

v. *Karmukasana*:

Sit in ordinary padmasana. Catch hold of the right toe with the right hand and the left toe with the left hand, thus making a cross of your hands at the elbow.

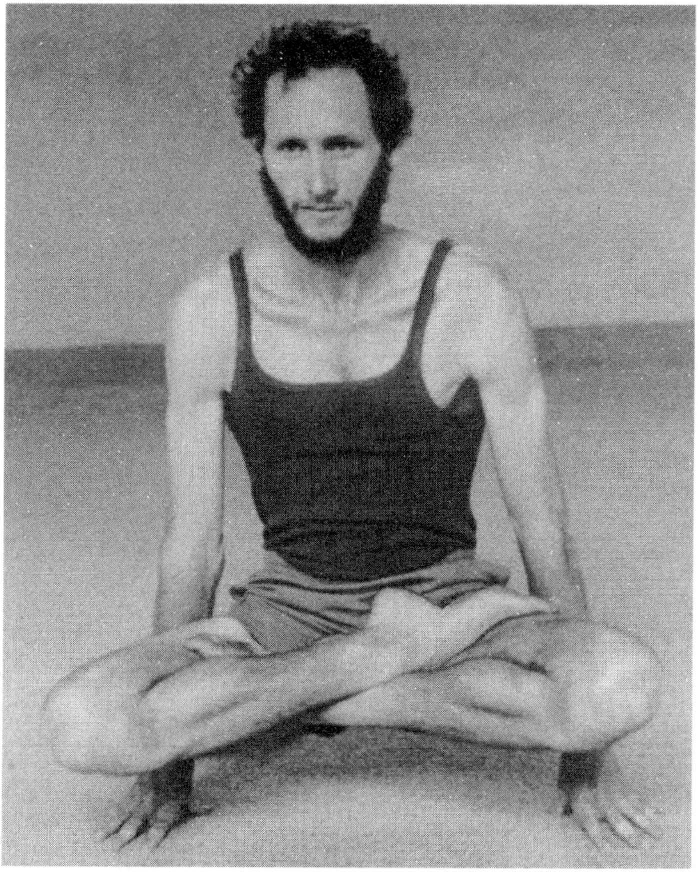

vi. *Utthita Padmasana*:

Sit in padmasana. Keep your palms on the ground by your sides. Slowly raise the body. There should be no jerks. The body should not be trembling. Retain the breath as long as you remain in that raised position. When you come down you can exhale. Persons who cannot perform kukkutasana can do this. The hands are kept by the sides in this asana, but the hands are kept between the thigh and calf muscles in kukkutasana. This is the difference.

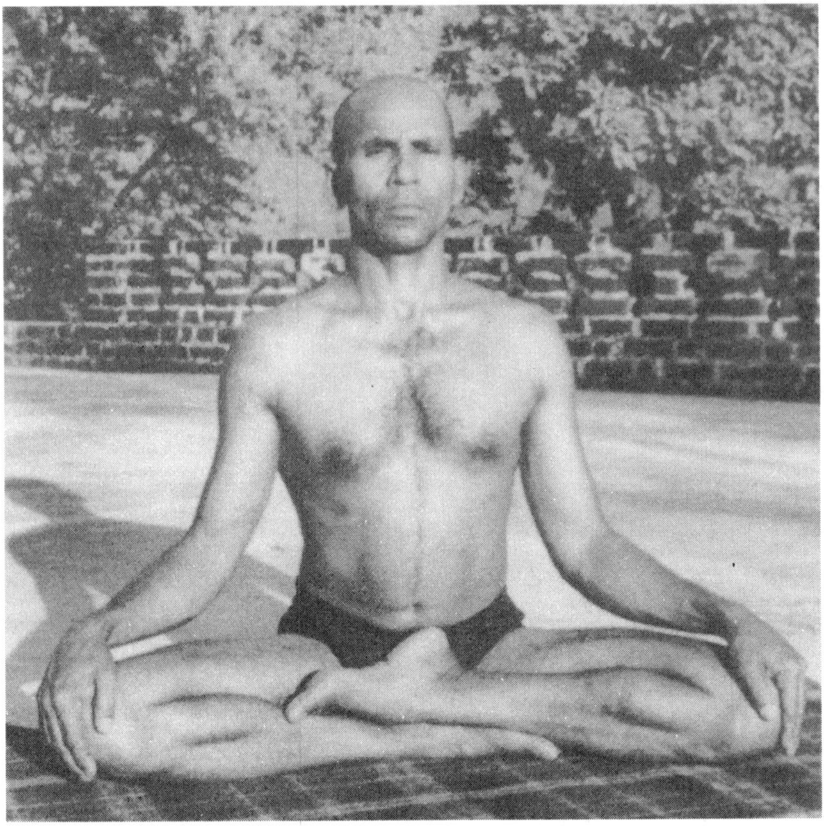

Siddhasana

Next to padmasana in importance comes siddhasana. Some eulogise this asana as even superior to padmasana for the purpose of meditation. If you get mastery over it you will acquire many siddhis (powers). It was practised by many siddhas (perfect yogis) of yore. Hence the name siddhasana.

Even fat persons with big thighs can practise this easily. In fact this is better for some persons than padmasana. Young brahmacharis who attempt to get established in celibacy should practise this. (Siddhasana is also known as sthirasana and muktasana.)

Technique: Place one heel at the anus, the terminal opening of the alimentary canal. Keep the other heel at the root of the generative organ. The feet or legs should be so nicely arranged that the ankle-joints should touch each other. Hands can be placed as shown in padmasana.

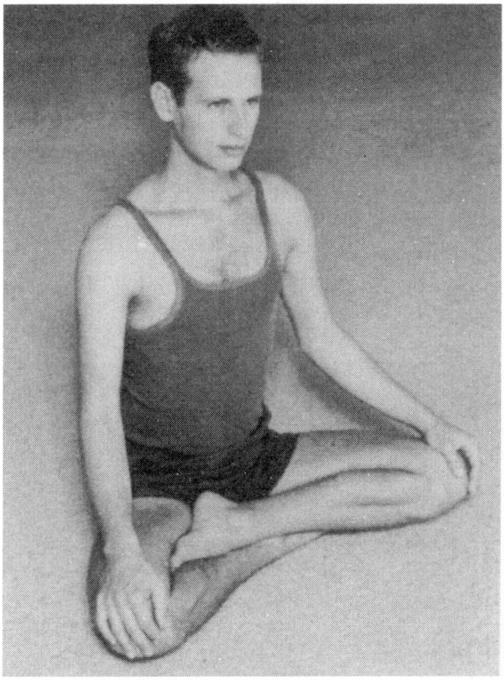

Varieties

i. *Guptasana (Hidden Pose)*:

The left heel is placed over the organ of generation. The right heel is also placed over it. The two ankles are in close opposition or contact. The right toes are thrust inside the hollow between the left thigh and left calf muscles. The left toes are covered by the right leg. Gupta means hidden. As this asana hides well the organ of generation it is called guptasana.

ii. *Vajrasana (Adamantine Pose)*:

The left heel is placed below the organ of generation. The right heel is placed over it. Vajra means adamantine. (There is also another variety of vajrasana. Instructions are given elsewhere.)

iii. *Kshemasana*:

When sitting in siddhasana if you raise your hands together up to your chest level, it is called kshemasana. It is meant that you are praying for the kshema (welfare) of the public. The palms must be facing each other.

Benefits of Padmasana and Siddhasana

Books on hatha yoga eulogise the merits and advantages of padmasana and siddhasana to a very high degree. He who sits in either of these even for 15 minutes daily with closed eyes, concentrating on God at the lotus of the heart, destroys all sins and gets moksha quickly. These asanas increase digestive fire and give good appetite, health and happiness. They remove rheumatism and keep the three humours — wind, bile and phlegm — in proper porportion. They purify and strengthen the nerves of the legs and thighs. They are suitable for keeping up celibacy.

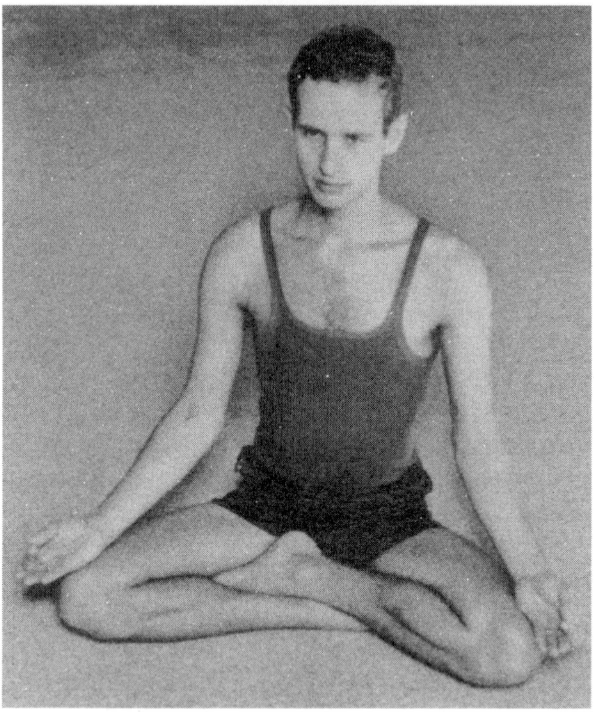

Svastikasana

Svastika is sitting at ease with the body erect. Spread the legs forward. Fold the left leg and place the foot near the right thigh muscles. Similarly, bend the right leg and push it in the space between the left thigh and calf muscles. Now you will find the two feet between the thighs and calves of the legs. This is very comfortable for meditation. Keep the hands as instructed in padmasana.

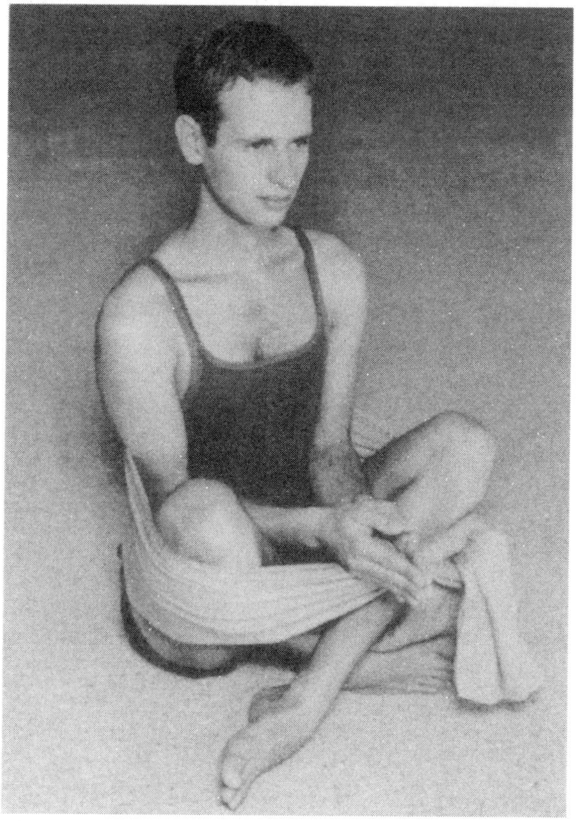

Sukhasana

Any easy comfortable posture for japa and meditation is sukhasana, the important point being that the head, neck and trunk should be in a straight line. People who begin japa and meditation after 30 and 40 years of age, generally are not able to sit in padma, siddha or svastikasana for a long time.

I will describe a nice form of sukhasana in which old persons can sit and meditate for a long time. This specially suits old people who are unable to sit in padma or siddhasana in spite of repeated attempts. Young people also can practise this.

Technique: Take a cloth 5 cubits long. (A cubit is the distance from the elbow to the tip of the middle finger — approximately 15 inches.) Fold it nicely lengthwise till the width becomes half a cubit. Sit on the floor and cross your legs, keeping the feet below your thighs. Raise the two knees to the level of your chest till you get a space of 8 or 10 inches between the two knees. Now take the folded cloth. Keep one end near the left knee; going to the back by the left side, touching the right knee, come to the starting point and make a knot of the two ends. Keep your palms face to face and place them on the support of the cloth between the knees. In this asana the hands, legs and backbone are supported, hence you will never feel tired. If you cannot do any other asanas, sit at least in this asana and do japa and meditation for a long time.

MUKHYA ASANAS

Sirshasana

Sirshasana is also known by other names: kapalyasana, vrikshasana (like a tree), viparita karani and topsy-turvy pose. It is the king of all asanas.

Technique: Spread a fourfold blanket. Sit on the two knees. Make a finger-lock by interweaving the fingers. Place it on the ground up to the elbow. Now, keep the top of your head cradled against this finger-lock or between the two hands. Slowly raise the legs till they become vertical. (Stand for five seconds in the beginning and gradually increase the period by 15 seconds each week to 20 minutes or half an hour.) Then slowly bring the legs down. Strong people can remain in this asana for half an hour within a period of two or three months' practice. Do it slowly. Do not be anxious. Be calm. Be cool. There is eternity before you. On this score do not be sluggish in your practice. Do this asana on an empty stomach. If you have time, do twice daily both morning and evening. Perform this asana very, very slowly and avoid jerks. While standing on the head, breathe slowly through the nose and never through the mouth.

Instead of making a finger-lock, you can place the hands on the ground, one on each side of the head, making an equilateral triangle. If you are fat you will find it easier to practise this method. When you learn balancing, then you can take to finger-lock method. This asana is nothing for those who can do balance in parallel bars on the ground. Ask your friend to assist you to keep the legs steady while practising, or get the help of a wall when you begin to learn this.

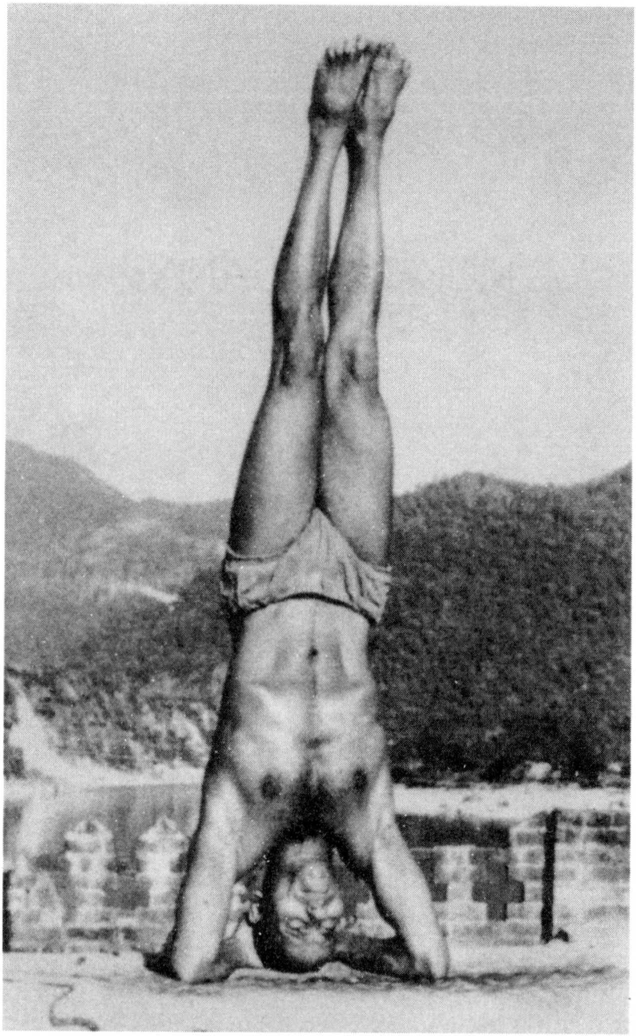

In the beginning, some may have some sensation during practice but soon this vanishes. It brings joy. After the exercise is over, take a little rest for five minutes and then take a cup of milk. Those who do this asana for a long time, say 20 minutes or half an hour, should take some kind of light refreshment, milk or anything, when it is over. This is very important. In summer do not practise this asana for a long time. In winter you can practise as long as you desire.

There are people who are doing this asana for two or three hours at one stretch. Pandit Raghunath Sastri at Badrinarayan was very fond of this asana and used to practise it for two or three hours. There was a yogi at Varanasi who entered into samadhi in this asana. Sri Jaspat Rai, P.V. Acharyaji Maharaj and others were doing this asana regularly for more than one hour daily at a stretch.

Benefits: This is very useful in keeping up celibacy. It makes you an urdhvaretas. The seminal energy is transmuted into spiritual energy. This is also called sex-sublimation. In an urdhvareto-yogi the seminal energy flows upwards into the brain for being stored up as spiritual force which is used for contemplative purposes (dhyana). When you do this asana, imagine that the energy is being converted into spiritual energy and is passing along the spinal column into the brain for storage. Sirshasana invigorates, energises and vivifies.

Sirshasana is really a blessing and a nectar. Words will fail to adequately describe its beneficial results and effects. In this asana alone the brain can draw plenty of prana and blood. It acts against the force of gravity and draws an abundance of blood from the heart. Memory increases admirably. Lawyers, occultists and thinkers will appreciate this asana. It leads to natural pranayama and samadhi by itself. If you watch the breath you will notice that it becomes finer and finer. In the beginning of practice there will be slight difficulty in breathing. As you advance in practice this vanishes entirely. You will find real pleasure and exhilaration of spirit in this asana.

Great benefit is derived by sitting for meditation after sirshasana. You can hear anahata sounds quite distinctly. Young, robust persons should perform this asana. The advantages that are derived from it are incalculable. Those who practise it should not have frequent copulation.

This is a panacea, a cure-all, a sovereign specific for all diseases. It brightens the psychic faculties and awakens kundalini shakti, removes all sorts of diseases of the intestines and stomach and augments mental power. It is a powerful blood-purifier and nervine tonic. All diseases of the eye, nose, head, throat, stomach, genito-urinary system, liver, spleen and lungs are cured, as are renal colic, deafness, gonorrhoea, diabetes, asthma, consumption, piles, syphilis, etc. It augments the digestive fire. Wrinkles and greyness will disappear. 'He who practises this for three hours daily conquers time.' — *Yoga Tattva Upanishad*. Many uterine and ovarian diseases are cured, and sterility disappears.

Asana, pranayama and japa should go hand in hand. Repeat the mantra of your chosen deity or the mantra given by your guru, during the practice of this asana.

Sri Prakash Jung had swelling of feet and disease of heart. The muscles of the heart were not able to contract and dilate properly in its function of pumping. That was the diagnosis of the doctors. He practised sirshasana regularly for a few days. All swelling disappeared. The heart functioned properly. There was no pain at all. He used to do this asana for half an hour daily.

Pandit Surya Narayan was doing this asana. His memory has considerably improved. The pain in the back and shoulders (chronic rheumatism) vanished completely.

Varieties

i. *Ardha Vrikshasana*:

As you stand in sirshasana, just fold the legs at the knee joint and keep them along the thighs.

ii. *Mukta Hasta Vrikshasana*:

Instead of making the finger-lock, keep the hands on the ground by the side of the head.

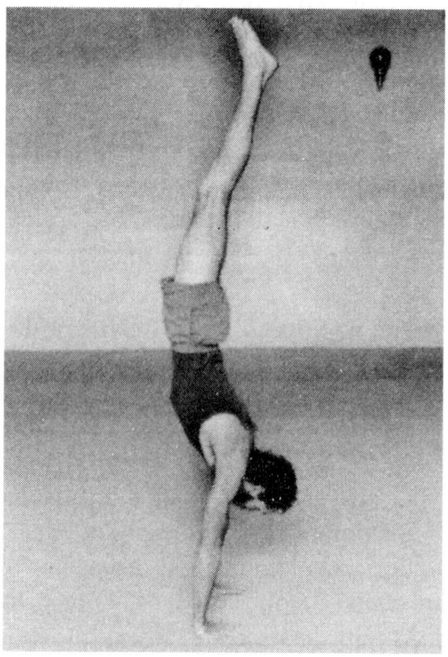

iii. *Hasta Vrikshasana*:

You will have to stand on the two hands alone in this asana. First throw your legs on the wall, standing on your hands only. Slowly try to take your legs away from the wall. In a few days you will learn balancing.

iv. *Ekapada Vrikshasana*:

After performing the sirshasana, slowly bend one leg at the knee and keep the heel over the other thigh.

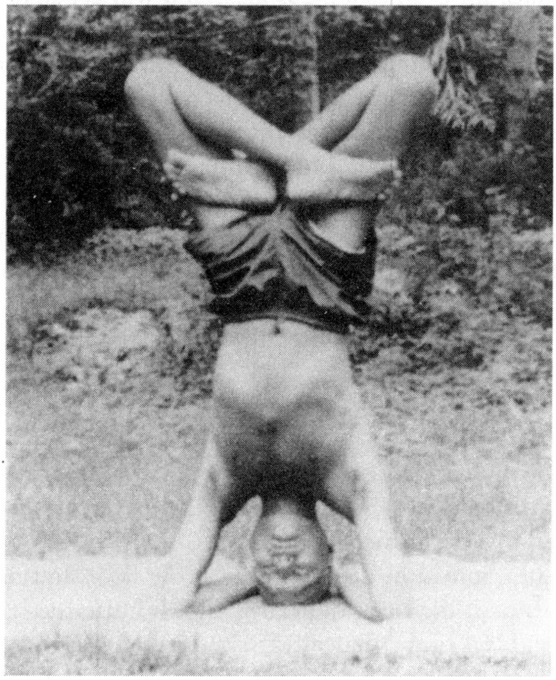

v. *Urdhva Padmasana*:

Perform sirshasana as mentioned before. Slowly bend the right leg and keep it on the left thigh and then the left leg and keep it on the right thigh. You must do this very carefully and slowly. If you can stand in sirshasana for more than ten or fifteen minutes, then alone you can attempt this. Otherwise you will have a fall. A gymnast who can balance himself on the parallel bars or on the ground can do it quite easily. The practice of this asana needs some strength. Breathe slowly through the nose and never by the mouth. Remain in the posture for five to ten minutes in the beginning and gradually increase the time.

Some persons will find it easy to do padmasana first and then they will raise the legs slowly. Experienced persons can bring down the padmasana to the ground and again they can raise the legs above as before. Those who practise this asana should take some light tiffin (snack), a cup of milk or fruit juice after finishing this asana. Practitioners of sirshasana and urdhva padmasana should keep up brahmacharya. Then only will they realise the maximum benefits.

Benefits: When any sort of prayer or japa is done during the course of asanas, it becomes a tapas also. You will get siddhis. In days of yore tapasvins used to stand on the head for a period of twelve years and repeat the mantra of the chosen deity or guru. You will find this in the *Mahabharata* in many instances. Japa or meditation in urdhva padmasana or sirshasana touches the heart of the Lord deeply. He showers His blessings quickly. Many difficulties will be obviated.

All the advantages of sirshasana are derived from this asana. He who practises this will have perfect control over the body. Judge Kedarnath could turn out double the work in courts and read books for many hours after the practice of this asana. You can also practise it regularly and sincerely, and get the full benefits and live long in perfect health.

Sarvangasana

This is a mysterious asana which gives wonderful benefits. It is termed 'all-members pose' because all the parts of the body are engaged when it is performed.

Technique: Spread a thick blanket on the floor and practise over the blanket. Lie on the back quite flat. Slowly raise the legs. Lift the trunk, hips and legs quite vertically. Support the back with two hands, one on each side. Rest the elbows on the ground. Press the chin against the chest and form a chin lock (jalandhara bandha). Allow the back shoulder portion and neck to touch the ground closely. Do not allow the body to shake or move to and fro. Keep the legs straight. In this the whole weight of the body is thrown on the shoulders. You really stand on the shoulders with the help and support of the elbows. Concentrate on the thyroid gland which lies on the front lower part of the neck. Retain the breath as long as you can with comfort, and slowly exhale through the nose. When the asana is over, bring the legs down very, very slowly with elegance and without any jerks. Do it very gracefully.

Practise this asana for two minutes in the beginning and gradually increase it to half an hour. You can do it twice daily, morning and evening. It should immediately be followed by matsyasana (fish-posture). This will relieve pains in the back part of the neck and intensify the usefulness of sarvangasana.

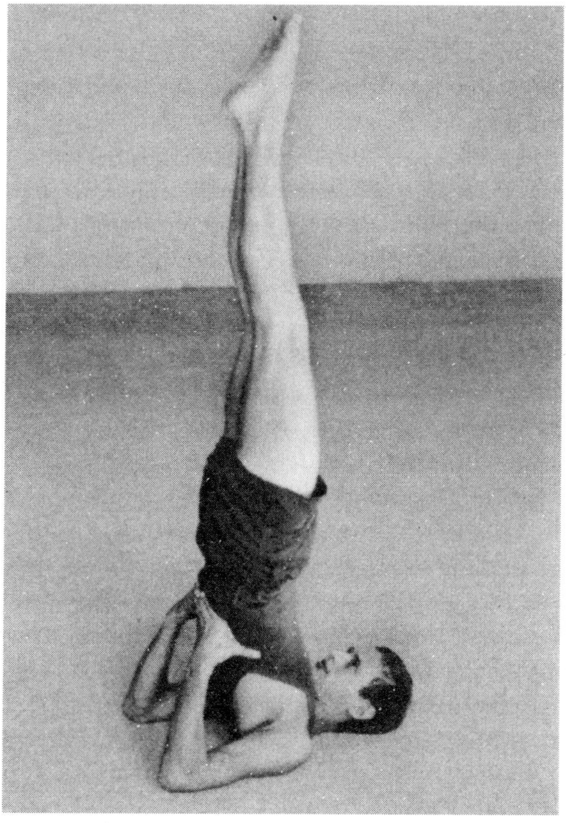

Benefits: The thyroid gland which plays a prominent part in metabolism, growth, nutrition and structure, is nourished properly. Healthy thyroid means healthy function of the circulatory, respiratory, alimentary, genito-urinary and nervous systems of the body. The thyroid operates in conjunction with the other ductless glands: pituitary, pineal in the brain, suprarenal above the kidneys, liver, spleen and testes. If the thyroid is diseased, all the other glands suffer. A vicious circle is formed. Sarvangasana keeps a healthy thyroid, which means healthy functioning of all the organs of the body.

Sarvangasana supplies a large quantity of blood to the spinal roots of nerves. It centralises the blood in the spinal column and nourishes it beautifully. But for this asana there is no scope for these nerve-roots to draw sufficient blood supply. It keeps the spine quite elastic. Elasticity of the spine means everlasting youth. It prevents the bones from early ossification, so you will preserve and retain your youth for a long time. This asana destroys the ravages of old age. It helps a lot in maintaining celibacy. Like sirshasana, it makes you an urdhvareto-yogi.

Sarvangasana acts as a powerful blood tonic and purifier. It tones the nerves. It is a cheap, readily available blood, nervine and digestive tonic, at your disposal at all times. It will reduce your doctor's bills. When you have not much time to practise a course of asanas, do this without fail daily along with sirshasana and paschimottanasana. It is useful in gonorrhoea and other diseases of bladder and ovaries. It removes sterility and diseases of the womb. Sarvangasana awakens kundalini and augments the digestive fire. It removes dyspepsia, constipation and other gastro-intestinal disorders of a chronic nature. It energises, invigorates and vivifies. A course of sirshasana and sarvangasana powerfully rejuvenates the whole body.

I have taught this asana to hundreds of persons. I invariably recommend sirshasana and sarvangasana combined with paschimottanasana to those who approach me. These three alone can keep you in perfect health. You need not take any long walk or physical exercise. All have unanimously reported to me the wonderful, mysterious, beneficial results of sarvangasana. As soon as you come down from it, it braces you up and gives a new vigorous, healthy tone. It is an ideal 'pick-me-up'.

Halasana (Plough Pose)

When this pose is practised it gives the exact appearance of a plough. 'Hala' means a plough in sanskrit.

Technique: Spread a blanket on the ground. Lie flat on your back. Keep the hands at the sides on the ground with the palms facing the ground. Join both your legs and lift them up very slowly, keeping the knees straight. Keep the hands on the floor, and do not bend the trunk. Make an obtuse angle. Then slowly lower the legs, folding them over the body until the toes touch the ground behind the head. Keep the knees quite straight and close together. Press the chin against the chest. Breathe slowly through the nose only and not through the mouth.

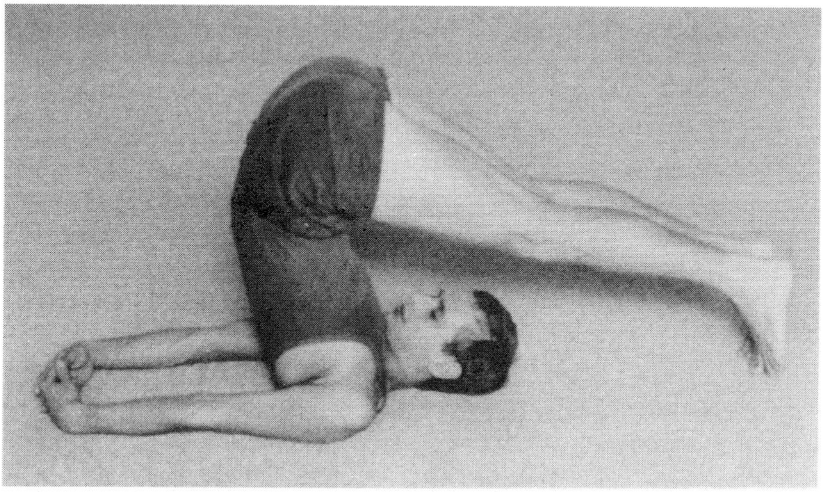

There is another variety of this asana. After the above posture is done, slowly bring the hands round and catch hold of the toes. This is also a better method. There should be no jerk in any way. When the asana is finished, very very slowly raise the legs and bring them to the original posture of lying flat on the ground.

Benefits: This asana tones the spinal nerves, the muscles of the back, the vertebral bones and the sympathetic nervous system that runs along the vertebral column on both sides. This asana fulfils and amplifies sarvangasana. A large quantity of blood is poured into the spinal roots of nerves, spinal cord, sympathetic ganglia, sympathetic nerves and muscles of the back. Hence they are well nourished. The muscles of the back are alternatively contracted, relaxed and then pulled and stretched. Hence they draw a good supply of blood by these various movements and are well nourished. Various sorts of myalgia (muscular rheumatism), lumbago, sprain and neuralgia are cured by this asana. This asana prevents the early ossification of the vertebral bones. Old age manifests quickly on account of early ossification, and bones become hard and brittle in the degenerative process. He who practises halasana is very nimble, agile and full of energy. A man who practises halasana can never become lazy.

The vertebral column becomes supple and elastic. It is twisted and rolled, as it were, like a piece of canvas sheet. The vertebral column is a very important structure. It supports the whole body. It contains the spinal cord, spinal nerve and sympathetic system. Therefore you must keep it healthy, strong and elastic by the practice of halasana. The muscles of the abdomen, the rectal muscles and the muscles of the thigh are also toned and nourished. Obesity and chronic constipation and congestion and enlargement of the liver and spleen, are cured by this asana.

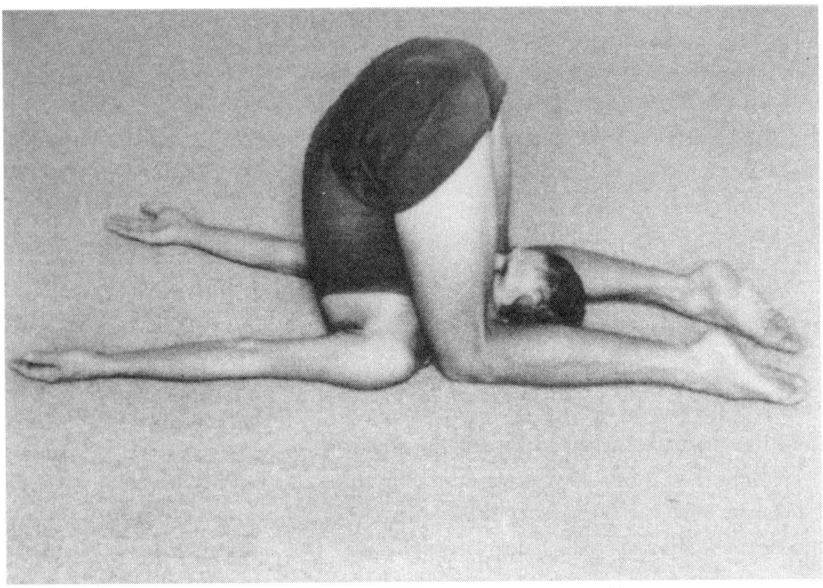

Varieties

i. *Karnapidasana*:

Perform halasana keeping the hands on the floor at the back. Now slowly bend the legs at the knees and bring the knees to touch your shoulders. In this asana the leg from the knees to the toes will be parallel to the ground.

ii. *Uttana Padasana*:

Lie down. Keep the legs straight and the hands by your sides, the palms facing the ground. Raise the two legs together about two feet from the ground without bending the legs and the knees. Slowly bring them down. Repeat this six times. Constipation, pain in the hips and thighs will be removed. (This is a preliminary exercise of sarvangasana.)

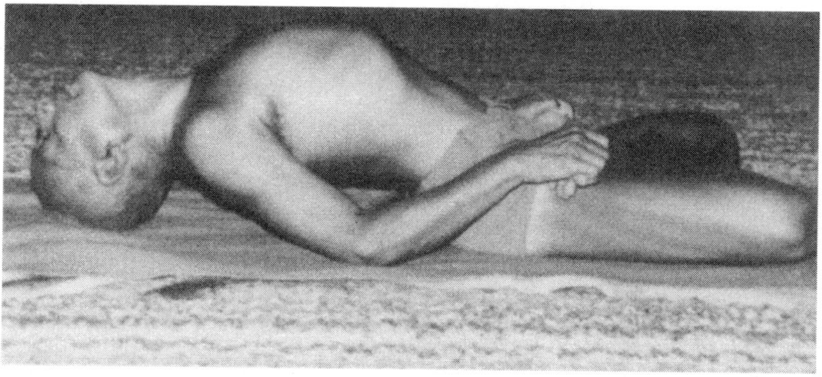

Matsyasana (Fish Pose)

As this asana will help one to float on water easily with plavini pranayama, it is called fish-pose, matsyasana.

Technique: Spread a blanket on the ground and sit on it with the legs stretched. Bend the right leg and place the heel on the left hip joint. Again bend the left leg and place the heel on the right hip joint. This is padmasana or foot lock. Fat persons with thick calves who find it difficult to do padmasana may simply sit in the ordinary way and then practise this asana.

Then lie on the back. The padmasana should not be raised from the ground. Rest the elbows or hands on the ground. Now lift the trunk and head. Rest the top of the head on the ground by arching the back and throwing the neck well behind. Then catch hold of the toes. This is matsyasana. Do it for 10 seconds to start with, and gradually increase it to 10 minutes.

When you have finished the asana, slowly release the head with the help of the hands and get up. Then unlock the foot-lock.

Practise padmasana first. Make it firm, easy and steady. Then take to matsyasana. You must practise this soon after sarvangasana. It will relieve stiffness of the neck and any crampy condition of the cervical region caused by long practice of sarvangasana. It gives natural massage, as it were, to the congested parts of the neck and shoulders. It affords the maximum benefits to sarvangasana; it supplements sarvangasana.

Benefits: Matsyasana is the destroyer of many diseases. It removes constipation. It brings down the accumulated faecal matter to the rectum. As the larynx or wind-box and trachea (wind-pipe) are thrown open widely, this asana helps deep breathing. It is useful in asthma, consumption, chronic bronchitis, etc. The apices of the lungs, which are located just behind and above the clavicular bone (or collar bone in common parlance), receive proper pure air and sufficient supply of pure oxygen. The cervical and upper dorsal nerves are nourished with a good quantity of blood and toned properly. The endocrine glands that are located in the brain — pituitary and pineal — are stimulated and toned also. These glands play a vital part in the physiological functioning of the various systems of the body.

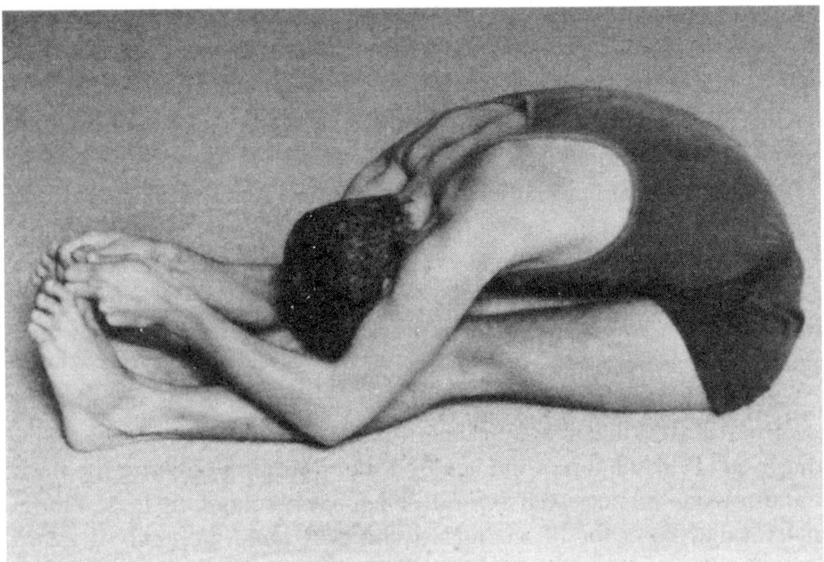

Paschimottanasana

Sit on the ground and stretch the legs still like a stick. Catch the toes with the thumb, index and middle fingers. While catching, you will have to bend the trunk forwards. Fat persons will find it rather difficult to bend. Exhale and slowly bend without jerks till your forehead touches your knees. You can keep the face between the knees also. When you bend down draw the belly back. This facilitates the bending forwards. Bend slowly by gradual degrees. Take your own time, there is no hurry. When you bend down, bend the head between the arms. Retain it on a level with them. Young persons with elastic spine can touch the knees with the forehead even in their very first attempt. In the case of adults with rigid spinal column, it will take a fortnight or a month for complete success in the posture. Hold the breath out till you take the forehead back to its original position, till you sit straight again. Then breathe.

Retain the pose for five seconds. Then gradually increase the period to ten minutes.

Those who find it difficult to do the full paschimottanasana can do half pose with one leg and one hand and then with the other leg and other hand. They will find this easier. After some days when the spine has become more elastic they can have recourse to the full pose. You will have to use common-sense while practising asanas. (Before you practise this, read the instructions on janusirshasana.)

Benefits: This is an excellent asana. It makes the breath flow through the sushumna, and rouses the gastric fire. It reduces fat in the abdomen. It is a specific for corpulence or obesity and for the enlargement of spleen and liver. Books on hatha yoga speak highly of this asana. Sarvangasana is for the stimulation of the endocrine glands and paschimottanasana for the stimulation of the abdominal viscera, such as kidneys, liver, pancreas, etc. It increases the peristalsis of the bowels. (Peristalsis is the vermicular movement of the bowels or intestines by which food and faecal matter are pushed from one portion of the bowels to another.) This asana relieves constipation, removes sluggishness of the liver, dyspepsia, belching and gastritis. Lumbago or stiff back and all sorts of myalgia and other diseases of the back muscles are cured. It cures piles and diabetes also. The hip, the muscles of the abdomen, the solar plexus of nerves, the epigastric plexus of nerves, bladder, prostate, lumbar nerves and sympathetic cord are all toned up and kept in a healthy, sound condition. Thanks to paschimottanasana, and to the rishis who first introduced these wonderful asanas to the students of hatha yoga!

Janusirshasana (Head-knee Pose)

Technique: Sit down on the floor. Press the perineal space with the left heel, stretching the right leg at full length. Keep it quite straight. Catch hold of the foot with both hands. Exhale. Draw the belly inwards. Slowly bend the head down and touch the right knee with the forehead. Keep that position for 5 to 10 seconds. (Gradually increase the period. You can do the asana even for half an hour by steady practise.)

Then slowly raise the head to its former, normal position. Take rest for a few minutes. Again practise this asana. Do it 5 or 6 times. Change the sides alternately. When you practise, draw the muscles of the anus upwards. Feel that the seminal energy is flowing upwards towards the brain as ojas shakti (spiritual energy). Use the bhavana shakti ('feeling' energy) of your mind. Those who practise this asana will find it easy to practise paschimottanasana.

Instead of taking the heel to the perineum you can put it on the thigh. This is a little more difficult than the previous one. Practise this asana after evacuating the bowels.

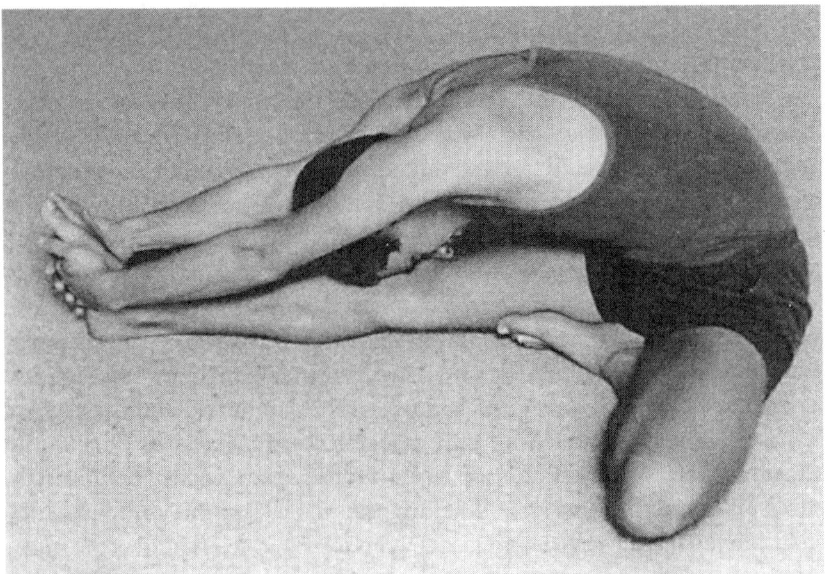

Benefits: This asana increases the digestive fire and helps digestion. It stimulates the solar plexus and helps you in keeping up celibacy. All urinary troubles are cured. It is very useful for intestinal colic. Kundalini is awakened. Laziness and weakness will vanish. The legs are strengthened. All other benefits mentioned in paschimottanasana can be derived from this asana also.

Mayurasana (Peacock Pose)

'Mayur' means peacock in sanskrit. When this asana is exhibited it resembles a peacock which has spread out the bundle of feathers at its back. This is a little more difficult than sarvangasana and matsyasana. It demands good physical strength. Gymnasts can do it very easily. It corresponds more or less to plank exercises on the parallel bars.

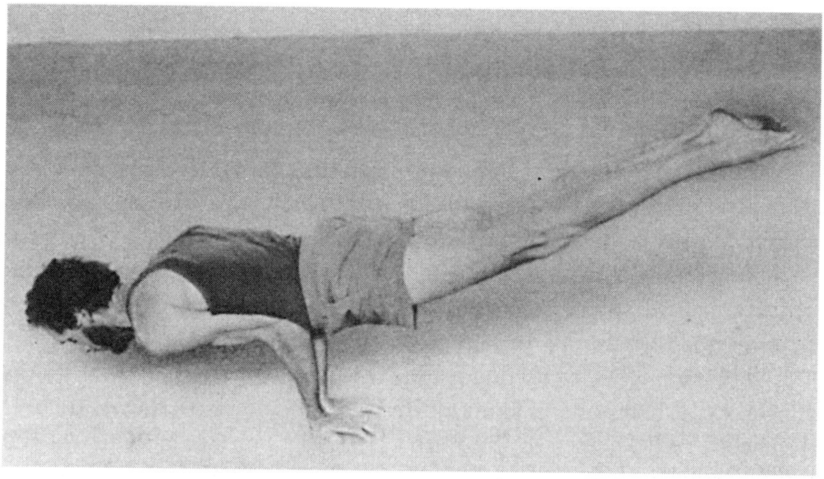

Technique: Kneel on the ground, and squat on the toes. Raise the heels up. Join the two forearms together. Place the palms of the two hands on the ground. The two little fingers must be in close opposition or juxtaposition. The thumbs should touch the ground. They should project towards the feet.

Now you have got steady and firm forearms for supporting the whole body in the ensuing elevation of the trunk and legs. Now bring down the abdomen slowly against the conjoined elbows. Support your body upon your elbows that are pressed now against the navel. This is the first stage. Stretch your legs and raise the feet straight on a level with the head, parallel to the ground. This is the second stage.

Beginners find it difficult to keep up the balance as soon as they raise the feet off the ground. Place a cushion in front. Sometimes you will have a fall forwards and you may hurt your nose slightly. Try to slip on the sides when you cannot keep up the balance. If you find it difficult to stretch the legs backwards at one stroke, slowly stretch one leg first and then the other. If you adopt the device of leaning the body forwards and head downwards, the feet will by themselves leave the ground and you can stretch them quite easily. When the asana is in full manifestation the head, trunk, buttocks, thighs, legs and feet will be in one straight line and parallel to the ground. This posture is very beautiful to look at.

Beginners can practise it by holding the sides of a cot. They will find it easy to practise this way. If you understand the technique of this asana and if you use your common-sense, you can easily keep up the balance without much difficulty. Fat people must be cautious to avoid falls and slips. Do not jerk the feet when you stretch them.

Practise this asana from 5 to 20 seconds. Those who have good physical strength can do it for 2 or 3 minutes.

Retain the breath when you raise the body. It will give you immense strength. Then breathe gently while you hold the posture. When you finish the asana, exhale slowly.

Benefits: Mayurasana has got a charm of its own. It braces you up quickly. It gives you full exercise within a few seconds. It serves like a hypodermic injection of adrenalin or digitalin.

This is a powerful asana for improving the digestion. It destroys the effects of unwholesome food and it increases the digestive power. It cures dyspepsia and diseases of the stomach — like chronic gastritis — and reduces splenic and liver enlargement by increasing the intra-abdominal pressure. The lungs and the whole abdominal viscera (organs) are properly toned and stimulated by the increase of intra-abdominal pressure. Sluggishness of the liver (hepatic torpidity) disappears. It tones the bowels, removes constipation (ordinary or chronic) and awakens kundalini. It gives wonderful appetite, removes all diseases caused by an excess of wind, bile or phlegm, cures diabetes and haemorrhoids, and strengthens the muscles of the arms. This one asana can give you maximum physical exercise in the minimum time.

Varieties

i. *Hamsasana*:

This is quite an easy asana. The preliminary portion of mayurasana is known as hamsasana. Here the toes are kept on the ground before the legs are raised for mayurasana.

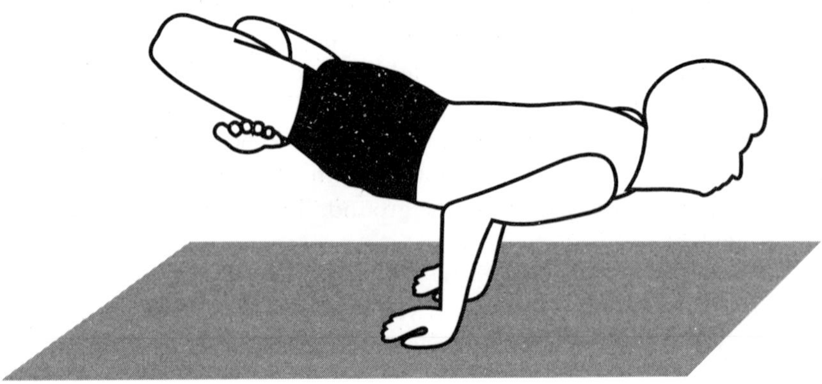

ii. *Lolasana*:

Form padmasana, sit in the first stage of mayurasana. Now the weight of your body will be on your knees and hands. Then slowly raise the lower part of your body forming the padmasana. This is a sort of swinging pose with padmasana. This is termed lolasana. It is a variety of mayurasana. The benefits of mayurasana are derived from this asana also.

Ardha-Matsyendrasana

Ardha means half. This is half a pose. It takes its name from the sage Matsyendra, who first taught this asana to the students of hatha yoga. Matsyendra is said to have been the disciple of Lord Siva. Once Siva departed for a lonely island. There he taught Parvati the mysteries of yoga. A fish that happened to be near the shore heard the teachings of Lord Siva. Siva came to know this. His heart being filled with mercy, he sprinkled water on this yogi-fish. Immediately, on account of Lord Siva's grace, the fish became a siddha yogi with a divine body. This yogi-fish was called by the name Matsyendra.

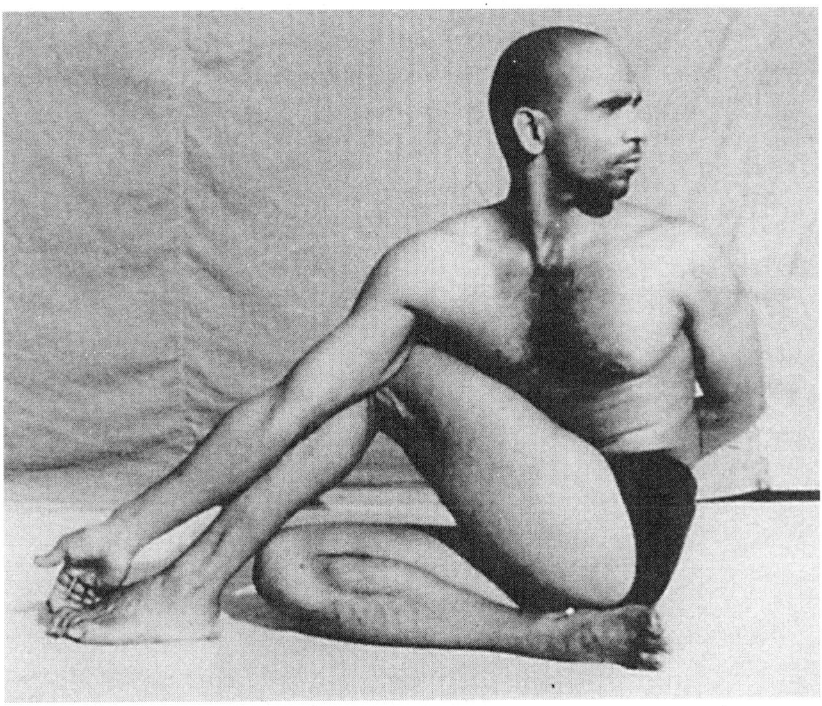

Paschimottanasana and halasana bend the spine forwards. Dhanurasana, bhujangasana and salabhasana are counterposes to bend the spine backwards. This is not sufficient. It must be twisted and bent from side to side also (lateral movements), then only perfect elasticity of the spinal column can be ensured. Matsyendrasana serves this purpose well, in giving a lateral twist to the spinal column. Some hatha yogis start with this asana when they give practical lessons to yoga students.

Technique: Place the left heel near the anus and below the scrotum. It can touch the perineum. Do not allow the heel to move from this space. (Perineum is the space between the anus and the external organ of generation.) Bend the right knee and place the right ankle at the root of the left thigh and rest the right foot well on the ground, close to the left hip joint. Place the left axilla or arm-pit over the top of the vertically bent right knee. Push the knee now a little to the back so that it touches the back part of the axilla. Catch hold of the left knee with the left palm. Then applying pressure at the left shoulder-joint, slowly twist the spine and turn to the extreme right. Turn the face also to the right as much as you can. Bring it in line with the right shoulder. Swing the right arm round behind the back. Catch hold of the left thigh with the right hand. Retain the pose from five to fifteen seconds. Keep the vertebral column erect. Do not bend. Similarly, twist the spine to the left side. This will complete the spinal twist.

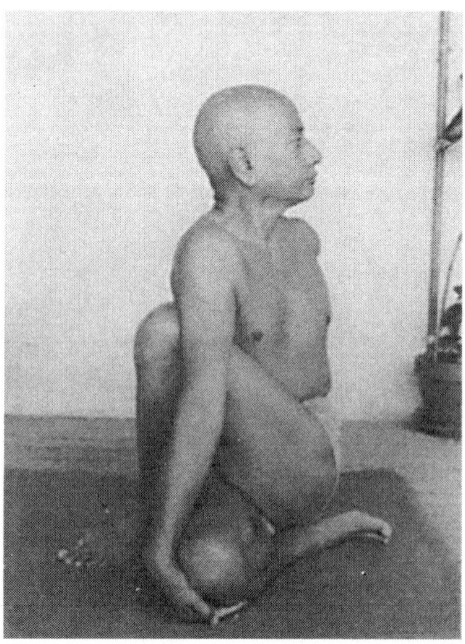

Benefits: This asana increases appetite by increasing the digestive fire. It destroys terrible diseases. It rouses kundalini and makes the chandra nadi (moon) flow steadily. (The moon is said to be located above the root of the palate. It drops the cool ambrosial nectar which is normally wasted by mixing with gastric fire. But this asana prevents it.)

It keeps the spine elastic and gives a good massage to the abdominal organs. Lumbago and all sorts of muscular rheumatism of the back muscles are cured. The spinal nerve-roots and sympathetic system are toned. They draw a good supply of blood. This asana is an auxilliary to paschimottanasana.

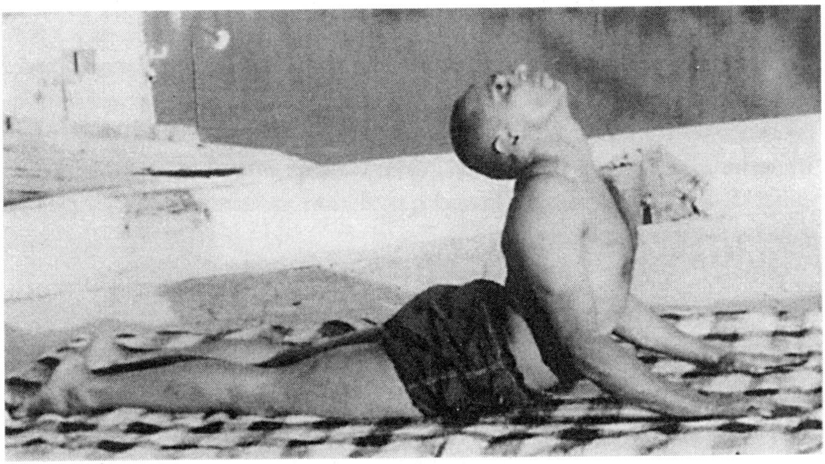

Bhujangasana (Cobra Pose)

'Bhujanga' means a cobra in sanskrit. When this pose is exhibited the raised head and trunk resemble the raised hood of a cobra. Hence this is called bhujangasana.

Technique: Spread a blanket on the ground. Lie face downwards on the ground, the chin pressed against the chest. Relax all muscles. Be at ease. Place the palms on the ground just below the shoulders. Let the body, from the navel downwards to the toes, touch the ground. Raise the head and upper portion of the body slowly just as the cobra raises its hood. Bend the spine backwards. Now the muscles of the back and lumbar regions are well contracted. The intra-abdominal pressure is also increased. Then slowly bring down the head to its original position. The chin-lock is formed. Repeat the process of raising the head and bringing it down half a dozen times, steadily. Breathe slowly through the nose. Retain the breath till you raise the head and bend the spine properly. Then you can slowly exhale. Then retain the breath while bringing the head down. As soon as the head touches the ground, breathe again slowly.

Benefits: Bhujangasana bends the spine backwards, while sarvangasana and halasana bend it forwards. This relieves hunchback, back pain, lumbago and myalgia of the back. It increases the intra-abdominal pressure and brings down the loaded faecal matter from the transverse colon to the rectum. Hence it relieves constipation. It increases bodily heat and destroys a host of ailments. It awakens the kundalini that is sleeping dormant in the muladhara chakra. It gives good appetite.

Bhujangasana is particularly useful for ladies in toning their ovaries and uterus. It is a powerful tonic. It will relieve amenorrhoea (absence of menstruation), dysmenorrhoea (painful or difficult menstruation), leucorrhoea (whites), and various other utero-ovarine diseases. It keeps up efficient blood circulation in those parts. Deliveries will be normal and easy.

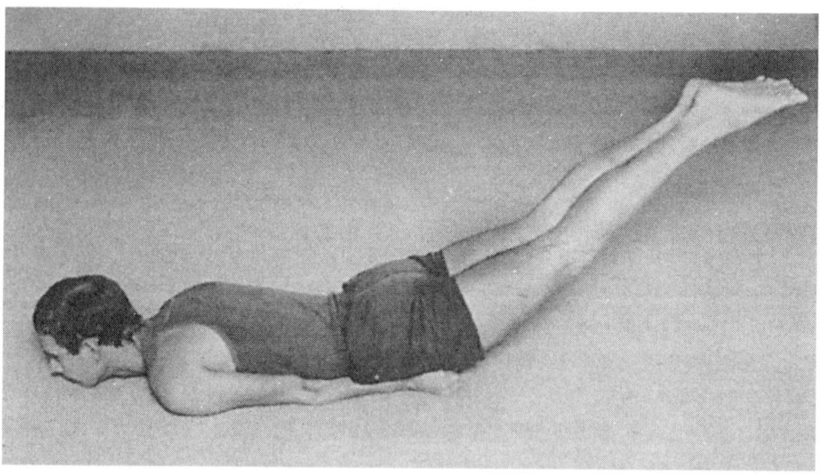

Salabhasana (Locust Pose)

When this pose is demonstrated it resembles a locust. Hence the name salabha or locust.

Technique: Lie on the ground, face downwards. Keep the arms by the sides. The palms should be turned up. You can place the hands underneath the belly — this is another way. Inhale slightly. Stiffen the whole body and raise the legs in the air one cubit high. Raise the head as in bhujangasana. Keep the thighs, legs and toes together. Turn up the soles of the feet. Lift up the legs, thighs and lower portion of the abdomen. Keep up this pose from 5 to 30 seconds. Bring the legs down slowly. Retain the breath till you finish the asana and then exhale slowly.

You can repeat the process 6 to 7 times.

Benefits: This asana bends the spine backwards. Like mayurasana, it increases the intra-abdominal pressure. It supplements bhujangasana. Bhujangasana develops the upper half of the body, while salabhasana develops the lower half of the body and the lower extremities also. It tones the muscles of the abdomen, back, thighs and legs. It brings down the accumulated matter to the ascending colon, from ascending colon to transverse colon or large intestines, from transverse colon to descending colon and from there to the rectum. (Read any book on elementary physiology. It will help you a lot.)

This asana gives good exercise for the abdomen. It relieves constipation, tones the abdominal viscera — liver, pancreas, kidneys, etc. — and removes several diseases of the stomach and bowels. It cures sluggishness of liver and hunchback. The lumbo-sacral bones are toned up and lumbago is removed. All forms of myalgia of the lumbar region (hips) are removed. The digestive fire is increased and dyspepsia is removed. You will have very good appetite.

Dhanurasana (Bow Posture)

When this asana is performed it resembles the bow (dhanura). The stretched arms and forelegs form the string of the bow. It bends the spine backwards. It supplements bhujangasana. We can say it is a combination of bhujangasana and salabhasana, with the addition of catching the ankles with the hands. Bhujangasana, salabhasana and dhanurasana form a valuable combination. They always go together. They form one set of asanas. This combination acts as a counter-pose to halasana and paschimottanasana, which bend the spine forwards.

Technique: Lie on your chest with the face downwards. Relax all the muscles. Keep the arms at the sides. Gently fold the legs at the back. Raise your hands backwards and catch hold of the ankles with the hands. Raise the chest and head. Expand the chest. Keep the arms and forelegs quite straight and stiff. Now a good convex arch is formed. If you stretch the legs you can raise your chest up. You should dexterously manipulate. Retain the breath in a mild manner and exhale slowly. Do this five or six times. You can retain the pose as long as you can comfortably keep it. Keep the knees close.

The whole body rests on the abdomen. This asana gives a good massage to the abdominal region. You must do it when the stomach is empty. You can give a good movement to the bow-shaped body from side to side and forwards and backwards. This will ensure a thorough massage to the abdomen. Swing, rock and rejoice. Mentally repeat OM, OM, OM.

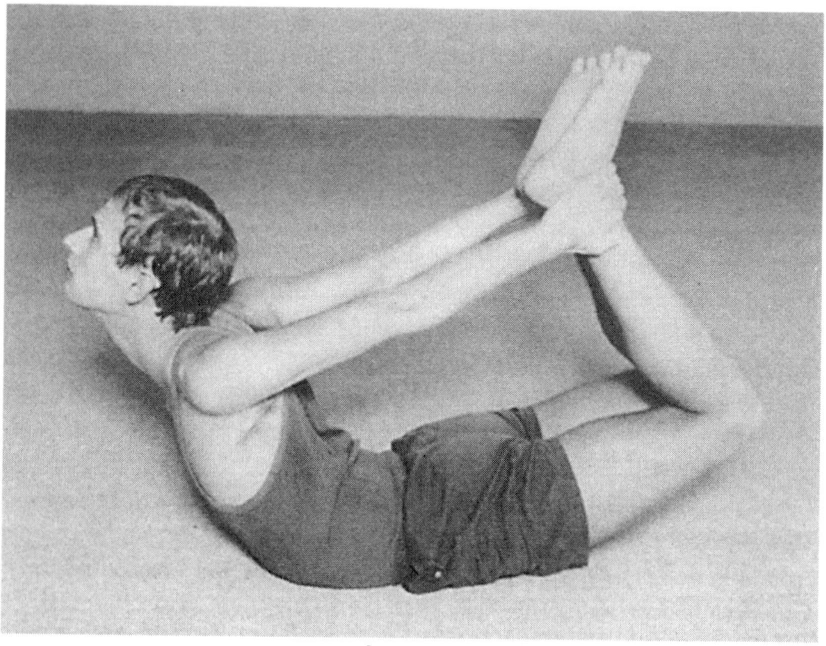

Benefits: This is useful in chronic constipation, dyspepsia and sluggishness of liver. It removes hunchback, rheumatism of legs, knee joints and hands. It reduces fat, energises digestion, increases peristalsis, invigorates the appetite and relieves congestion of blood in the abdominal viscera and tones them also.

Dhanurasana is a blessing for people who suffer from gastro-intestinal diseases. Like halasana, it keeps the spine elastic. It prevents premature ossification of bones. He who does halasana, mayurasana and dhanurasana can never become lazy. He is full of energy, vigour and vitality.

i. *Ushtrasana (Camel Pose)*:

Lie on the ground face downwards. Turn the legs and keep them over the thighs. Catch the toes or ankles with your hands. You can raise the head a bit above. This is similar to dhanurasana but the thighs are kept on the ground in this asana. The benefits of dhanurasana and salabhasana can be had in this pose.

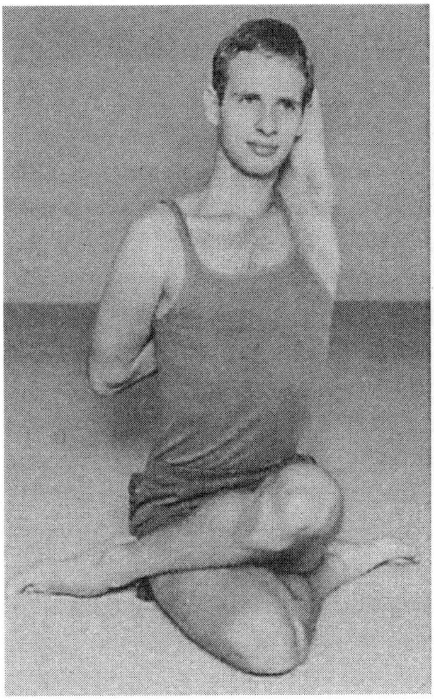

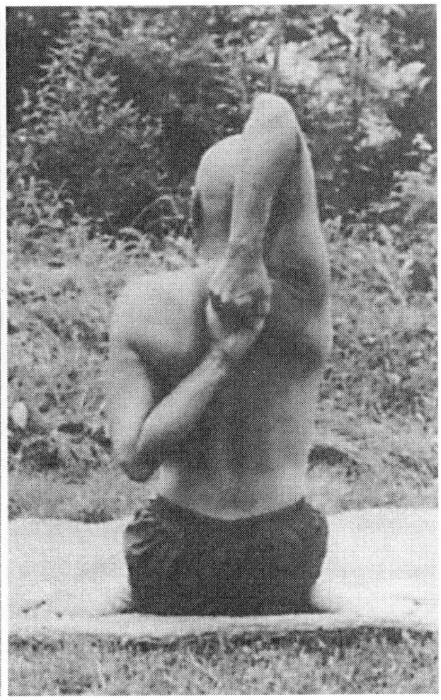

Gomukhasana (Cow-Face Posture)

When this asana is demonstrated it will look like the face of a cow. Hence this significant name. (Gomukha means 'cow-face'.)

Technique: place the heel of the left leg under the left part of the anus. Bring the right leg in such a way that the right knee will be above the left knee and the right sole along the side of the left thigh in close contact. By gradual practise you will have to bring the right heel to touch the left buttock. Sit quite erect. Now you will have to make a finger-lock of the two index-fingers at the back dexterously, of course with a little difficulty in the beginning. Take the left hand to the back, raise the left index-finger upwards. Bring the right hand over the right shoulder and down the back, with the index-finger downwards, and firmly catch hold of the left index-finger. Make a finger-lock now. If it slips, try again, and keep the lock for two minutes. Breathe slowly. The asana will now look like the face of a cow. When you make the finger-lock, do not turn the body; do not bend the heel and chest. Keep the trunk quite straight. Change the arms and legs alternately. Fat people will find it difficult to do this asana, to adjust the heels and thighs and to make the finger-lock; but continual practice will make them alright.

If you find a little congestion of blood in the thighs, massage them with your hands as soon as you release the posture.

Benefits: This asana removes rheumatism in the legs, sciatica, piles or haemorrhoids, neuralgia of the legs and thighs, indigestion, dyspepsia, muscular pain in the back and sprain in the forearms. This helps in maintaining brahmacharya and good health. Mula bandha comes by itself and can be kept up with ease. Hence, this asana is suitable for the practice of pranayama. Ordinarily you can sit at all times in this asana without having a finger-lock.

You can sit in this asana for long meditation also. Lean persons with thin thighs and legs will like it very much. Yogi Swami Swarupananda of Jwalapur, Hardwar, was a votary of this asana. He used to sit in it always. It was his favourite.

Variety

i. *Vama Janvasana*:

Keep the legs as in gomukhasana, but have the hands can be kept near your chest or on the lap or knees.

Vajrasana (The Admantine Pose)

Those who sit in this asana have a steady, firm pose. They cannot be easily shaken. The knees are rendered very hard. The spinal column becomes firm and strong. This asana resembles more or less the namaz pose in which the Muslims sit for prayer.

Technique: Sit back on the heels with the soles of the feet on both sides of the anus. The part from the toes to the knee should touch the ground. The whole burden of the body is put on the knees and ankles. In the beginning of practice you may feel a slight pain in the knee and ankle joints, but it passes off very quickly. Massage the paining parts and the two joints with the hands. You can use a little Iodex or Amritanjan for rubbing. After fixing the feet and the knees, put both the hands straight on the knees. Keep the knees quite close. Sit like this, keeping the trunk, neck and head in one straight line. This is the most common asana. You can sit in this for a very long time comfortably. Yogis generally sit in this asana.

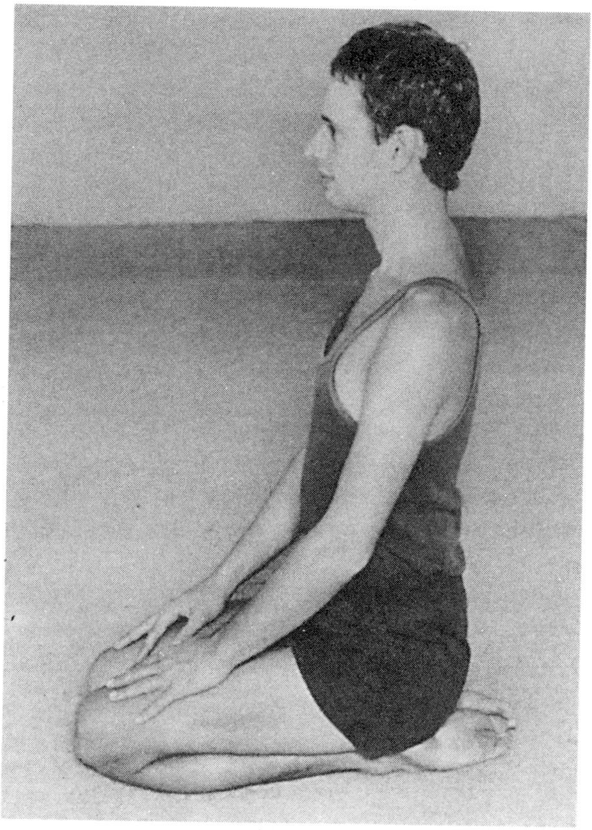

Benefits: If you sit in this asana for about half an hour immediately after food, the food will be digested well. Dyspeptics will derive much benefit. The nerves and muscles of the legs and thighs are strengthened. Myalgia in the knees, legs, toes and thighs disappears. Sciatica vanishes. Flatulence is removed. The stomach works vigorously. The practice of vajrasana exercises a stimulating, beneficial influence on the *kanda, which is situated above the anus and from which the 72,000 nadis spring.

* See Kundalini section

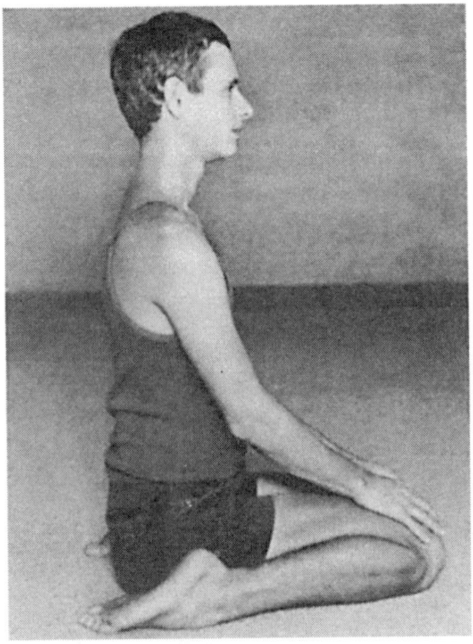

Varieties

i. Some people will keep the heels quite separate, while the anus and the buttocks are kept between the two heels and the legs by the side of the two thighs.

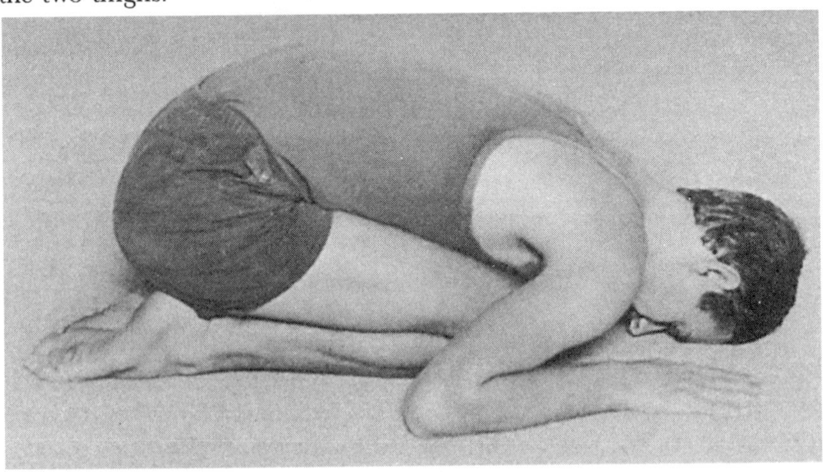

ii. *Ardha Kurmasana*:

Sit in vajrasana and stretch your hands to your face level, and slowly bend forward so that the chest rests on the thighs and the face is on the ground, hands touching the ground.

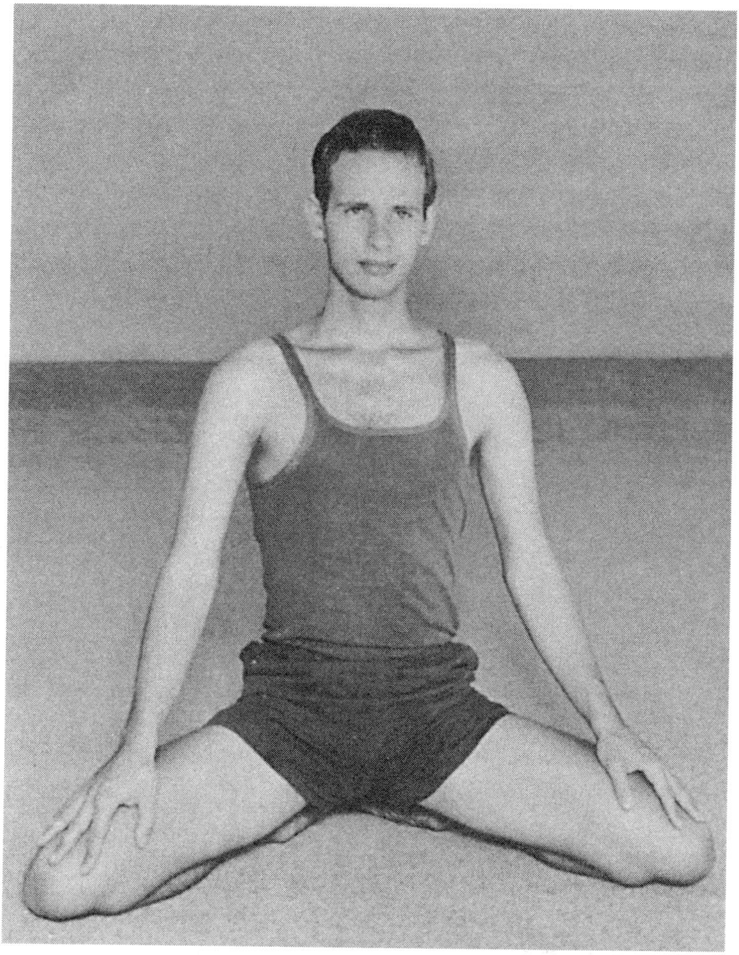

iii. *Mandukasana (Frog Pose)*:

Take the feet towards the back. Let the toes touch each other. Spread the knees apart. Keep the hands on the knees. This is called mandukasana.

iv. *Parvatasana*:

Sit in vajrasana posture. Raise your body and bring the hands above your head very slowly. This is called parvatasana. A better variety of parvatasana is described elsewhere.

v. *Ananda Mandirasana*:

Sit in vajrasana and catch hold of the heels with the two hands.

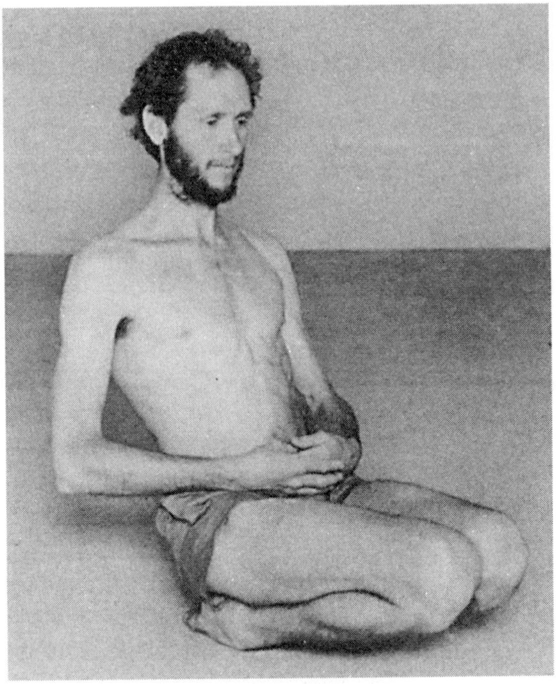

vi. *Angushthasana*:

This is an important asana for keeping up brahmacharya. While sitting in vajrasana slowly raise you knees.

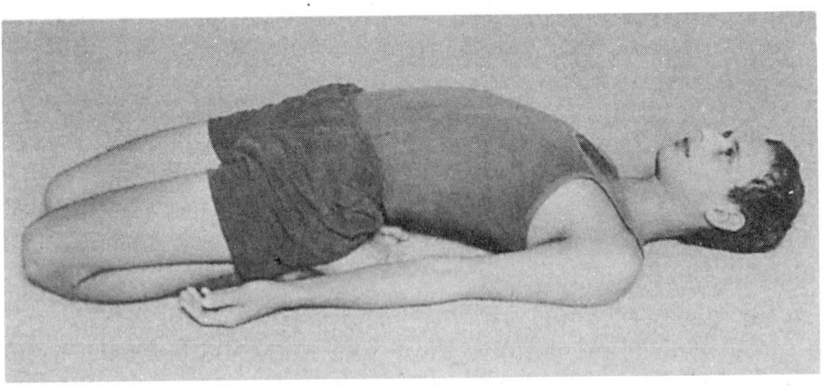

vii. *Supta Vajrasana*:

This is sleeping pose and vajrasana combined. It is sometimes called ardha savasana. First you must be perfect in doing vajrasana.

Then you can take to this asana. More strain and force come to the knees in this asana than in vajrasana. Sit in vajrasana and then lie down on the back. Make a finger-lock. Allow the head to rest on the palms, or, you can place the arms alongside the body. In the beginning the entire portion of the back may not touch the ground. The lower portion will remain raised up. With a few days' practice you will be able to do this asana quite satisfactorily.

In this you will get all the advantages of vajrasana. Hunchback is removed as the spine is bent backwards. The spine gets elastic also. He who does this asana will find it easy to do chakrasana.

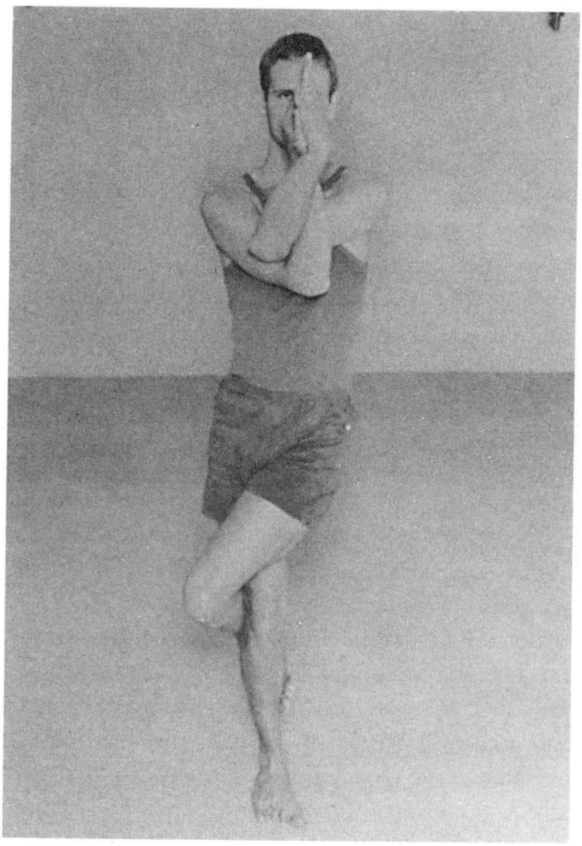

Garudasana (Eagle Pose)

When this asana is demonstrated it resembles the appearance of Garuda, the eagle. Hence it is called garudasana.

Technique: First stand up quite straight. Raise up your left leg and take it round the right leg. The left thigh should cross the right thigh. Just as the creeper encircles or winds round a tree, so also the left leg should wind around the right leg. Keep arms also likewise, one arm winding round the other. The palms of the hands should touch each other. Make the fingers like the beak of an eagle. Keep the hands just in front of the face. Change the legs and hands alternately.

When you stand as instructed above, steadily bend and try to touch the ground with the toe of the leg that encircles. Then alone can you get the maximum benefit of this asana. You can take the help of somebody when you bend down. Both the legs have to be bent. You can do basti (cleansing the bowels with water) in this asana.

Benefits: The whole weight of the body comes on one leg, whereas in kukkutasana the whole weight of the body comes on the two hands. The nerves and bones of the legs and hands are strengthened. The hands and legs are lengthened. A man may grow tall by the practice of this asana. The nerves of the kidneys also are strengthened. Sciatica, rheumatism of the legs and hands are cured. The bones of the vertebral column get developed and strengthened. Hydrocele and swelling of the testicles are cured. The muscles of the calves get developed. The nerves of the legs and hands are strengthened.

Padangushthasana

Fat people will find it a little difficult to practise this asana. They are tossed about, either from side to side or forwards and backwards. A little steady practise will make matters alright. Rishis of yore prescribed this asana along with sirshasana and sarvangasana for brahmacharis for the preservation of virya or the vital energy.

Technique: Put the left heel in the centre of the anus or perineum, the space between the anus and the external organ of generation. Put the whole weight of the body on the toes, particularly the left big toe. Place the right foot over the left thigh near the knee. Sit carefully now keeping up balance. If you find it difficult to practise this asana independently, you can take the help of a bench by placing your hands on the bench or sit by the side of a wall. Place the hands on the hips. Retain the breath as long as you can do it comfortably. Breathe slowly. Gaze steadily at any black or white spot in front of you. Repeat your guru mantra or Ram Ram while practising the asana.

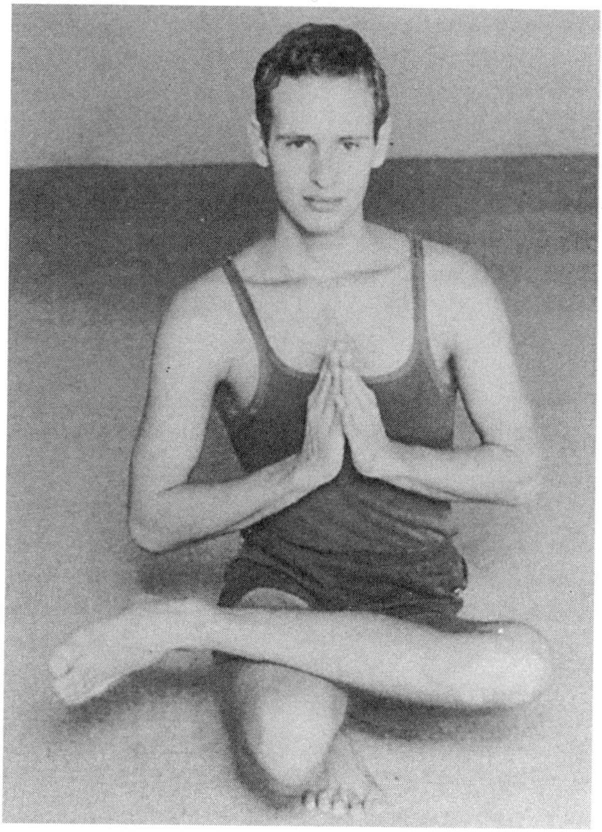

Benefits: The perineal space is four inches in breadth. Underneath this space lies the spermatic duct that carries the semen or vital energy from the testes. By pressing this with the heel, the flow of semen outside is checked. A steady practice of this asana removes wet-dreams or spermatorrhoea and makes one an urdhvareto-yogi or a yogi in whom the semen flows upwards to the brain and gets stored up there as ojas shakti or spiritual power. A combination of asanas such as sirshasana, sarvangasana, siddhasana, bhujangasana and padangushthasana is very conducive to keeping up brahmacharya. Each has its own specific action. Siddhasana and bhujangasana act on the testes and its cells and prevent the formation of semen. Sirshasana and sarvangasana help the flow of semen towards the brain. Padangushtasana acts on the spermatic duct effectively.

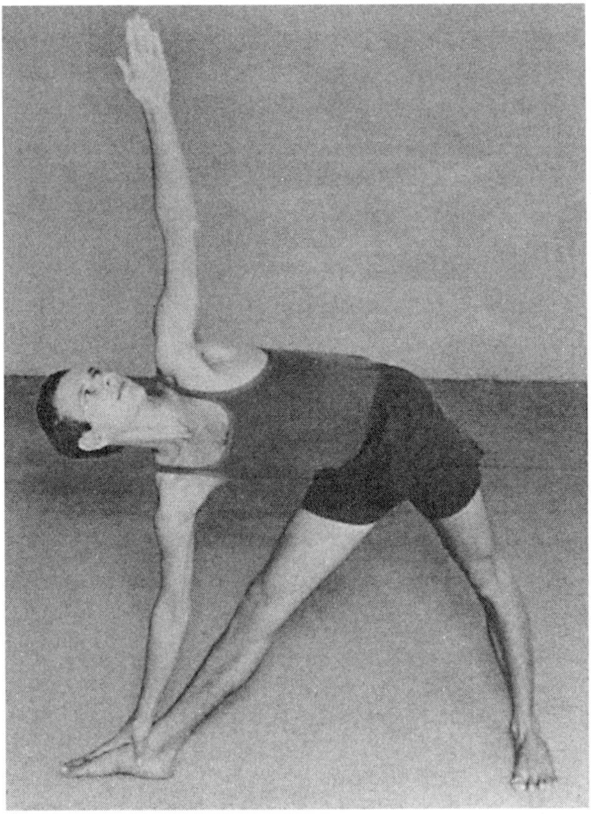

Trikonasana (Three Angle Pose)

Technique: Stand erect. Keep your legs two feet apart. Now stretch your arms wide on the sides in a line with the shoulders. The arms must now be quite parallel to the ground. (You might have done this portion of the exercise in your drill class in the school.) Now bend slowly to the right. Keep the left knee stiff and erect. This is important. Touch the right toe with the fingers of the right hand. Bend the neck slightly to the right. It may touch the right shoulder. Now stretch the left arm above. Retain the posture for two or three minutes. Breathe slowly. Again you can practise on the left side. Let the fingers of the left hand touch the left toe. Stretch the right arm in the air. Do three or six times on each side.

Benefits: This asana gives very good lateral movements to the spine. It is an auxiliary to ardha matsyendrasana. It amplifies and fulfils the matsyendrasana. If you have a healthy spine you can sit in your meditation in one asana for many hours without fatigue. For a yogi the spine is most important as it is connected with the spinal cord and the sympathetic system. It is the spine that contains the important sushumna nadi which plays a vital part in the movement of kundalini. This asana tones the spinal nerves and the abdominal organs, increases peristalsis of the bowels and invigorates appetite. Constipation is relieved. The body becomes light. Those who suffer from shortening of the leg due to fracture of hip or thigh bone (femur) or bones of the leg (tibia or fibula) will be benefited by this asana. It lengthens the legs. Krishna Kumar Bhargava practised this asana for three months. His leg became lengthened and he was able to walk for one or two miles.

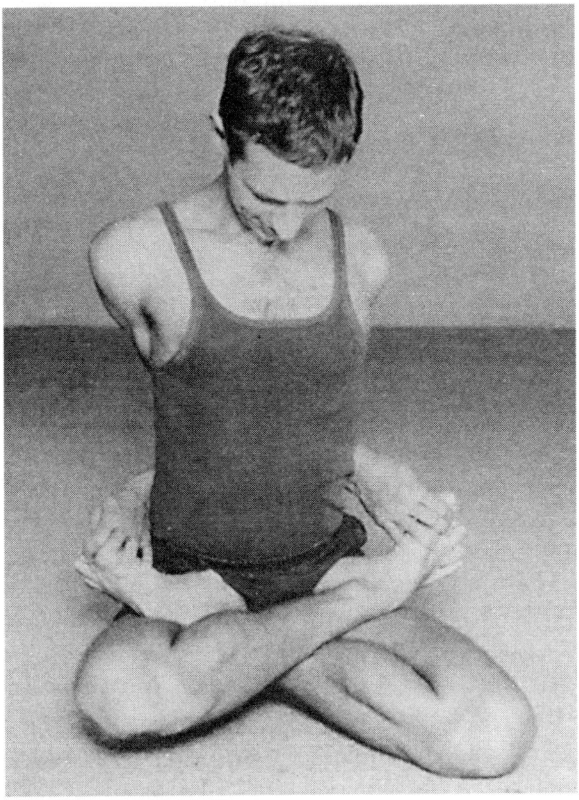

Baddha Padmasana (Locked-up Lotus Pose)

This is a variety of padmasana (lotus pose).

Technique: Sit in padmasana with legs crossed. The heels should touch the lower part of the belly or abdomen. Take your right hand behind the back. Catch hold of the toe of the right foot with the forefinger and middle finger of the right hand. Then take your left hand behind the back and catch hold of the toe of the left foot with the forefinger and middle finger of the left hand. Now press the chin against the chest. Look at the tip of the nose, (nasikagra drishti). Breathe slowly.

Some people find it difficult to catch hold of the two toes at a time. They can practise ardha baddha padmasana (half-pose) to start with for a month. Afterwards they can take to the purna baddha padmasana (full-pose). Practise this half-pose on the right side. Then do alternately on the left side also. During the half-pose, catch hold of one toe with one finger. Change the side afterwards. The half-pose is a preparatory stage for the full pose. In doing the full pose, use a little skill. Catch one toe first, and when you attempt to catch the other one slightly bend the body forwards. This will make matters easy in catching the other toe.

This is not an asana for meditation. This is chiefly intended for improving the health, vigour and vitality of the body to a considerable degree. The benefits of padmasana are derived in this asana to an enormous extent. This must be practised regularly at least for six months, then only maximum advantages can be realised. You cannot expect the full benefits by merely sitting for a couple of minutes. You must practise this at least for half an hour. If you can do it for an hour or an hour and a half, you will doubtless derive immense benefit. There are persons who do it for full three hours. How tenacious and patient these people are! They keep wonderful health and vigour and a high standard of vitality.

Many diseases are cured by this asana. Chronic diseases of the stomach, liver, spleen and intestines that are pronounced incurable by allopaths and ayurvedic practitioners are cured by a steady practice of this asana. There is no doubt of this. Diseases of the stomach such as chronic gastritis, dyspepsia, flatulence, colic, dysentery, ascites, constipation, acidity, belching and chronic lumbago are removed. As it keeps the spinal column erect, hunchback is removed. The nerves of the waist, hip, feet and legs are purified. Enlargement of the spleen and liver is cured. Torpidity of the liver disappears. This asana exercises a potent influence over the surya chakra (solar plexus of nerves) behind the navel and stimulates it. You draw a great deal of energy.

While in the asana, draw the belly backwards and upwards. Repeat OM or Ram mentally. Imagine that the seminal energy flows towards the brain for being stored up as ojas shakti. Do this special practice for ten minutes daily. This process is a great help for keeping up brahmacharya.

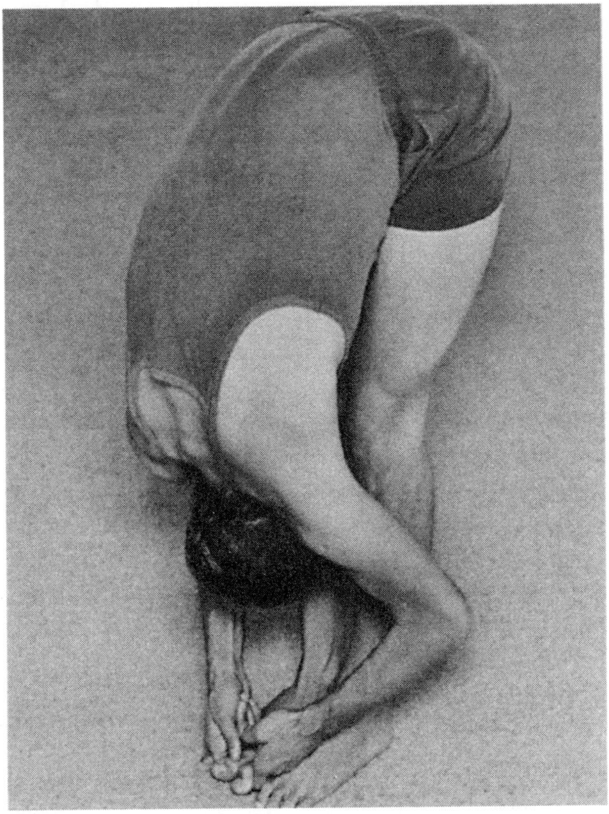

Padahastasana

This can be styled as 'standing paschimottanasana', as the technique is the same. The only difficulty is that you will have to do this while standing. Some people call this hastapadasana.

Technique: Stand erect. Let the hands down closely by the sides. Keep the heels close and toes apart. Raise the hands above the head. Slowly bend the body downwards. Keep the knees stiff and erect. Do not bend the legs at the knees. Slowly bring the hands down without bending at the elbows and catch hold of the toes with your thumb, index and middle fingers only. When you bend down, slowly exhale and draw the belly backwards. Keep the forehead between the knees. The face is buried between the hollow of knees, or the head can be pushed further between the two thighs.

(There are some varieties in this asana by interchanging the feet and hands. There is no space here for a detailed description. They are not of much use.) Retain the pose from 2 to 10 seconds. Fat people will find it difficult to practise this asana in the beginning. With patience and perserverance they will be able to do it perfectly in a short time. When you draw the abdomen back you will have to contract the abdominal muscles and rectum.

If you find it difficult to catch hold of the toes, owing to the stiffness of the muscles of the hips and excess of fat in the abdomen, bend the knees slightly. After catching hold of the toes, straighten and stiffen the legs. That is common sense. You can drink a small quantity of water before you do this asana.

Benefits: There are manifold benefits of this asana. You will feel much invigorated after the exercise is over. The body is rendered light as much tamas is dispelled. Adiposity disappears. Any shortening of the legs owing to fracture of the leg or thigh-bones is rectified. You will get slight lengthening of the leg by practice of this for about three months and by rubbing the thighs and legs with mustard oil to which a little salt is added. (Salt increases penetration of the oil.) This asana helps free passage of apana vayu downwards. The sushumna nadi is purified and strengthened. The benefits of paschimottanasana are derived from this asana also.

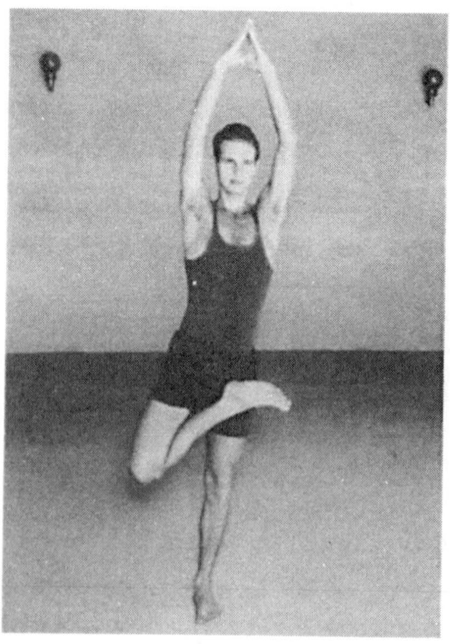

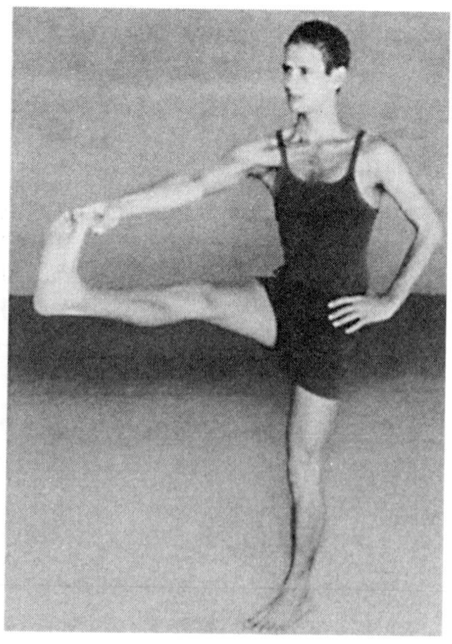

Varieties

i. *Padahastasana (Second Variety)*:

Stand erect. Slowly raise your left leg and catch hold of the toe with your fingers. Keep the right hand on your hip. Do not bend the legs. Some people call this variety padahastasana.

ii. *Tadasana (Tree Pose)*:

This is a familiar exercise among the school students in the drill class. Raise one hand above the head very quickly. Do not bend the head. Then bring it to the former position. Again do the same with the other hand. Repeat this as many times as you can. Instead of taking directly above the head at one stretch, you can stop for a while when the hand comes to your shoulder level, parallel to the ground. You can take the two hands together also. When this asana is over, shampoo the muscles of the hands, shoulders, etc. This asana is also called vrikshasana. (Sirshasana is also called vrikshasana.) Stand erect on one leg keeping the other leg at the root of the other thigh. This is also a variety of vrikshasana.

iii. *Purna Padasana*:

If you keep your hands at your sides and stand erect, it is called purna padasana.

Matsyendrasana (Full Pose — Spine Twist)

Those who have practised ardha matsyendrasana for some time are ready now for taking up this full pose. The full pose is a little more difficult than the half pose. The late Sri Madhavadasji Maharaj of Malsar (Gujerat), a famous hatha yogi, used to teach his students this pose straightaway.

Technique: Sit erect with legs stretched. Place the left foot on the joint of the right thigh, with the heel at the navel. Let the right foot touch the ground by the side of your left knee. Place the left hand outside the right knee and press the knee to the left side. Get hold of the right toe with the fingers (thumb, index and middle fingers) of the left hand. The right foot should remain firm. Bring the right arm behind the back and catch hold of the left heel. The face and body are turned back towards the right side. Twist the spine. Gaze at the tip of the nose. Breathe slowly. Retain the pose for 20 seconds. You can keep it for two or three minutes also by gradual practise. Repeat the process several times. The technique appears to be difficult. If you give careful attention and think with concentration, then it is very clear and easy.

Or watch when your friend does this asana.

This should be practised both by the right side and left side by turns; then only maximum benefits of the asana will be derived. First do the half pose for 2 or 3 weeks and then attempt this. Then the muscles and joints will be more elastic and flexible. If you find it difficult to keep up your balance, instead of bringing your hand towards the back you can keep the palm on the ground. This will give you good support and make matters easy. Slowly you can take the hand away and turn it towards the back.

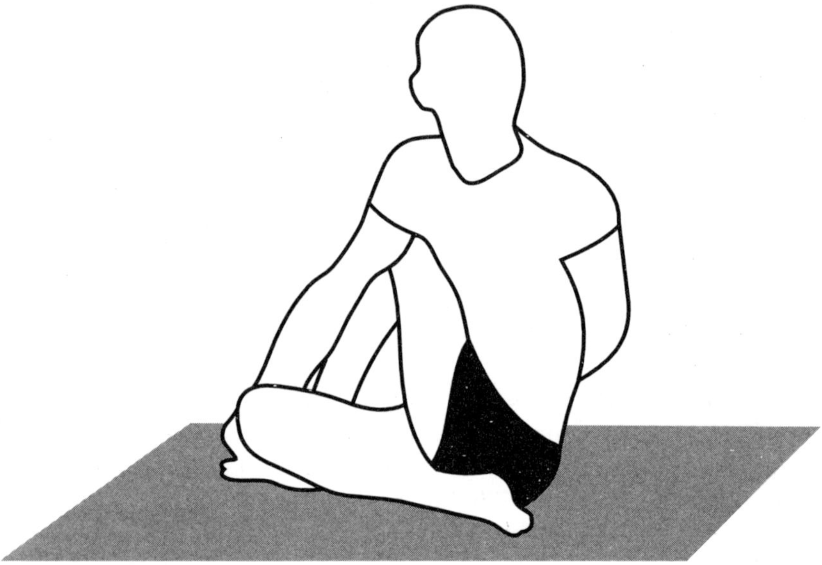

Benefits: The advantages that are derived from the half pose will be derived in this full pose to a greater extent. The synovial fluid of the joints increases and the joints become very active. All the adhesions in the joints that are caused by rheumatism are removed. It bestows beautiful health. It augments the prana-shakti (vigour and vitality) and consequently removes innumerable diseases. The pressure of the heel on the navel forces blood towards the back which nourishes well all the nerves of the back, particularly the prana *nadis of the back. It awakens the *kundalini and brings peace of mind. Hail, hail to yogi Matsyendra who first introduced this asana amongst the hatha yoga students.

* See Kundalini section

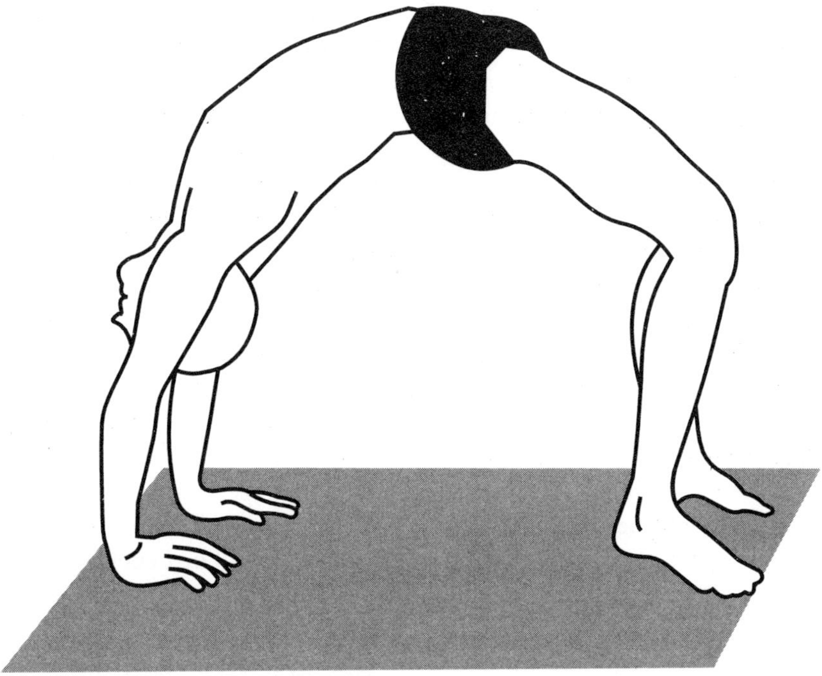

Chakrasana (Circle Pose)

Many acrobats demonstrate this asana in the streets. It resembles a circle. Hence the significant name 'chakrasana'. In fact, it resembles more a bow than a circle. Young boys can do it very easily because their spine is very elastic. When the bones become rigid and ossified in advanced years, bending of the spine becomes difficult.

Technique: Stand up. Raise the hands above the head. Slowly bend towards the back making a curve of the body. When the hands come to your hip level at the back, slowly bend your legs at the knee. This will help you to bend further and to touch the ground with your hands. Do not be in a hurry. Do it slowly by adjusting balance, otherwise you will have a fall. Practise this asana on a thick folded blanket. In the beginning, you can do it by the side of a wall or you can ask your friend to catch hold of your hips firmly, and then bend.

There is another way of doing this which is suitable for old people. There is no danger of falling at all. Lie down on the back. Keep the soles of the feet on the ground. The palms must be kept by the side of your head and the elbows above. Now bring your heels near to your hips on the ground and raise your body up, thus making a curve of your spine. By continuous practice one can render the spine very elastic. Elasticity of spines means everlasting youth. A man with a rigid spine can form a semicircle at the outset. In course of time all the rigid parts will become elastic. You can catch hold of the heels with the hands when you do this asana. If you find it difficult to hold this posture for a long time, repeat it a couple of times, with a short rest in between. When you raise yourself in this asana the body will be light. You will get exhilaration of spirit at once. You will be ready for active work. If there is any pain in the neck and shoulders after the practice of sarvangasana do this immediately for a few minutes. It will relieve the pain, as it bends the neck backwards and thus it is a counter-pose to sarvangasana.

Benefits. He who practises this will have perfect control of his body. He will be agile and nimble. He can turn out more work in a short space of time, and all the parts of the body will be benefited by it. All the other benefits of bhujangasana, salabhasana and dhanurasana are derived from this asana.

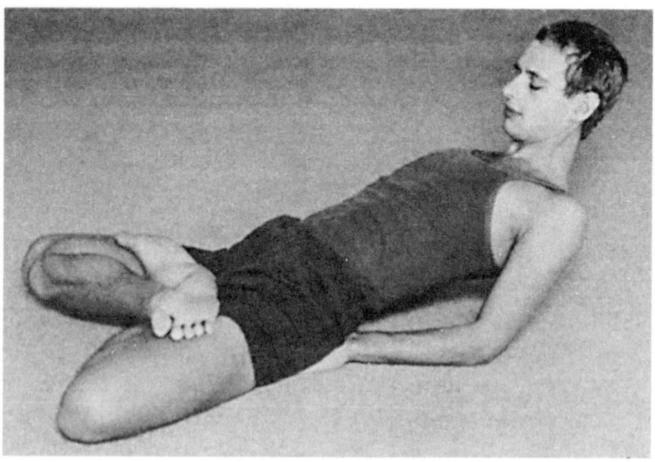

Tolangulasana (Weighing Scale Pose)

This asana resembles the form of a weighing scale. Hence this is called tolangulasana.

Technique: Lie down in padmasana as in matsyasana. Place the palms of the hands underneath the buttocks. If you find it difficult to keep the palms below the buttocks, slowly rest on your two elbows by gradually reclining. Raise the head and the upper part of your body above the ground. Now the whole body will be resting on the buttocks and forearms. Press the chin against the chest. (This is jalandhara bandha, which can be done in this asana). Retain the breath as long as comfortable and then slowly exhale. You can do this for five to thirty minutes.

Benefits: This asana removes flatulence. The spine is expanded and developed. Owing to the tension of the abdomen the faecal matter is pushed down to the rectum from the colon. As the chest considerably expands, the pigeon chest is slowly removed and you will have a broad fine chest. You will obtain the benefits of padmasana. The muscles and the nerves of the arms get increased supply of blood. Therefore they will become strong.

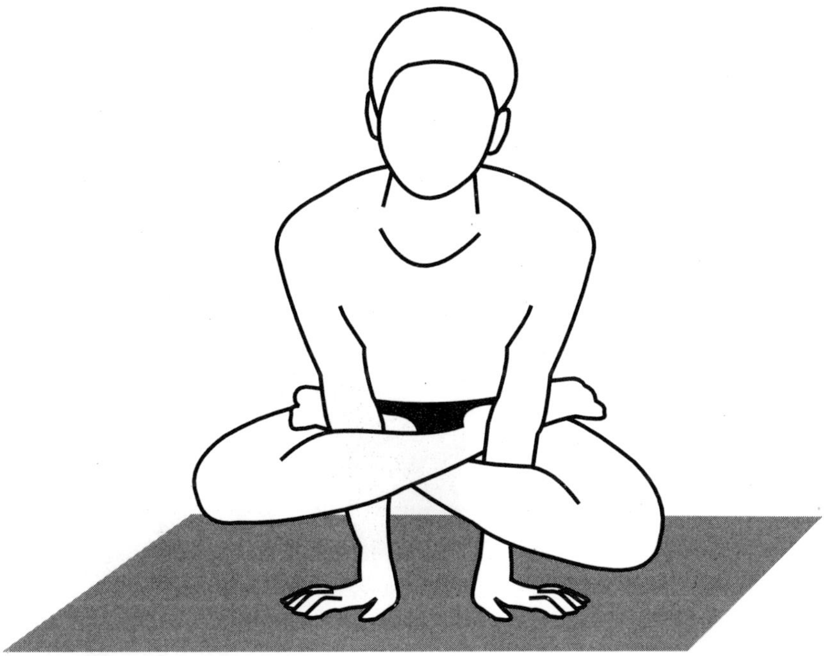

Kukkutasana (Cock Pose)

In Sanskrit, kukkuta means cock. When the asana is demonstrated it resembles a cock.

Technique: First do padmasana. Introduce your two arms, one by one as far as the elbow joint into the space between the calves and the thighs. Place the palms on the ground, fingers pointing forwards. Raise the body from the ground. The lock of the feet should come as far as the elbow joint. If you raise the padmasana a bit, it will be easy to introduce the hands. (Fat persons will find it difficult to insert the hands between the thigh and calf muscles.) Remain in this asana as long as you can.

Benefits: All the benefits of padmasana can be derived from this asana to a maximum degree. Laziness vanishes. The nadis get purified. Biceps of the arms, deltoid of the shoulders, pectoralis major and minor, etc., become well developed. The chest becomes broad.

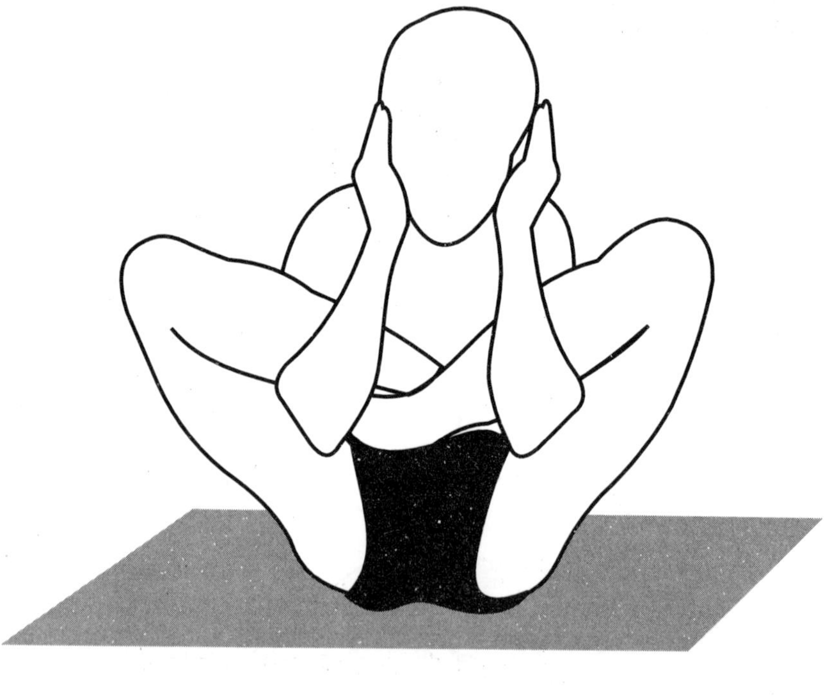

Garbhasana (Child-in-the-Womb Pose)

When this asana is demonstrated it resembles the position of the child when it is in the womb. Hence this is called garbhasana.

Technique: As described in kukkutasana, introduce both hands in the space between the thighs and calves. Bring the elbows out through the legs. Catch hold of the right ear with the right hand and the left ear with the left hand. You should perform the last stage of this asana with great care, because when you try to catch hold of the ears with the hands you may fall down backwards. You will not have hands to support the body and you will be helpless. But by practice you can slowly balance the body on the buttocks. The body will remain steady after a few days' practice. If you find it difficult to perform the asana, you can do it without the padmasana. Catch hold of the ears or neck by introducing the arm behind the thighs. In this modified pose the leg will be stretching downwards. Remain in the asana for two or three minutes. Repeat it five times.

Benefits: The digestive power is augmented. Appetite increases. The bowels become quite free. You will get clear motions. Many intestinal diseases are removed. Hands and legs will become strong.

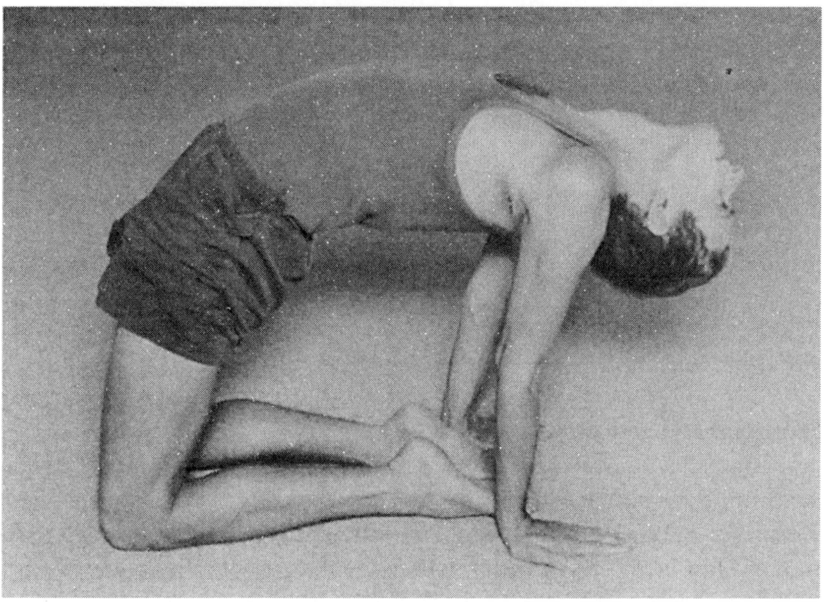

Sasangasana

Bend the legs and kneel on your toes and knees. Keep the palms by the side of the soles. Make a perfect curve of the back and let your head hang backwards towards the ground. Do not bend the arms. Keep them straight. This is similar to dhanurasana. You can call it dhanurasana in a kneeling posture. The benefits of dhanurasana are derived in this pose.

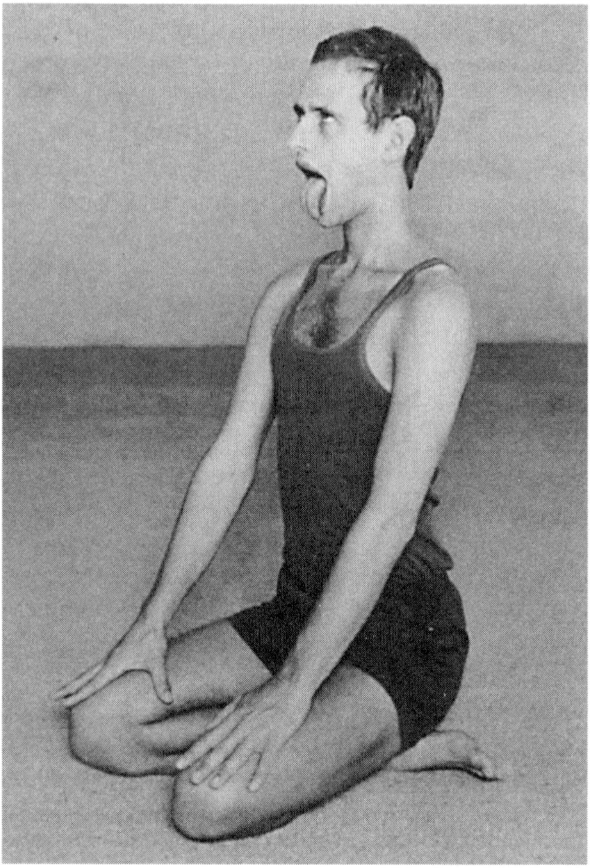

Simhasana (Lion Pose)

Place the two heels under the scrotum or between the anus and the scrotum, the left heel on the right side and the right heel on the left side. Keep the hands on the knees. Spread out the fingers. Open your mouth. This is the destroyer of diseases. This is practised by yogis. The bandhas can be nicely practised in this asana.

Gorakshasana

Turn the feet upward and place them in a hidden manner between the thigh and calf muscles. Cover the heels by the hands. Do jalandhara bandha. Have nasikagra drishti. This asana gives success to the yogis.

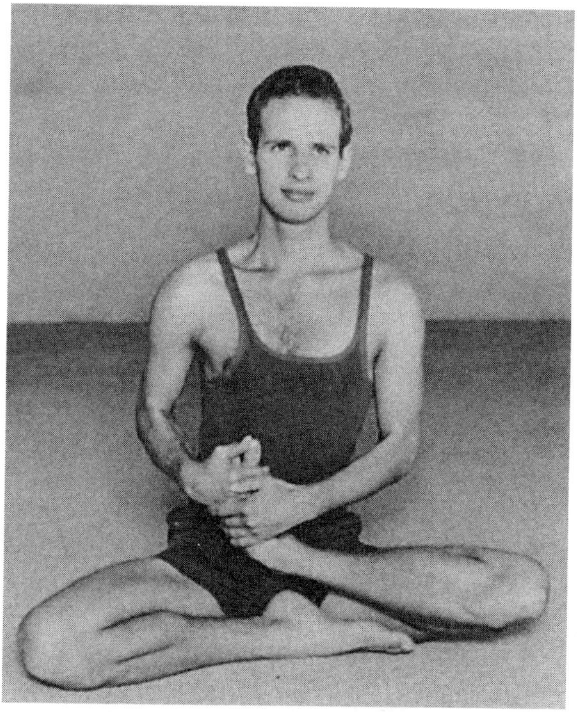

Kandapidanasana

Technique: This asana is a bit difficult for people with big thigh and calf muscles. Lean persons can do it very beautifully. Sit on the ground, heels and the toes together. That is, the soles must be facing each other. Slowly twist the feet and place the heels at the perineum and the toes towards the back at the anus. Now the body will rest only on the two knees and the sides of the feet. Keep the hands on the knees. Sit erect.

There is another way of doing this asana. Sit on the ground with the soles of the feet in close opposition. They also must be facing each other. Take hold of the toes of one foot with both the hands and slowly attempt to take the foot to the belly. In a similar manner bring slowly the other foot also to the belly. When you are able to do this asana with each foot separately, then try to do it with both the feet at one stroke. Practise this asana gradually with great care. If you do it quickly with force, you will get pain in the legs, knees, toes, etc. When the asana is complete, the soles will be diverging and the dorsal (back) sides of the feet will be facing each other.

Benefits: All sorts of knee troubles, rheumatism of the legs, sciatica, gout of the toes will be cured. The nerves of the calves and legs will be toned. Fat people will find it difficult to practise this.

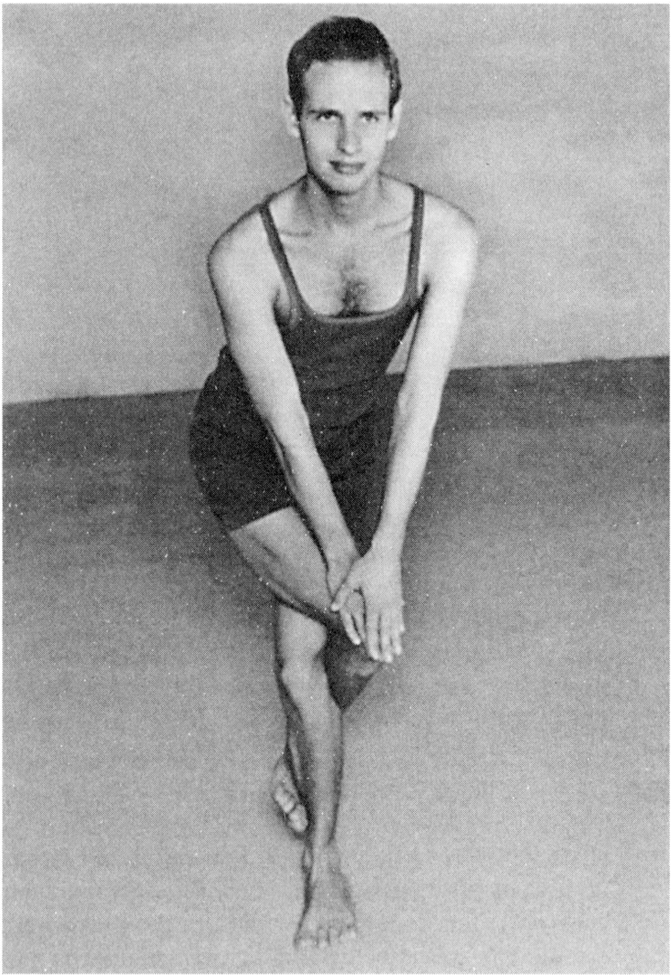

Sankatasana

Stand on the left foot. Raise the right leg and surround it over the left. Keep the hands on the knees. This is sankatasana. Garudasana posture also is called by this name.

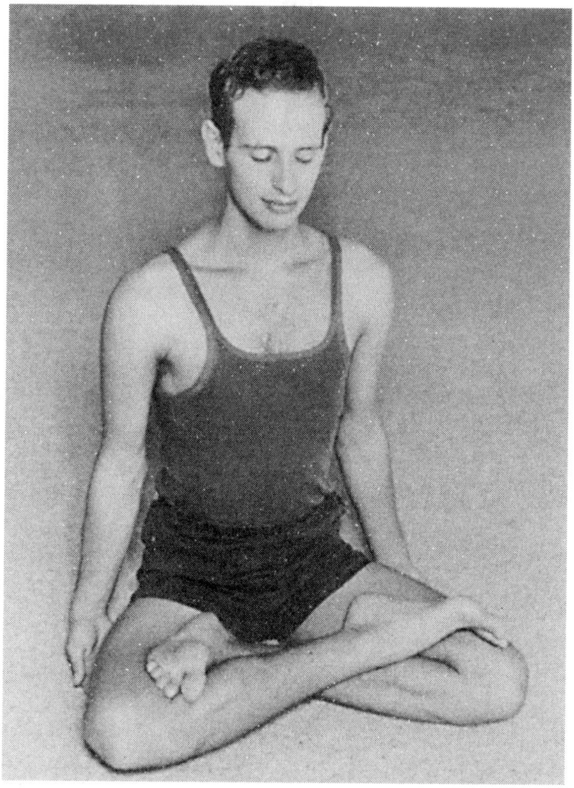

Yogasana

Keep the right foot on the left knee and the left foot on the right knee, soles turning upwards. Place the hands on the ground by your sides, palms facing upwards. Gaze at the tip of the nose, and meditate for a long time.

Utkatasana

Stand up. Keep the feet close together. Keep the hands on the hips, one on each side. Then slowly lower the body. You will experience a little difficulty when you lower the body down. In the beginning you can catch hold of the sides of a door at your hip level and then with that support, lower the body. You can take the help of the two arms of a chair also. He who practises pranayama can practise this asana very easily. It does not require much strength. One should know balancing of the body. A thin man with a wiry body can do this very beautifully.

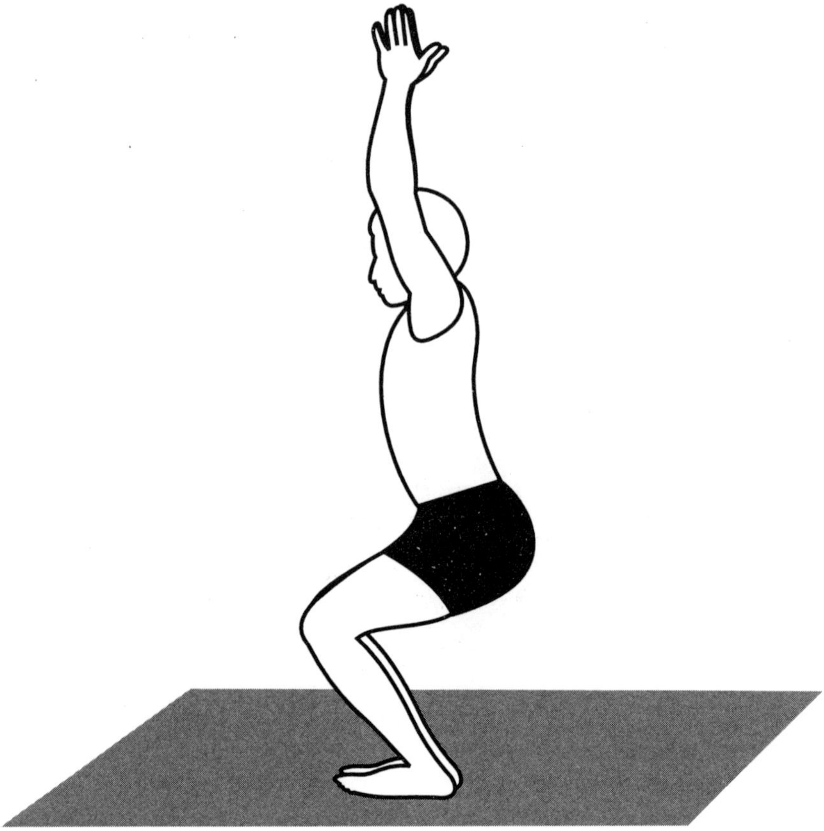

When you lower the body you may lose the balance and the body may be tossed either laterally or anterio-posteriorly; but a few days' practice will enable you to keep up the posture steadily. When you perform it perfectly, your legs from toes to knees and the part of the body from the buttocks to the head will be in a perpendicular line to the ground and your thighs will be in a parallel line with the ground. In the beginning when you practise it you can sit on a chair. Slowly raise the body two or three inches above the chair and try to keep up the balance. After a few days, ask your friend to carefully remove the chair and try to keep up the balance. Then sit on the toes. The whole burden of the body is placed on the toes only. The buttocks will touch the heels. Lumbago is cured. Wrists and toes are strengthened. This is very useful for elephantiasis. You can lower the body still further; this pose is used for basti kriya.

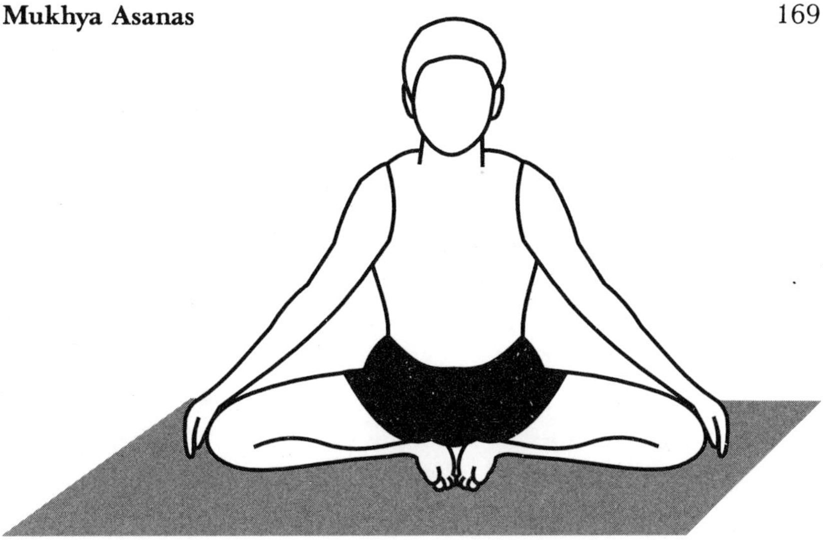

Bhadrasana (Gentle Pose)

Sit at ease. Keep the body erect. Press the two heels firmly against the sides of the perineum or at the anus. Fix the gaze at the tip of the nose. This destroys all diseases and the effects of poison.

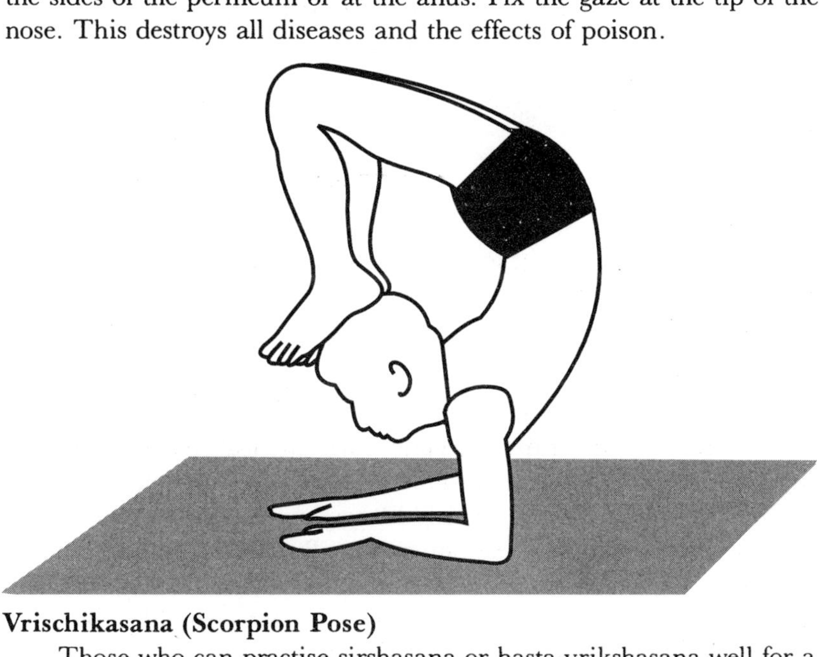

Vrischikasana (Scorpion Pose)

Those who can practise sirshasana or hasta-vrikshasana well for a long time, can attempt this. Keep the hands and elbows on the ground.

In the beginning, practise it by the side of a wall. Now throw the legs on the wall, and then try to keep up the balance after taking the feet two inches away from the wall. Do this for a few days. When you are able to keep up the balance, slowly bend the legs at the knees and hips towards the back, and place your soles or toes on your head. All the benefits of sirshasana, chakrasana and dhanurasana can be had in this posture to a maximum degree.

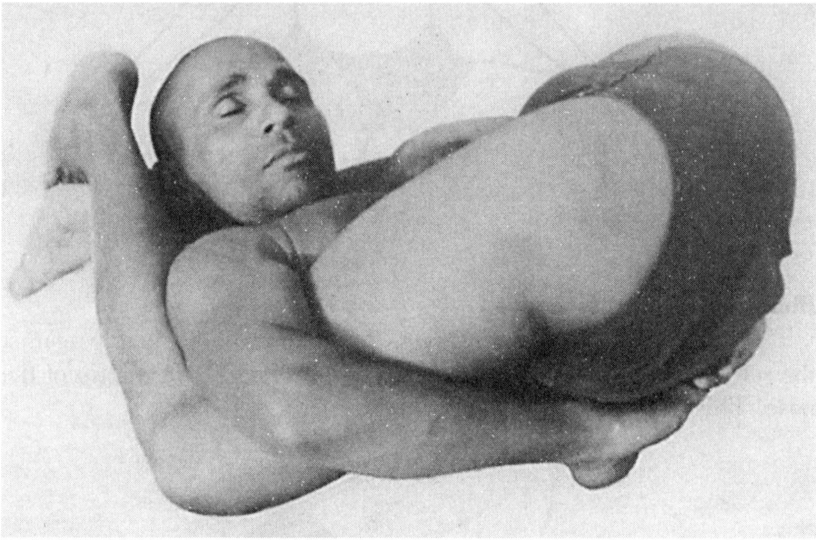

Yoga Nidrasana

Lie down as in savasana. (Fat people cannot do this. They need not try it.) Take hold of the legs and fix the feet below the neck or head. Then slowly raise the buttocks and keep the palms on the ground below the buttocks or hips.

Physical Culture in Bed

There is a general misconception that physical culture is only for the youth and that the more aged men and women should just helplessly watch old age set in. No. Even middle-aged people have benefited by a regular practice of asanas and pranayama. By gradual practice one can thoroughly master all the important asanas and pranayama. Patience and perseverance are required. They can start with the following simple exercises which they can do regularly in bed as soon as they wake up in the morning. The entire series of exercises will not take up more than fifteen minutes; and these fifteen minutes will bestow on them greater fitness for the day's activities, and longevity also.

Sit up in bed cross-legged.

Exercise no. 1: Catch hold of your left wrist with your right hand, behind your back. Now bend forward and try to touch the bed with your forehead.

Release the hold on the left wrist and in one backward motion swing back, resting the two palms on the bed.

Keep the right palm on the bed and swing the trunk to the right and touch the bed on the right side with the left palm also. Twist the trunk to the left side and place both the palms on the bed on the left side. Do this on both sides.

Exercise no. 2: Stretch the legs forward. Catch hold of the toes with your hands. Try to bend forward and touch the knees with your forehead, without bending the knees.

Exercise no. 3: Sit cross-legged again. Breathe out completely and slowly. Draw the belly in (uddiyana bandha). Release the abdomen. Breathe normally.

Exercise no. 4: Now, draw the belly in and release it in rapid succession. Do not hold the breath. Do not shake the body violently also. This is an exercise exclusively for the abdomen. This is called agnisara.

Exercise no. 5: Close the fist and raise the forearm, bending at the elbows. Throw the arms forward; then again draw the forearm backward, bending at the elbows. Repeat this three or four times. Stretch the arms sideways, and resume the normal position. Similarly, stretch the arms upwards and bring them back to the normal position.

RELAXATION

The practice of relaxing the muscles of the body will bring rest to the body and to the mind also. The tension of the muscles will be relieved. People who know the science of relaxation do not waste any energy. They can meditate well.

Savasana (Corpse Pose)

This is an asana for relaxation of all muscles, nerves, etc. It should be performed at the very end of your asana practice. (Mritasana is another name for this pose.)

Technique: Spread a soft blanket. Lie flat on your back. Keep the hands on the ground by the sides. Stretch the legs quite straight. Let the feet drop outwards. Close the eyes and breathe slowly. Relax all the muscles, nerves, organs, etc. Start the relaxation process from the toes. Then proceed to the calf-muscles, muscles of the back, chest, arm, forearm and hands, neck, face etc. See that the abdominal organs, heart, chest and brain are also relaxed. Relax the plexus of nerves also. Now repeat OM, OM, OM. Think of Atman. Meditate gently with a feeling of purity. Do not sleep. Continue the meditation for 15 minutes. You will enjoy perfect peace, ease, comfort and relaxation. Every one of you should enjoy it. Words are imperfect, they cannot adequately describe the feeling.

Benefits: Savasana combines pose and meditation. It gives relief, comfort and ease. After 15 minutes relaxation you will be wonderfully refreshed and rejuvenated. You will be more efficient and effective in whatever you do.

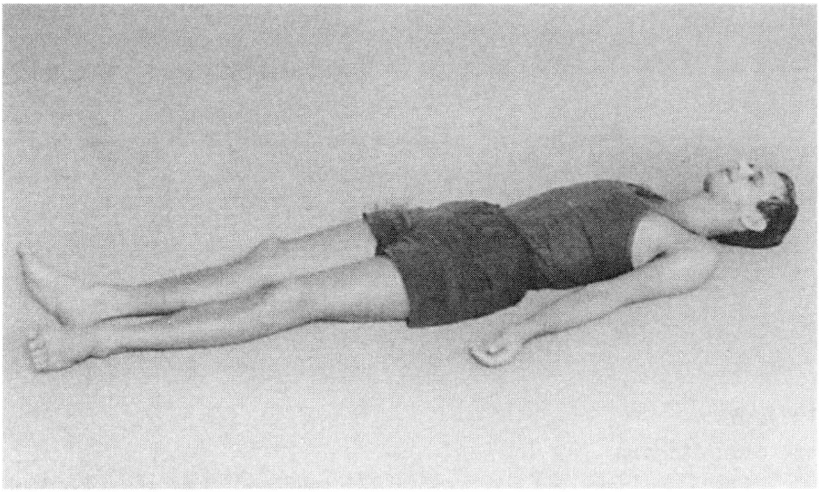

Relaxation is a very important factor in muscular exercises. The muscles that are put under severe strain demand relaxation and rest. It is savasana that promptly and efficiently ensures complete relaxation and rest. In halasana, sarvangasana, paschimottanasana, dhanurasana and ardha-matsyendrasana you know pretty well that all the muscles of the back — lattissimus dorsi, psoas magnus and quadratus lumborum —the abdominus rectus, pectoralis major of the chest, biceps, triceps, the deltoid of the arm and sartorius of the thighs are all stretched and contracted to an enormous degree. During intense muscular activity the metabolism is increased. Metabolism is the anabolic and catabolic changes that take place in the body (wear and tear in the system). Anabolic changes are constructive and catabolic changes are the destructive ones. During metabolism all the muscular tissues are supplied with fresh oxygenated blood or plasma through capillary oozing, and carbon-dioxide is taken back through the veins to the right auricle of the heart. This is termed tissue respiration. Just as interchange of oxygen and carbon-dioxide takes place in the lungs, so also interchange of carbon-dioxide and oxygen takes place in the tissues also. Mark the wonderful creation and working of the internal mechanism of the body! How marvellous is the machinery. Can a scientist make a single atom, a single cell, a single organ of the body? Bow with folded hands before the Creator of this wonderful mechanism of the body. Repeat OM, OM. Enter into silence. Meditate. The whole mystery of creation will be revealed unto you through His grace.

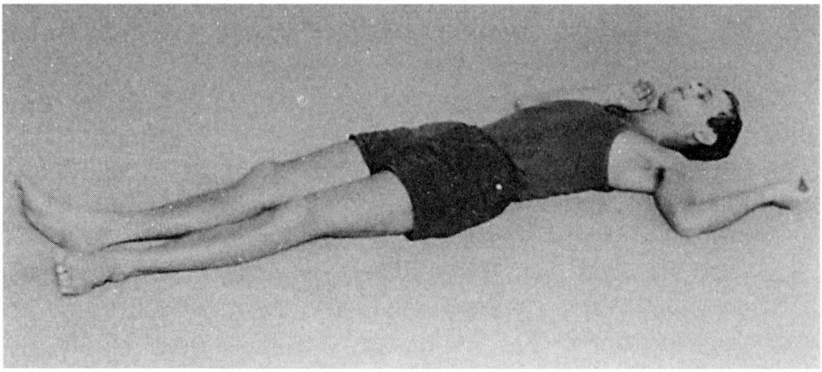

Varieties

i. *Jeshthikasana*:

This is an exercise for relaxation like savasana. This must be done at the end of all the asanas. In this the hands are kept on the ground by the sides of the head, while in savasana the hands are kept at the sides.

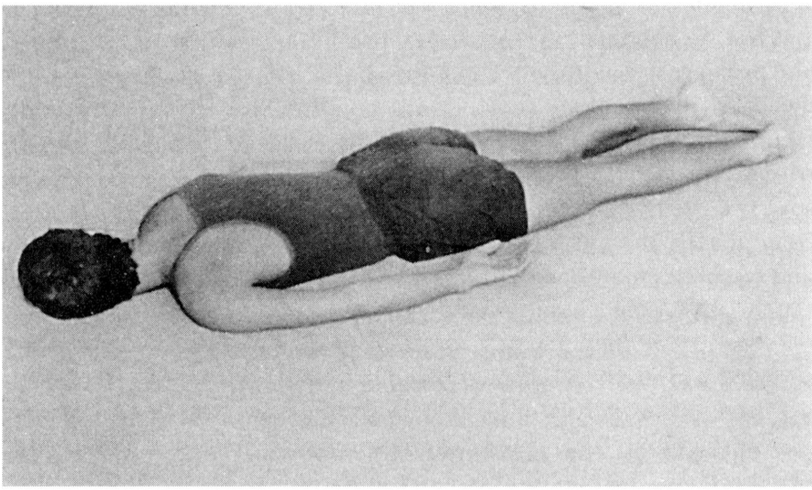

ii. *Adhvasana*:

Lie down quite flat, keeping the belly and chest on the ground. The hands will be at sides, palms facing upwards. Stretch the body well. This is a reverse pose of savasana with the same benefits. For some time keep the right cheek on the ground and for some time the left cheek.

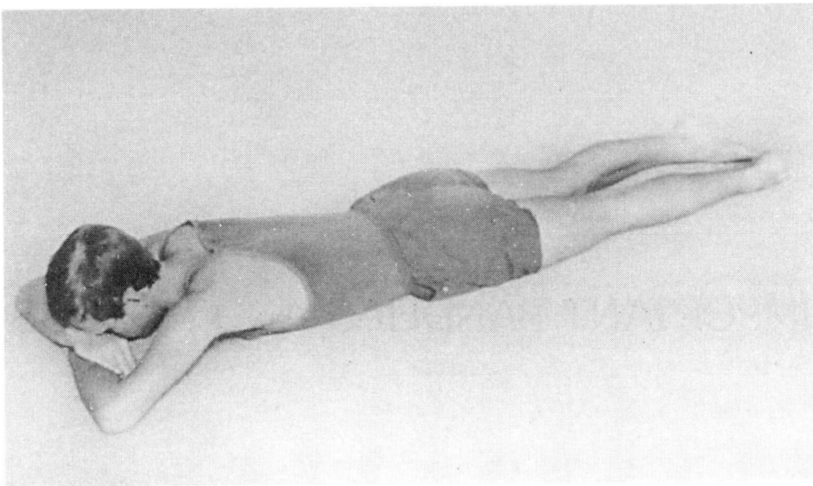

iii. *Makarasana (Dolphin Pose)*:

Lie on the ground face downwards as in adhvasana. Rest the forehead on the crossed wrists.

Mental Relaxation

Mental poise and calmness may be brought about by the eradication of worry and anger. Fear really underlies both worry and anger. Nothing is gained by worry and anger, but on the contrary much energy is wasted by these kinds of lower emotions. If a man worries much and if he is irritable, he is indeed a very weak man. Be careful and thoughtful. All unnecessary worries can be avoided. Relaxation of the muscles reacts on the mind and brings rest to the mind also. Body and mind are intimately connected.

Sit for 15 minutes in a relaxed and easy comfortable position. Close your eyes. Withdraw the mind from outside objects. Still the mind. Silence the bubbling thoughts. Think that the body is like a coconut shell and you are entirely different from the body. Think that the body is an instrument in your hands. Identify yourself with the all-pervading spirit or Atman. Imagine that the whole world and your body are floating like a piece of straw in this vast ocean of spirit. Feel that you are in touch with the Supreme Being. Feel that the life of the whole world is pulsating, vibrating and throbbing through you. Feel that the ocean of life is gently rocking you on its vast bosom. Then open your eyes. You will experience immense mental peace, mental vigour and mental strength.

IMPORTANT BANDHAS AND MUDRAS

There are several varieties in mudras and bandhas: jalandhara bandha, uddiyana bandha, mula bandha and maha mudra; maha vedha; nabho, khechari, viparita karani, yoni, jambhavi, asvini, pasini, matangi, kaki, bhujangini and yoga mudras.

Among these I will give you a short description of the few important ones. You can select that which suits you well and practise regularly. Cough, asthma, enlargement of the spleen and liver, venereal disease, consumption, chronic constipation, leprosy and all sorts of incurable diseases are also cured. Sex-sublimation is attained. These mudras and bandhas will bestow on you all that you want. There is nothing in this world like the mudras and bandhas for giving success.

Mula Bandha

Press the perineum with the left heel. Contract the anus. Put the right heel on the organ of generation. Forcibly draw the *apana vayu slowly upwards. This requires much practice. This is called mula bandha, destroyer of decay and death.

*Prana manipulates the physical body, and fills the whole physical sheath. It ever fluctuates and renders the mind unsteady.

Yoga teaches the methods to control prana and attain blissful union with the Lord through such control. Through the practice of pranayama and bandhas, the prana is brought under control. Siddhi or perfection in the practice of pranayama is attained through the help of band-

* See Pranayama chapter

has. The practice of this mula bandha helps brahmacharya, gives nerve vigour, relieves constipation and increases the gastric fire. He who practises mula bandha will keep up everlasting youth. No grey hairs will manifest.

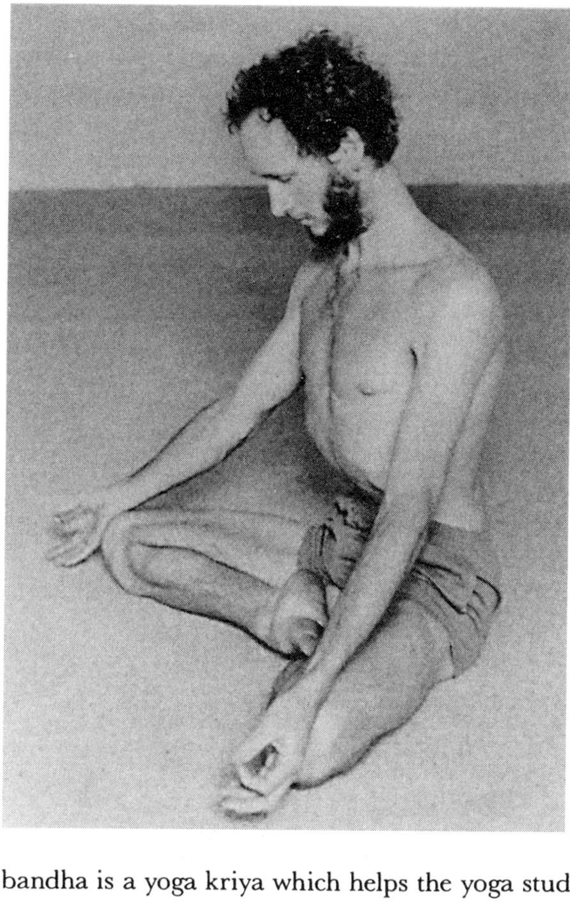

Mula bandha is a yoga kriya which helps the yoga student to take the apana and the sex-energy upwards. The yoga student sits in siddhasana and takes the apana and sex-energy upwards by contracting the anus and practising kumbhak or retention of breath. By long practice the downward seminal flow is checked and semen is sublimated into ojas shakti or spiritual energy which helps contemplation. This bandha helps in maintaining brahmacharya.

The apana vayu which does the function of ejection of excreta has a natural tendency to move downwards. Through the practice of mula bandha the apana vayu is made to move upwards by contracting the anus and by forcibly drawing it upwards. The prana vayu is united with the apana and the united prana-apana is made to enter the sushumna nadi or Brahma nadi. Then the yogi attains perfection in yoga. This is a secret in yoga. Then the yogi is dead to the world. He drinks the nectar of immortality. He gets all divine glories and powers.

When the apana is united with prana, the anahata sounds or different kinds of nadas (mystical inner sounds) are heard very distinctly by the yogi, because the outside worldly sounds are shut out. He has deep concentration. Prana, apana, nada and bindhu unite now. The yogi reaches perfection in yoga.

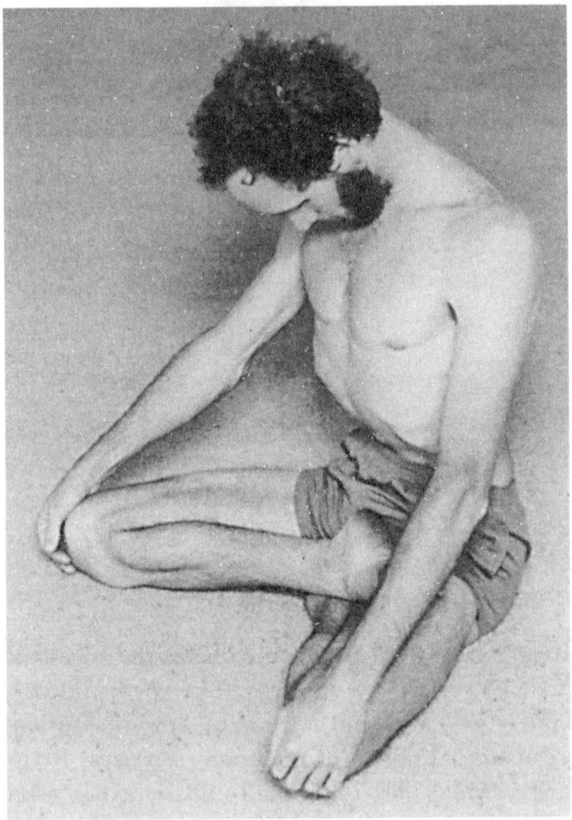

Jalandhara Bandha

Contract the throat. Press the chin firmly on the chest. This bandha is practised at the end of puraka (inhalation) and beginning of kumbhaka (retention of breath). By the practice of this bandha the prana moves in the right path. It is united with the apana. Ida and pingala nadis are shut out. The gastric fire which is situated in the region of the navel consumes the nectar which exudes out of the sahasrara through the hole in the palate. The yoga student should practise this bandha in order to prevent the nectar being thus consumed. The yogi drinks the nectar and attains immortality.

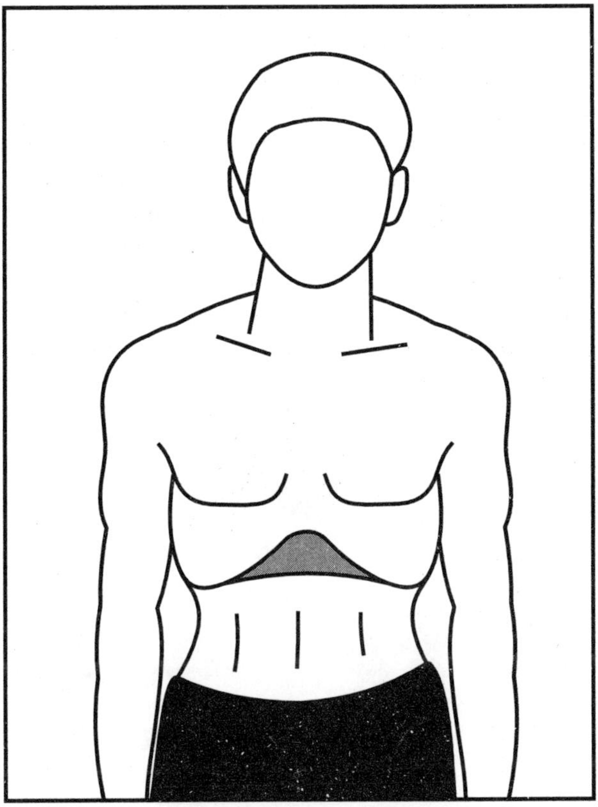

Uddiyana Bandha

Empty the lungs by a strong and forcible exhalation. Now contract and forcibly draw up the intestines and also the navel towards the back, so that the abdomen rests against the back of the body high up in the thoracic cavity. He who practises this bandha constantly, conquers death and becomes young. This helps a lot in keeping up brahmacharya. All bandhas awaken the kundalini. Uddiyana is practised at the end of kumbhaka and beginning of rechaka. When you practise this bandha, the diaphragm — the muscular portion between the thoracic cavity and abdomen — is raised up, the abdominal wall is drawn backwards. Bend your trunk forwards when you do uddiyana. Uddiyana can be done in sitting and standing postures. When you practise in the standing posture, place your hands on the knees or a little above the knees. Keep the legs a little apart.

Uddiyana is a blessing to humanity. It imparts beautiful health, strength, vigour and vitality to the practitioner. When it is combined with nauli kriya, which consists in churning the contents of the abdomen, it serves as powerful gastro-intestinal tonic. These are two potent weapons of the yogi to combat constipation, weak peristalsis of the intestines and the gastro-intestinal disorders of the alimentary system. By these two yoga exercises alone you can manipulate and massage all the abdominal viscera and tone them up.

Those who want to practise nauli should practise uddiyana in the beginning. Uddiyana reduces fat in the belly. For abdominal exercises nothing can compete with uddiyana and nauli. They stand unique, unrivalled and unprecedented amongst all systems of physical exercises in the east and west.

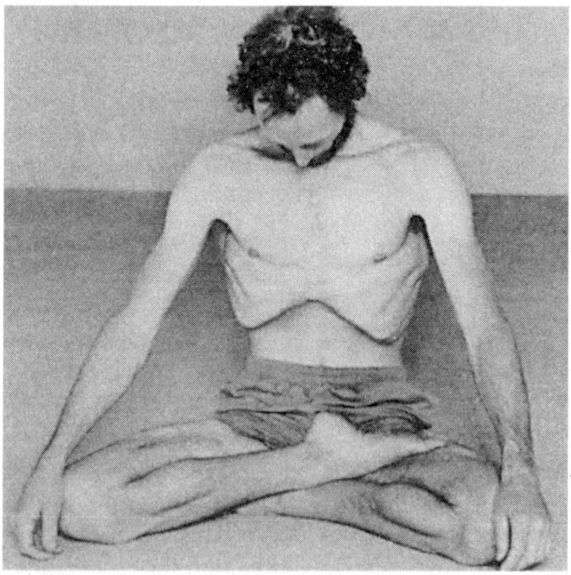

Maha Bandha

Press the anus with the left heel. Place the right foot upon the left thigh. Contract the anus and muscles of the perineum. Draw the apana vayu upwards. Draw the breath in slowly and retain it by jalandhara bandha (pressing the chin to the chest) as long as you can. Then exhale slowly. Fix the mind on *sushumna. Practise first on the left side and then on the right side. Generally the yogi does maha mudra, maha bandha and maha vedha together. This is a good combination. Then only maximum benefits are derived. The yogi achieves all his desires and obtains siddhis.

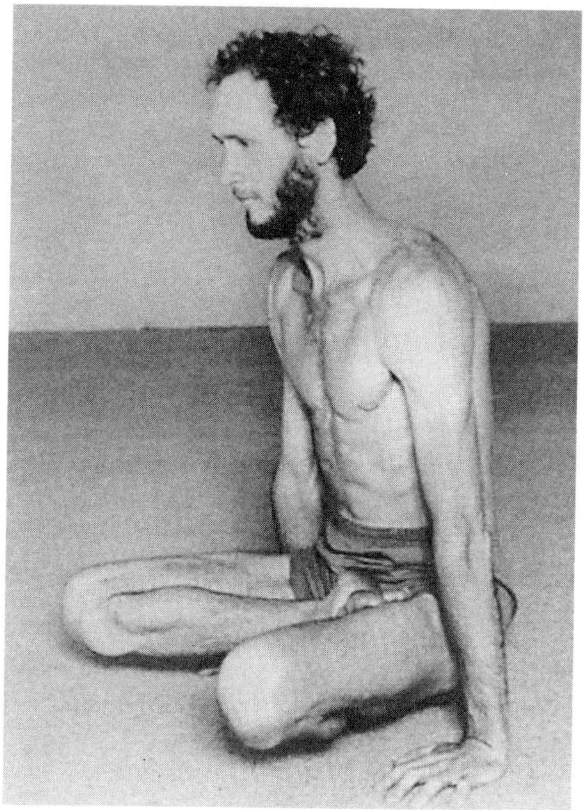

Maha Vedha

Sit in maha bandha posture. Draw the breath in slowly. Retain the breath. Press the chin against the chest. Place the palms on the ground. Rest the body on the palms. Raise the buttocks slowly and strike them gently against the ground. The asana must be intact and firm when you raise the buttocks. This kriya destroys decay and death. The yogi gets control over the mind and conquers death.

---

* See Kundalini Section

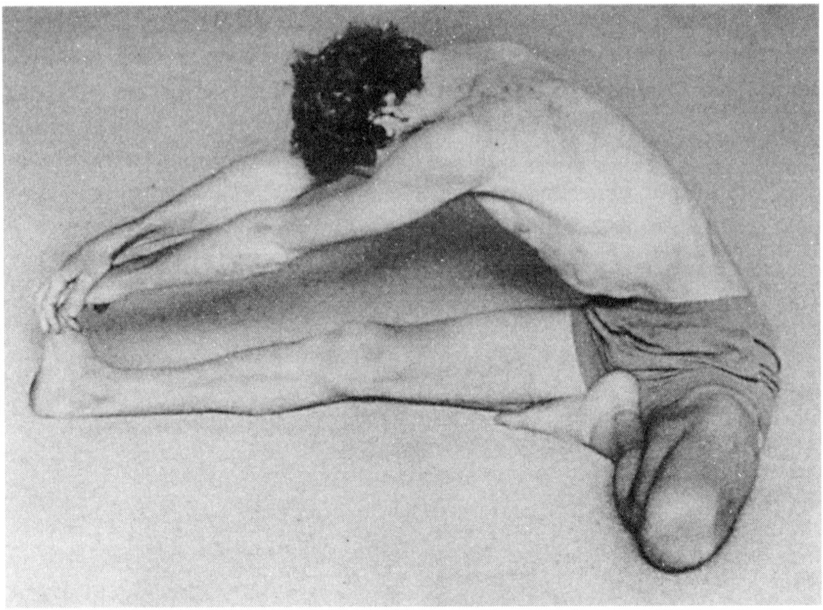

Maha Mudra

Press the anus carefully with the left heel. Stretch out the right leg. Take hold of the toe with the two hands. Inhale and retain the breath (kumbhaka). Press the chin against the chest firmly in jalandhara bandha. Fix the gaze at the space between the eye-brows. Retain the posture as long as you can. Practise first with the right leg and then with the left leg. This cures constipation, haemorrhoids or piles, enlargement of spleen, indigestion, chronic gastritis, leprosy, constipation, fever, etc. Life is increased. It confers great siddhis on the practitioner. When you do this mudra the posture will be almost similar to janusirshasana.

Yoga Mudra

Sit in padmasana. Place the palms on the heels. Exhale slowly and bend forwards and touch the ground with the forehead. If you retain the pose for a long time you can breathe in and out as usual, or come to the former position and inhale. Instead of keeping the hands on the heels you can take them behind your back. Catch hold of the left wrist with your right hand. This pose removes all kinds of disorders in the abdomen.

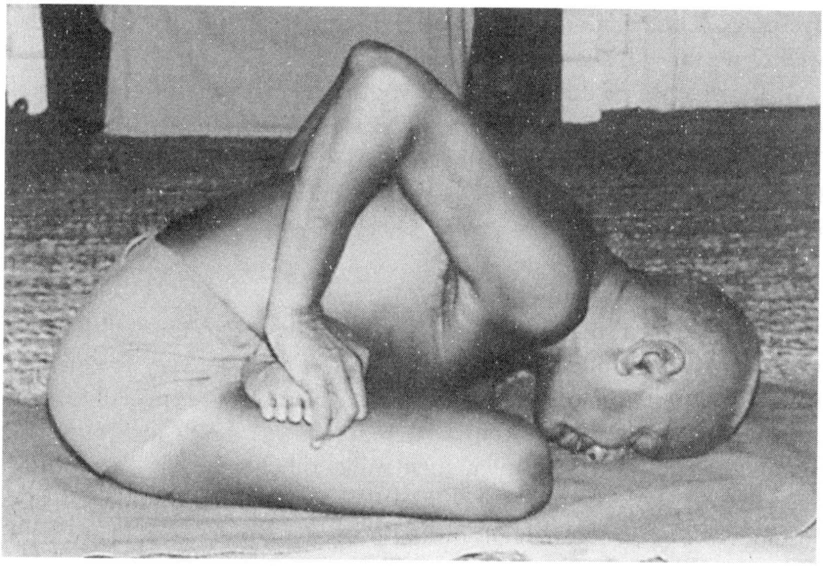

Yoga Mudra

Khechari Mudra

Khe means 'in sky' and chari means 'to move'. The yogi moves in the sky. Hence this is known as khechari mudra.

This mudra can be performed by a man only if he has undergone the preliminary exercise under the direct guidance of a guru who is practising khechari mudra. The preliminary portion of this mudra is in making the tongue so long that the tip of the tongue might touch the space between the two eyebrows. The guru will cut the lower tendon of the tongue with a bright, clean knife, little by little every week. By sprinkling salt and turmeric powder, the cut edges may not join together again. The tongue is rubbed with fresh butter and drawn out. Then the tongue is held with the fingers, and moved to and fro. 'Milking the tongue' means taking hold of it and drawing it as the milkman does the udder of the cow during milking.

Cutting the lower tendon of the tongue should be done regularly, once a week for a period varying from six months to two years. By all these means the tongue can be lengthened to reach the forehead. This is the preliminary portion of khechari mudra.

Then, sitting in siddhasana, turn the tongue upwards and backwards so as to reach the palate and close the posterior nasal opening with the tongue. The gaze is then fixed at the space between the two eyebrows. The respiration will stop. The tongue is on the mouth of the well of nectar. This is khechari mudra.

By practise of this mudra the yogi is free from fainting, hunger, thirst and laziness. He is free from diseases, decay, old age and death. This mudra makes one an urdhvareto-yogi. As the body of the yogi is filled with the nectar, he will not die even by virulent poison. This mudra gives kaya siddhi to yogis. Khechari is the best of all mudras.

Vajroli Mudra

This is an important yogic kriya in hatha yoga. You will have to work hard to get full success in this kriya. There are very few people who are experts in this act. Through a silver tube (a specially made catheter) passed into the urethra (urinary canal) for 12 inches inside, yoga students draw first water, then milk, oil, honey, etc. They draw mercury in the end. Later on they can draw these liquids directly through the urethra without the help of the tube. This kriya is of immense help in the establishment of brahmacharya. On the first day you should send the catheter inside the urethra for one inch only, the second day two inches, third day three inches, and so on. You must gradually practise till you are able to send 12 inches of the catheter inside. (Raja Bhartrihari could do this kriya very dexterously.)

Not even a drop of semen comes out of the yogi who practises this mudra. (But even if it is discharged he can draw it back through this mudra.) The yogi who draws his semen up and preserves it conquers death. A good smell emanates from his body. (Lord Krishna was a skilled expert in this mudra. That is the reason why he was called a nitya-brahmachari though he was amidst several gopis.)

Viparita Karani Mudra

Lie on the ground. Keeping the legs straight, slowly raise the legs and hips off the ground. Support the buttocks with the hands. Rest the elbows on the ground. Remain steady. On the first day do it for a minute, and gradually increase the period to three hours. After six months wrinkles on the face and grey hairs will disappear. The yogis who practise this for three hours daily conquer death. As the gastric fire is increased, those who practise this for a long time should take some nourishment such as milk, etc., as soon as it is over. (Sirshasana posture is also called viparita karani mudra.)

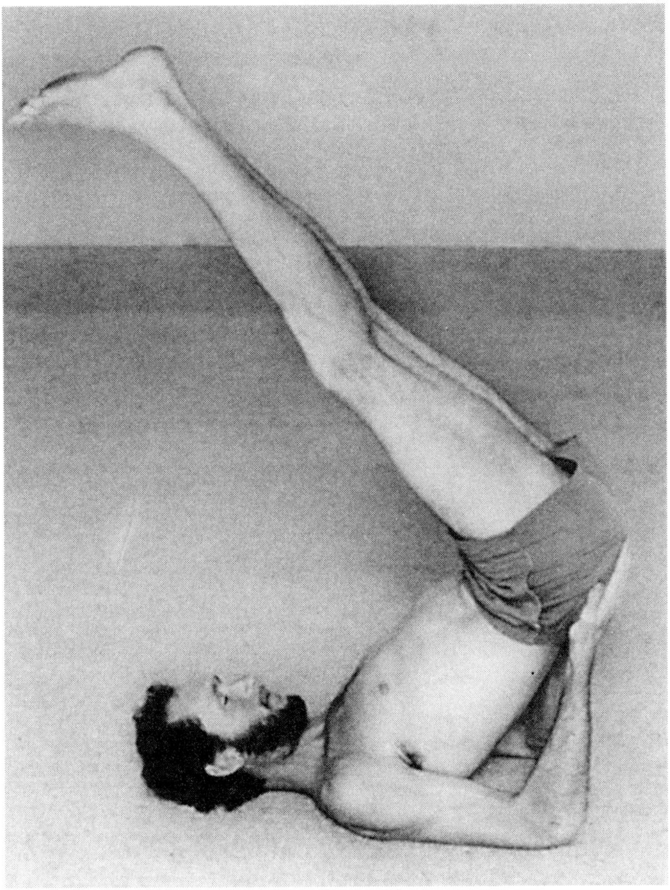

Above: Viparita Karani

Shakti Chalana Mudra

Sit in a secluded room in siddhasana. Draw in the air forcibly and join it with apana. Do mula bandha till the vayu enters the sushumna. By retaining the air, the kundalini, being suffocated, awakens and finds its way through sushumna to the brahmarandhra. Through the practice of this mudra one can become a siddha.

Sit in siddhasana. Take hold of the foot near the ankle and slowly beat the kanda with the foot. This is tadana kriya. By this method also kundalini can be awakened.

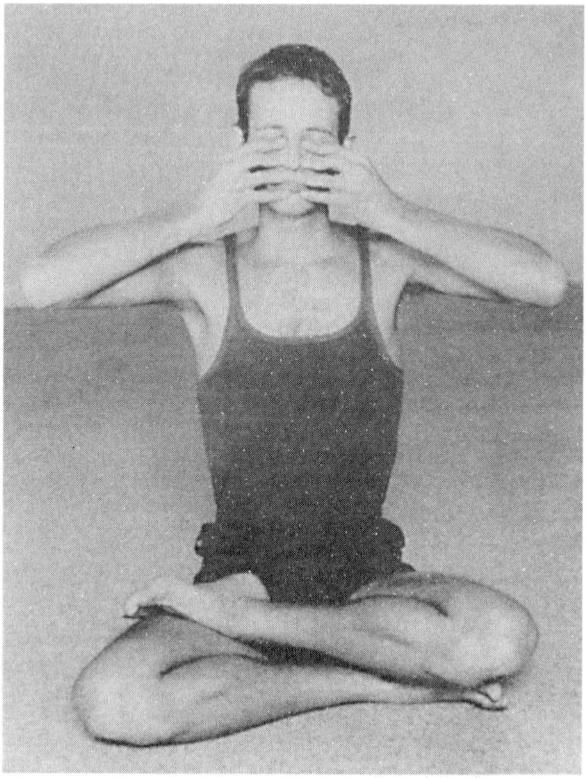

Yoni Mudra

Sit in siddhasana. Close the ears with the thumbs, eyes with the index-fingers, nostrils with the middle fingers, the upper lips with the ring-fingers and the lower lips with the little fingers.

Dive deep and meditate on the chakras and kundalini. This is more difficult than the other mudras. You have to exert much to get success in this. You must be perfectly established in brahmacharya if you want sure success in this mudra. It is said to be 'very difficult to be obtained, even by devas'. Therefore realise the importance of this mudra. Practise it very cautiously.

SHAT—KRIYAS

Those who are of a flabby and phlegmatic constitution should practise at first these six kriyas to prepare themselves for the practice of pranayama.

Success comes easily. These six kriyas are:

1. Dhauti
2. Basti
3. Neti
4. Tratak
5. Nauli
6. Kapalabhati

Dhauti

Take a clean piece of muslin cloth 4 fingers wide and 15 feet long. The borders of the cloth should be nicely stitched on all sides and no pieces of thread should be hanging loose. Dip it in tepid water. Then slowly swallow it and draw it out again. Swallow one foot the first day and increase it daily, little by little. This is called vastra-dhauti. In the beginning you may have slight retching. It stops on the third day. This practice cures diseases of the stomach such as gastritis, dyspepsia and belching, fever, lumbago, asthma, diseases of the spleen, leprosy, skin diseases and disorders of phlegm and bile. You need not practise it daily. You can practise it once a week or once a fortnight. Wash the cloth with soap and keep it always clean. Drink a cup of milk after the practice is over; otherwise, you will feel a dry sensation inside.

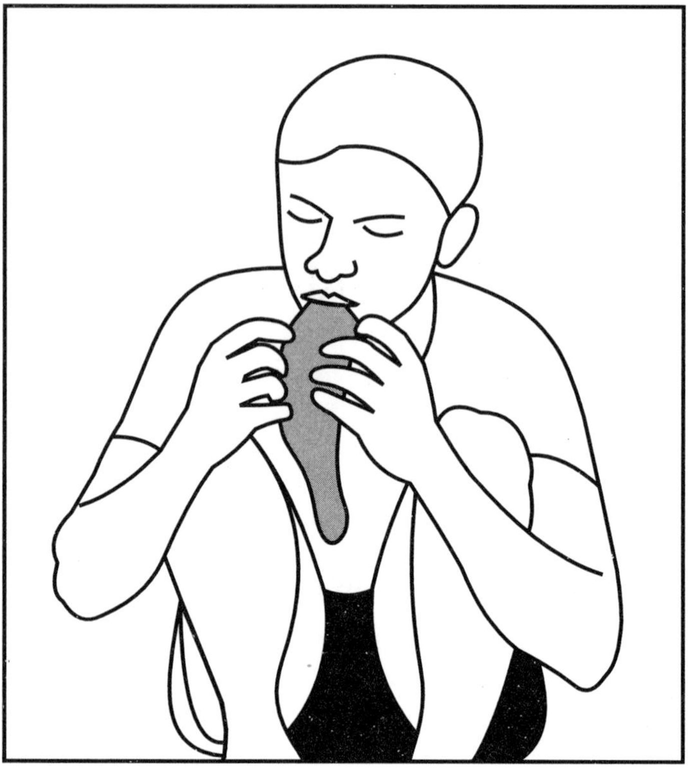

Basti

This can be practised with or without a bamboo tube, but it is better to have a bamboo tube. Sit in a tub of water. The water should cover your navel. Assume the uttkatasana posture by resting your body on the forepart of your feet, the heels pressing against the posterior. Take a small bamboo tube, 6 fingers long, and insert four fingers of its length into the anus after lubricating the tube with vaseline or soap or castor oil. Then contract the anus. Draw the water into the bowels slowly. Shake well the water within the bowels and then expel the water outside. It is known as jala-basti. It cures urinary disorders, dyspepsia, myalgia, dropsy, disorders of digestion, diseases of the spleen and bowels, diseases arising from the excess of wind, bile and phlegm. This kriya should be done in the morning when the stomach is empty. Drink a cup of milk or take your meal when it is over. It can be practised while standing in a river.

There is another way of doing basti without the help of water. It is called sthala basti. Sit in paschimottanasana on the ground and churn the abdominal and intestinal portions slowly with a downward motion. Contract the sphincter muscles. This removes constipation and all the abdominal disorders. This is not as effective as jala basti.

Neti

Neti is intended for the purification of the nostrils. The nostrils must be always kept clean. Unclean nostrils will lead to irregular breathing.

Take a fine piece of waxed thread about 12 inches long. There should not be any knot in the thread, nor should it be too thin or weak. Insert one end of it into the right nostril and catch hold of the other end firmly. Make a forcible, continuous inhalation and pass it inside. Then slowly pull it out. Again in the same way pass it through the left nostril and take it out slowly. Do not injure your nostrils through violent pulling. After some practice, pass the thread through one nostril and take it out through the other. In the beginning you will begin to sneeze profusely when you insert the thread into the nose. This passes off after three or four attempts. This can be practised when you find that your nostril is blocked from cold.

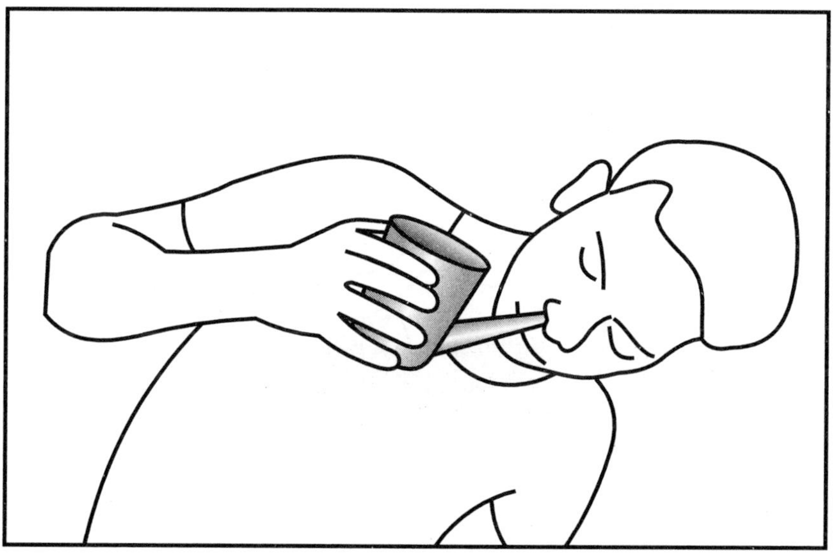

There is another easier method of cleaning the nostrils. Take some water in your hand or in a wide-mouthed cup. Draw the water slowly through the nose and expel it forcibly through the nose. Or, you can use a 'neti pot', and slowly pour the water through first the nostril which is clearest, and then through the other nostril. Keep the head tilted as in the illustration. There are many people who can do this easily. After one or two attempts some persons may suffer from slight cold and cough when they begin to learn this. As soon as they are all right again, they can practise.

This kriya purifies the skull and produces clear and keen sight. Rhinitis and coryza are cured.

Tratak (Gazing)

Gaze steadily without winking with a concentrated mind at any small object, until tears begin to flow. By this practice all diseases of the eye are removed. Unsteadiness of the mind vanishes. Sambhavi siddhi is obtained. Will-power is developed. Clairvoyance is induced.

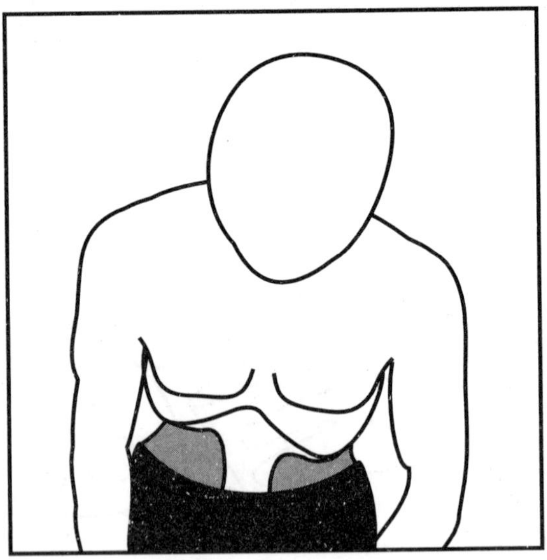

Nauli

This is abdominal churning with the help of the rectus muscle of

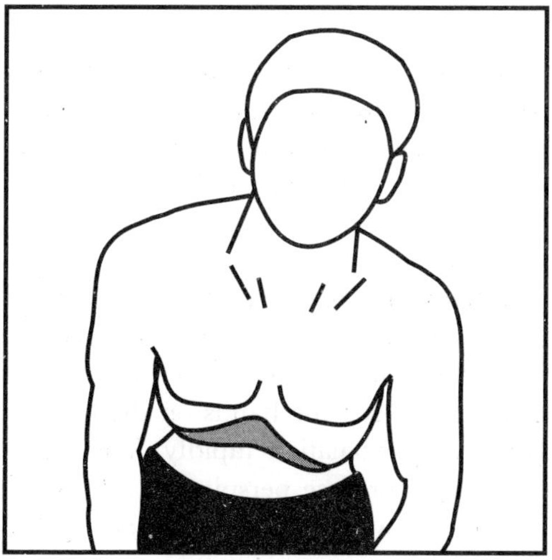

the abdomen. For this practice you should be proficient in uddiyana bandha.

Method: Stand up, keeping the feet a foot apart. Rest your hands on your thighs, thus making a slight curve of the back. Then do uddiyana bandha. Do this for one week before proceeding to the next stage.

Now keep the centre of the abdomen free by contracting the left and right sides of the abdomen. You will have all the muscles in the centre in a vertical line. Keep it as long as you can with comfort. Do only this for a few days.

Here you contract the right side of the abdomen, keepng the left side free. You will have the muscles on the left side only. Again, contract the left side muscles and allow the right side free. By having such gradual practices you will understand how to contract the muscles on the right, central and left of the abdomen. Practice this stage for a week.

Keep the muscles in the centre. Slowly bring to the right side and then to the left side in a circular way. Do this several times from right to left and then from left to right. You should turn the muscles in a circular manner slowly. When you advance in the practice it can be done quickly, but you can derive full benefits when you do it slowly and gradually. This last stage of nauli will appear like 'churning'.

Beginners will feel slight pain in the abdomen in the first few attempts. They need not fear and stop the practice. The pain will vanish in a few days. This exercise is not possible for those with a barrel-like belly.

Benefits: Nauli kriya eradicates chronic constipation, dyspepsia and all other diseases of the gastro-intestinal system. The liver and pancreas are toned. The kidneys and other organs of the abdomen function properly. Nauli is a blessing to humanity.

Kapalabhati

'Kapala' is a Sanskrit word; it means skull. 'Bhati' means shine. The term 'kapalabhati' means an exercise that makes the skull shine. This kriya cleanses the skull. So this is taken as one of the shat-karmas.

Sit in padmasana. Keep the hands on the knees. Close the eyes. Perform inhalation and exhalation rapidly. This should be practised vigorously. One will get profuse perspiration. This is a good form of exercise. Those who are well-versed in kapalabhati can do *bhastrika very easily.

There is no retention in this pranayama. Exhalation plays a prominent part. Inhalation is mild, slow and long (deergha). The exhalation should be done quickly and forcibly by contracting the abdominal muscles with a backward push. When you inhale, release the abdominal muscles. (Some people naturally make a curve of the spine and bend their heads also. This is not desirable. The head and the trunk should be erect.) Sudden expulsions of breath follow one another as in bhastrika. To start with, you can have one expulsion per second. Gradually you can have two expulsions per second. To begin with do one round in the morning consisting of ten expulsions only. In the second week, do one round in the morning and two rounds in the evening. Thus every week, gradually and cautiously increase ten expulsions to each round till you get 120 expulsions for each round.

It cleanses the respiratory system and the nasal passages and removes the spasm in bronchial tubes. Consequently asthma is relieved and also cured in course of time. The apices of the lungs get proper oxygenation, and do not, thereby, afford favourable breeding grounds for tubercule bacilli. Consumption is cured by this practice and the lungs are considerably developed. Carbon dioxide is eliminated on a large scale and impurities of the blood are thrown out. The tissues and cells absorb a large quantity of oxygen. The practitioner keeps up good health. The heart functions properly and the circulatory and respiratory systems are toned to a considerable degree.

---

* See page 223

SPECIAL INSTRUCTIONS

1. Asanas should be practised in a well-ventilated room where there is free movement of fresh air. The floor must be even and clean. Asanas can be practised on the sandy bed of rivers, open airy places and by the seaside also. If you practise them in a room, see that the room is not congested, so as to allow free movement of hands, legs and of the body.

2. Asanas should be done on an empty stomach in the morning or at least three hours after food. Morning time is best for doing asanas.

3. It is always best to start japa and meditation in the early morning at 4 a.m., as soon as you get up from bed. At this time the mind is quite calm and refreshed. You can catch the meditative mood now quite easily. Meditation is very important. In the early morning, as soon as you get up from bed, the mind is like a clean slate, free from worldly thoughts. The mind will enter into the meditative mood without any effort or struggle.

4. The vast majority of persons waste their precious time in the early morning in answering calls of nature for half an hour and washing their teeth for another half an hour. The sun rises before they sit for meditation. This is bad. Aspirants should try to defaecate within five minutes and cleanse their teeth within five minutes. If the bowels are constipated, have vigorous practise of salabhasana, bhujangasana and dhanurasana for five minutes as soon as you get up from bed. If you are habituated to answer the calls of nature late in the day, you can do so after finishing asanas and pranayama, japa and meditation.

5. Before starting the practice of asanas, take a dose of worm powder, Santonin, 1 or 2 grams at bed time, and 2 oz. castor oil early in the next morning. Float the oil in peppermint water, tea or pepper water and then take. Take oil alone if you like. Thorough cleaning of the bowels is necessary when you take to yoga practices.

6. Drink water through the mouth, send it to the stomach and small intestines and make it pass through the anus at once as in enema. This is termed shankha prakshalana kriya in hatha yoga. (Even the smoke of a cigarette can be passed through the anus. Brahmachari Shambhunathji of Kishkindha did this. Yogi Trilinga Swami of Varanasi was very clever in this kriya.) The help of nauli and basti kriya is needed in this. There is no difficulty at all in the path of yoga for sincere practitioners.

7. Drink ten glasses of water through the mouth or nose. Keep it for 20 seconds. Then bring it out slowly. This is kunjara kriya or kunjara yoga. This is a cleansing process of the stomach. All the decomposing matter that undergoes fermentation in the stomach will come out. You will have no disease of the stomach. Do it occasionally. Do not make it a habit. This is a hatha yoga kriya.

8. Those who suffer from chronic constipation can practise ganesha kriya, the removal of excreta by introducing the middle finger, lubricated with oil or soap, into the rectum. Occasional douching will be beneficial to empty the loaded stomach.

9. Spread a blanket on the floor and practise the asanas on the blanket. Use a pillow or fourfolded blanket for practising sirshasana and its varieties.

10. Wear a kowpeen or langotee or suspendary bandage when you practise asanas. You can have a shirt on the body.

11. Do not wear spectacles when you do asanas. They may be broken and may injure the eyes.

12. Those who practise sirshasana etc. for a long time, should take light tiffin or a cup of milk after finishing the asana.

13. If you can devote half an hour or more to sirshasana alone, you can cut short the time for other asanas.

14. Be regular in the practice. Those who practise by fits and starts will not derive any benefit.

15. 'Without observing moderation of diet, if one takes to the yoga practices, he cannot obtain any benefit but gets various diseases.' *Gheranda Samhita* (V:10)

16. Start with minimum time of doing asanas and then gradually increase the period. You can do the asanas as long as you can comfortably keep up the posture.

17. Asana is the third anga or limb in ashtanga yoga. When you are established in asana, then only will you derive the benefits of pranayama.

18. Maximum benefits can be achieved if japa also is done during the practice of asanas and pranayama.

19. If the foundation of a building is not properly laid, the superstructure will fall down in no time. Even so, if a yoga student has not gained mastery over the asanas, he cannot successfully proceed in his higher courses of yoga practices.

20. Regularity in the practice is very necessary if one wants to realise the maximum benefits of asanas. Generally people practise for two months in the beginning with great interest and enthusiasm and leave off the practice. This is a sad mistake. They want a yoga teacher always by their side. They have got the effeminate leaning mentality. They are lazy, torpid and slothful.

21. Nowadays outdoor games have become very costly. Nets, rackets, balls and inflators have to be purchased again and again. No expense is needed for the practice of asanas.

22. Physical exercises draw the prana out. Asanas send the prana in, and distribute it quite evenly throughout the body and different systems. Asanas are not only physical but also spiritual, as they awaken the serpent power that is sleeping in the muladhara chakra.

23. Asanas are not mere physical exercises alone. They are something more than that. They have a spiritual basis. They help a long way in controlling the senses, mind and body. Body, nerves and muscles are purified (sarira shuddhi and nadi shuddhi). Asanas awaken the kundalini, which gives bliss, power and yoga samadhi to the aspirant. If you do dand and bhaitaks (Indian physical exercises) 500 times a day, or pumping marches on the parallel bars 50 times a day for five years, they will not in any way help in the awakening of this mysterious power, kundalini. Do you see the difference?

24. Ladies should also practise asanas. They will have healthy and strong children. If mothers are healthy and strong, children also will be healthy and strong. Regeneration of the young ladies means the regeneration of the whole world. If ladies practise a course of asanas systematically with interest and attention, they will have wonderful health

and vitality. There is no doubt of this. I hope they will give patient hearing to my earnest and sincere prayer and start practising these asanas from the very day they read these yoga lessons. Glory to these new yoga lady students who tread the path of yoga. Children born of yoginis will also be yogis.

25. Japa and pranayama should go hand in hand with yoga asanas. Then it becomes a real yoga.

26. In the beginning you cannot perform some of the asanas perfectly. Regular practice will bring perfection. Patience and perseverance, earnestness and sincerity are needed.

27. Sirshasana, sarvangasana, paschimottanasana, dhanurasana and mayurasana are a good combination. Sirshasana, sarvangasana and paschimottanasana are the trinity asanas. You can reduce the number of asanas if you cannot spare time. These three asanas will give you all the advantages and benefits of all other asanas.

28. Four asanas are prescribed for japa and meditation, viz., padmasana, siddhasana, svastikasana and sukhasana. Padmasana is the best for the vast majority. Those who attempt to keep up brahmacharya should practise siddhasana.

29. Select a course of a few asanas to suit your temperament, capacity, convenience, leisure and requirement. Never change the asanas. Adhere to one set tenaciously. If you do one set of asanas today and some other tomorrow and so on, you cannot derive much benefit.

30. The more steady you are on the asana, the more you will be able to concentrate and make your mind one-pointed. You cannot get on well in your meditation without having a steady posture.

31. Common sense should be used throughout the practice. If one kind of food is not agreeable to your system, change it after due consideration or consultation with your guru. If a particular asana is not suitable, select something else. This is yukti (skill). Where there is yukti there is siddhi, bhukti and mukti (perfection, enjoyment and liberation).

32. If you cannot perform a particular asana quite satisfactorily do not lose heart. Where there is a will, there is a way. Rome was not built in a day. Remember the story of Bruce and the spider. Try, try, try again. Continuous practice will make you all right.

33. Mild kumbhaka (retention of breath) during the practice of asanas augments their efficacy and gives increased power and vitality to the practitioner.

34. No samadhi or super-conscious state is possible without awakening the kundalini. Kundalini can be awakened by various ways: asanas, mudras, bandhas, pranayama, devotion, grace of guru, japa, strong analytic will and the power of enquiry. Those who attempt to awaken the kundalini should have perfect purity in thought, word and deed; they should have mental and physical brahmacharya — then only can they enjoy the benefits of samadhi. When kundalini is awakened the old samskaras are loosened and the hridayagranthi (heart knot of ignorance) will be cut asunder. You will be freed from the wheel of samsara (birth and death) and will eventually attain the immortal state of satchidananda (existence, knowledge, bliss absolute).

35. Those who practise japa can repeat the mantra during the practice of asanas. When you recite the mantra for six months a habit will be formed and this will keep up the uninterrupted practice even during the performance of asanas. There will be no difficulty. Business people who have very little time at their disposal can have japa during their practice of asanas. It is something like getting four fruits by throwing one stone only. You will get many siddhis.

36. Nauli and uddiyana alone cannot give you moksha. It is a means for keeping good health. Do not make it the be-all and end-all. The summum bonum of life is realisation of Atman. Purify your mind, concentrate and meditate.

37. The practise of asanas before starting japa and meditation is very good and conducive. It removes laziness and drowsiness of the body and mind. It steadies the mind. It fills the mind with new vigour and peace.

38. If you are careful about your diet, asanas and meditation, you will have fine lustrous eyes, fair complexion and peace of mind in a short time. Hatha yoga ensures beauty, health, strength and long life to the yoga students.

39. Avoid unnecessary worry. Be not troubled, be not anxious. Do not be idle, do not waste time. Do not worry yourself if there is delay in your progress. You are bound to succeed if you are sincere.

40. Never miss a day in your sadhana or spiritual practices.

41. Do not shake the body unnecessarily. By shaking the body very often, the mind also is disturbed. Do not scratch the body every now and then. The asana should be as firm as a rock.

42. Breathe slowly. Do not change seat very often. Sit in the same place at the same time every day. Have the right kind of mental attitude

as taught by your guru.

43. The subtle desires that have arisen through many hundreds of lives never perish, except through the practice of yoga for a long time.

44. Never care for siddhis. Shun them ruthlessly. They will bring your downfall.

45. Yama and niyama are the foundations of yoga. If you are fully established in these, samadhi will automatically follow.

46. You must not give leniency to the mind. If you allow the mind to take one luxury today, it will demand two tomorrow. Luxuries will increase daily. It will become like an over-fondled child. 'Spare the rod and spoil the child' applies to the mind also. It is worse than a child. You will have to punish it by fasting for every serious mistake it does. Mahatma Gandhiji did this, so he had become pure, he had made his will pure, strong and irresistible. By practice, get a concentrated mind.

47. If you have a careful eye over your defects, if you are sincere and if you struggle, they are sure to vanish sooner or later. Destroy the impurities one by one, little by little, completely.

48. People do not want to remove impurity by selfless service, and tossing of the mind by worship. They at once jump to awaken the kundalini. They will only break their legs. Serve and worship. Exert. Jnana or moksha will come by itself. Kundalini will be awakened by itself.

49. A man can sit motionless on one asana for thirteen hours at a stretch, and yet be full of desires. This is a mere physical practice like an acrobatic or circus feat. Without closing the eyes, without winking, without turning the eyeballs, a man can practise tratak for three hours and yet be full of desires and egoism. This is also another kind of physical exercise which has nothing to do with spirituality. People are deceived when they see persons who can do the above practices.

50. Sow the seed of spirituality when you are young. Do not waste the virya (semen). Discipline the sense organs and mind. Do sadhana (spiritual practice). Concentrate. Purify. Meditate. Serve. Love. Be kind to all. Realise. When you become old you will be free from anxiety and fear of death, but it is very difficult to do any rigid sadhana in old age. Therefore, be on the alert during your teens.

51. Do not think any more of your worldly concerns than is necessary to determine your duty. Do your duty and leave the rest to God.

52. You will see for yourself in a short time the particular benefits you derive from particular kinds of sadhana.

53. If a man wishes to prosper in life, he must give up gambling, drinking, excessive sleep, drowsiness, fear, anger, indolence and procrastination.

54. You have got all the materials inside for wisdom, for becoming a yogi or jnani. Practise. Develop. Assert. Realise.

55. When you advance in spiritual practice you must observe strict mauna (vow of silence) for twenty-four hours continuously. This must be continued for some months.

56. Observe moderation in eating, drinking, sleeping and in everything. The middle path is always good and safe. Observe the golden medium. Then you can become a yogi soon.

57. Pure conduct, right enquiry and good company are necessary during the practice of yoga.

58. Abandon all acid, bitter and saltish food, take delight in drinking milk, practise celibacy, be moderate in eating.

59. Sattvic food is necessary when you practise asanas and pranayama. Take milk, ghee, sweet curd, fruits, almonds, cream, etc. Give up garlic, onions, meat, fish, smoking, liquors, sour and pungent articles. Over-loading must be avoided. Take moderate diet. Be regular and punctual in taking meals. Eating all sorts of things at all times is highly dangerous for a yogi.

60. You must use only a few selected things for your food, such as dhal, ghee, wheat flour, potatoes or milk and fruits.

61. You must have restraint in your food. Control of the tongue means control of the mind. You must not allow the tongue to run riot.

62. Practice of celibacy is very necessary. Food must be sattvic. Chillies, tamarind, hot curries and chutneys should be avoided.

63. He who is attached to his sons, wife, lands and wealth will not derive even an iota of benefit. He is only wasting his precious life and energy. Those who are engaged in endless sadhana are godly men.

64. Man thinks that he is imperfect if he has not got a wife. After he gets married he again thinks that he is imperfect so long as he has not got a son and a daughter. However much a man may gain materially there is always some sort of discontent and dissatisfaction. This is a universal experience.

65. Should we not try, therefore, to attain the thing more satisfying and eternally lasting? Or should we be content to lead a life of slavery and bondage obeying the impulse of our physical nature? This question will ultimately arise in everybody's heart.

PRANAYAMA

What is Prana?

Prana is the universal principle of energy or force. It is vital force. It is all-pervading. It may be either in a static or dynamic state. It is found in all forms from the highest to the lowest, from the ant to the elephant, from the unicellular amoeba to a man, from the elementary form of plant life to the developed form of animal life.

It is through the power of prana that the ears hear, the eyes see, the skin feels, the tongue tastes, the nose smells and the brain and the intellect do their functions. It is the prana that pumps the blood from the heart into the arteries; it is prana that carries out the processes of digestion, excretion and secretion; it is prana that shines in your eyes.

The smile in a young lady, the melody in music, the power in the emphatic words of an orator, the charm in the speech of one's beloved, are all due to prana. Fire burns through prana; wind blows through prana; rivers flow through prana; the aeroplane moves in the air through prana; the steam engine works through prana; trains and motor cars move through prana; radio waves travel through prana. Prana is the electron. Prana is force. Prana is magnetism. Prana is electricity. This working of prana is seen in the systolic and diastolic actions of the heart when it pumps the blood into the arteries; in the action of inspiration and expiration during the course of breathing; in the digestion of food; in the excretion of urine and faecal matter; in the manufacture of semen, chyle, chyme, gastric juice, bile, intestinal juice and saliva; in the closing and opening of the eyelids; in walking, playing, running, skipping, talking, thinking, reasoning, feeling and willing.

All forces, all powers and prana spring from the fountain or common source, 'Atman'. The Self is the master; the vital force is the servant. Just as the personal staff of the king will have to be on duty as long as the king is working, so also the senses cannot cease to function so long as the vital force or prana, their lord, is functioning. All physical forces and all mental forces come under the category 'prana'. It is force on every plane of being, from the highest to the lowest. Whatever has life is but an expression or manifestation of prana. Ether also is an expression of prana. Pranavadins or hatha yogis consider that prana-tattva is superior to manas-tattva, the mind-principle. They say that prana is present even when the mind is absent during sleep. Hence prana plays a more vital part than the mind.

Prana is expended by thinking, willing, acting, moving, talking, writing, etc. A healthy strong man has an abundance of prana (or nerve force or vitality). The prana is supplied by food, water, air, solar energy, etc. The supply of prana is taken up by the nervous system. The prana is absorbed by breathing. The excess of prana is stored in the brain and nerve centres. When the seminal energy is sublimated, or transformed, it supplies abundance of prana to the system. It is stored up in the brain in the form of 'ojas'. Ojas is nothing but prana.

The yogi stores an abundance of prana by regular practice of pranayama, just as the storage battery stores electricity. The yogi who has stored up a large supply of prana radiates strength and vitality all around. He is a big power-house. Those who come in close contact with him imbibe prana from him and get strength, vigour, vitality and exhilaration of spirits. Just as water flows from one vessel to another, prana actually flows like a steady current from a developed yogi towards weak persons. This can be actually seen by the yogi who has developed his inner yogic vision.

If you go through the parables in *Kaushitaki* and *Chhandogya Upanishads*, where all the indriyas, mind and prana fight amongst themselves as to their superiority, you will find that prana is regarded as the highest of all. Prana is the oldest, for it starts its functioning from the very moment the child is conceived. On the contrary, the organs of hearing, etc., begin to function only when their special abodes, the ears, etc., are formed. Prana is called oldest and best in *Upanishads*. It is through the vibrations of psychic prana that the life of the mind is kept up and thought is produced. You see, hear, talk, sense, think, feel, will, know, etc., through the help of prana, and therefore scriptures declare: 'Prana is Brahman'.

The energy in the body is prana. By controlling the motion of the lungs or respiratory organs we can control the prana that is vibrating inside. By control of prana the mind can be easily controlled, because the mind is fastened to the prana like the bird to the string. Just as the bird that is tied to a post by a string, after flying here and there, finds its resting place on the post, so also this mind-bird, after running hither and thither in various sensual objects, finds its resting place in prana during deep sleep.

Prana is related to mind, and through mind to will, and through will to the individual soul, and through this to the Supreme Being. If you know how to control the little waves of prana working through the mind, then the secret of subjugating universal prana will be known to you. The yogi who becomes an expert in the knowledge of this secret will have no fear from any power, because he has mastery over all the manifestations of powers in the universe.

What is commonly known as power of personality is nothing more than the natural capacity of a person to wield his prana. Some persons are more successful in life, more influential and fascinating than others, due to the power of this prana. Such people manipulate every day, unconsciously of course, the same influence which the yogi uses consciously by the command of his will. There are others who by chance tumble unaware on the prana and use it for lower purposes.

Prana is verily the life of all beings, therefore it is called the universal life force. It is the link between the astral and physical body. When the slender thread-like prana is cut off, the astral body separates from the physical body and death takes place. The prana that was working in the physical body is withdrawn into the astral body.

This prana remains in a subtle, motionless, unmanifested, undifferentiated state during the cosmic dissolution. When the vibration is set up, prana moves and acts upon space, and brings forth the various forms. The macrocosm and microcosm are combinations of prana (energy) and akasha (matter).

The Functions of Prana

Though the prana is one, it assumes different forms with different functions. The five most important are: prana, apana, samana, udana and vyana. Of these five, the prana and the apana are the chief agents.

The seat of prana is the heart, of apana the anus, of samana the region of the navel, of udana the throat, while vyana is all pervading — it moves all over the body.

Prana, the most important, works in the following regions: the facial region, nostrils, navel and about the heart. It is the cause for sound, utterance, breath, shortness of breath and cough.

Apana circulates in the region of the anus, penis and at the sides; it also vibrates in the thighs, testicles and in and below the navel cavity. It activates the above organs and parts of the body and helps urination, defaecation and excretion.

Vyana controls the functions not attended to by prana and apana in their respective regions. It circulates in the eyes, ears, waist, nostrils and private parts.

Samana pervades all over the body and circulates in all the 72,000 nadis and carries with it the fire of hunger. It helps digestion and the using up of all the food consumed by an individual.

Udana's field of action is represented by all the joints and the throat. It helps the various limbs to function.

There are five subdivisions of prana: naga, kurma, krikara, devadatta and dhananjaya. *Naga* controls speech, while *kurma* is in charge of the winking of the eyelids, *krikara* is behind hunger and thirst, *devadatta* is concerned with expansion such as yawning, and *dhananjaya* causes the sound in ears (heard when we plug the ears.)

The Colour of Pranas

Prana is said to be of the colour of blood, red gem or coral. *Apana* is of the colour of indragopa (an insect of white or red colour). *Samana* is of the colour between that of pure milk and crystal or of an oily and shining colour, i.e. of something between both prana and apana. *Udana* is of pale white colour and that of *vyana* resembles the colour of a ray of light.

The Length of the Air-Currents

This body of vayu (air) is 96 digits (6 feet) in length as a standard. The ordinary length of the air-current when exhaled is 12 digits (9 inches). In singing its length becomes 16 digits (1 foot), in eating it comes to 20 digits (15 inches), in sleeping 30 digits (22½ inches), in copulation 36 digits (27 inches) and in doing physical exercise it is much more than that. By decreasing the natural length (9 inches) of the expired air-currents, life is prolonged; and by increasing the current, duration of life is decreased.

Cleansing

We have seen above the importance of the proper functioning of prana by virtue of its being linked with every activity of ours. So, we should always keep the body — physical and astral — clean, and help the flow of prana through the astral channels, otherwise there will be a stoppage of the corresponding functions that will lead to a diseased condition of the body.

The art of cleansing the physical body and mind with the help of prana is composed of the three stages: rechaka (exhalation), puraka (inhalation) and kumbhaka (retention).

Method: Sit in padmasana and do uddiyana bandha. Exhale the air slowly and naturally, without making sound or using any extra force. Exhalation should be slowly done without jerking. It helps to burn all sins and effects a charming personality. This is rechaka.

Puraka means filling up. The yogi fills the entire body with prana even as he inhales air from outside. Care should be taken to see that every part of the body is filled with prana while doing this. Puraka also should be done slowly without haste or jerk. This act of filling the body with air (prana) should be done till it is felt near the crown of the head. This gives manliness, courage, strength, growth and fulfilment and a radiant personality.

Next comes retention of the inhaled breath. Try to retain the breath without fear, without shaking the body. This is called kumbhaka. (If you are disturbed in this act, slowly and steadily exhale without any fear or anxiety.) You should use your will power to retain the air inhaled and do not force the air inside by continuing the act of inhalation. This sort of retention burns the poison within the system, digests the food and kills all bad humours.

The practice of kumbhaka should be taken during the second month of practice, and not before. The first month should be fully devoted to mere exhalation and inhalation. The nadis get purified by that and become fit for doing kumbhaka.

The Centering of the Prana

By inhaling the prana from outside and filling the stomach with it, centering the prana with the mind in the middle of the navel, at the tip of the nose and at the toes (during sunrise and sunset, or at all times) the yogi is freed from all diseases and fatigue. By centering his prana at the tip of the nose he obtains mastery of the elements of the air; by centering at the middle of his navel, all diseases are destroyed; by centering at the toes, his body becomes light. He who drinks air through the tongue destroys fatigue, thirst and many other diseases. For him who drinks the air with his mouth during sunrise and sunset and the last two hours of the night, within three months the auspicious Saraswati (Goddess of Speech) is present in his speech i.e., he becomes eloquent and learned. In six months he is free from diseases. Drawing the air at the root of the tongue, the wise man, thus drinking nectar, enjoys all prosperity.

Breath and Prana

Breath is the external manifestation of prana, the vital force. Breath is gross; prana is subtle. By exercising control over the breath you can control the subtle prana inside. The breath resembles the important fly-wheel of an engine. Just as the other wheels stop when the driver stops the flywheel, so also other organs cease working when the yogi stops the breath. If you can control the fly-wheel you can easily control the other wheels. Likewise, if you can control the external breath you can easily control the inner vital force, prana. Then you can completely control all the forces of the universe, mental and physical.

Prana and mind are intimately related to each other. Mind cannot operate without the help of prana. It is the vibration of prana that produces thoughts in the mind. Just as water is in union with the milk, so also prana is in union with the mind. It is prana that sets the mind in motion. If you control prana, the mind will also be controlled. If you control the mind, the prana will be automatically controlled.

The yogi can also control the omnipresent manifesting power out of which all energies take their origin, whether concerning magnetism, electricity, gravitation, cohesion, nerve currents and vital forces, as well as thought vibrations — in fact the total forces of the universe.

What is Pranayama?

Pranayama is an exact science. It is the fourth limb of raja yoga. Pranayama removes all sorts of diseases, improves health, energises digestion, invigorates the nerves, steadies the mind, augments the gastric fire, destroys rajas, removes all laziness, makes the body light and healthy and awakens the *kundalini. He who practices pranayama will have good appetite, cheerfulness, handsome figure, strength, enthusiasm, courage, vigour and vitality and good concentration.

Just as the goldsmith removes the impurities of gold by heating it in the hot furnace by strongly blowing the blowpipe, so also the yoga student removes the impurities of the body and the senses by practising pranayama. As the turbulent horses of a chariot are kept under restraint by the driver, so also the prana and the mind should be kept under perfect control by the yoga practitioner. Only that mind whose impurities have been removed by the practise of pranayama can rest permanently in Brahman. Therefore practise pranayama daily, under the guidance of your guru.

The chief aim of pranayama is to unite the prana with the apana and take the united prana-apana slowly towards the head. The effect or fruit of pranayama is awakening of the sleeping kundalini.

Through the practice of pranayama the prana leaves the passages of *ida and *pingala and forces itself through the mouth of the *sushumna and enters therein. Sushumna is the only passage through which, when the prana passes, the light of jnana (wisdom) is kindled. When the prana moves through the sushumna the mind enters a thoughtless region. All the seeds of karma of the yogi are thereby burnt away. All the pranas are united during kumbhaka or retention of breath. The yogi offers the oblations of the senses into the fire of prana.

The Qualified Person

One who has a calm mind, who has subdued his senses, who has faith in the words of the guru and scriptures, who believes in God, who is moderate in eating, drinking and sleeping and who has an eager longing for deliverance from the wheel of birth and death, is a qualified person for the practice of pranayama or any other yoga practice. Such a man can easily get success in the practice. Pranayama should be practised with care, perseverance and faith.

Those who are addicted to sensual pleasures or who are arrogant, dishonest, untruthful, diplomatic, cunning and treacherous; those who disrespect sadhus, sannyasins and their gurus or spiritual preceptors, and take pleasure in vain controversies or are of a highly talkative nature; those who are disbelievers, who mix much with worldly-

---

* See section on Kundalini

minded people, who are cruel, harsh and greedy and do much useless worldly activity, can never attain success in pranayama or any other yoga practice.

There are three types of spiritual aspirants (adhikaris): good (uttama), middle (madhyama) and inferior (adhama), according to innate tendencies, intelligence, degree of dispassion, discrimination and longing for liberation; and the capacity for sadhana.

You must approach a guru who knows the science of yoga and has mastery over it. Sit at his lotus feet, serve him. Clear your doubts through sensible and reasonable questions. Receive instructions and practise them with enthusiasm, zeal, attention, earnestness and faith, according to the methods taught by the teacher.

A pranayama practitioner should always speak kind and sweet words. He must be kind to everybody. He must be honest. He must speak the truth. He must develop dispassion, patience, faith, devotion, mercy, etc. He must observe perfect celibacy. A householder should be very moderate in sexual matters during the practice.

The Five Essentials

Five things are necessary for practising pranayama. First, a good place; second, a suitable time; third, moderate, substantial, light and nutritious food; fourth, patient and persistent practice with zeal, ease and earnestness, and lastly the purification of nadis.*

The Place

Select a solitary, beautiful and pleasant spot, where there are no disturbances; on the bank of a river, lake or sea or the top of a hill where there is a nice spring and grove of trees, and where milk and articles of food are easily procurable. Build a small hut. Have one compound. In the corner of the enclosure, sink a well. It is impossible to get an ideal place that can satisfy you from all view-points.

The banks of Narmada, Jamuna, Ganga, Kaveri, Godavari and Krishna are very suitable for building huts. You must select one such spot where there are some other yoga practitioners in the neighbourhood. You can consult them in times of difficulties. You will have faith in the yogic kriyas. When you see others also who are devoted to such yoga practices you will diligently apply yourself to your

* See section on Kundalini

practice as you will get an impetus and you will strive to excel them. Nasik, Rishikesh, Jhansi, Prayag, Uttarkashi, Vrindaban, Ayodhya, Varanasi, etc. are good places. You can fix a spot in a place far from the crowded localities. If you build a hut in a crowded place people out of curiosity will molest you. You will have no spiritual vibrations there. You will be without any protections if you build your cottage in a thick forest. Thieves and wild animals will trouble you. The question of difficulty for food will arise. In *Svetasvatara Upanishad* it is said: 'At a level place, free from pebbles, fire and gravel and pleasant to the eyes, protected from the wind, let a person apply his mind to God.'

Those who practise in their own houses can convert a room into a forest. Never allow anyone to enter the room. Keep it sacred. If you cannot afford to have a special room for contemplative purposes and for practising pranayama, have a place in the corner of a quiet room, set apart for this purpose. Have it screened. Place the photo of your guru, favourite saint or tutelary deity in the room in front of your seat. Do puja (worship) daily to the picture, physically and mentally, before you start meditation and pranayama. Burn incense in the room. Keep some sacred books there such as *Ramayana*, *Srimad Bhagavatam*, *Bhagavad Gita*, *Upanishads*, *Yoga Vasistha*, etc. for your daily study. Spread a fourfold blanket and over it a piece of soft white cloth. This will serve the purpose of a seat. Or spread a seat or mat of kusa grass and over it spread a deer skin or tiger skin and then a soft white cloth. Sit on this for practising pranayama and meditation. You can have a raised platform made of cement. Over this you can spread your mat. Then small insects, ants, etc. will not molest you.

The Time

The practice of pranayama should be commenced in spring or autumn, because in these seasons success is attained without any difficulty or trouble. In the summer do not practise pranayama in the afternoon or evening. In the cool morning hours you can have your practice.

Pranayama should not be practised just after taking meals or when one is very hungry. A pranayama practitioner should take his food when pingala is working *(i.e. when the breath flows through the right nostril), because pingala is heating and digests the food quickly.

---

* See Swara Yoga section

Yogic Diet

One proficient in yoga should abandon articles of food detrimental to the practice of yoga. He should give up salt; mustard; sour, hot, pungent and bitter things; asafoetida; worship of fire; women; too much walking; bathing at sunrise; emaciation of the body by fasts, etc. During the early stages of practice a diet of milk and ghee is ordained; also food consisting of wheat, green pulse and red rice is said to favour the progress.

Posture

Correct posture is indispensably requisite for the successful practice of pranayama. An easy comfortable posture is asana. That pose is the best which continues to be comfortable for the greatest length of time. Chest, neck and head must be in one vertical line, then the spinal cord that lies within the spinal column will be quite free. You should not bend the body either forwards or backwards or to the right or left side. You should not sit crooked, nor allow the body to collapse. By regular practise the mastery over the pose will come by itself. Fat people will find it difficult to practise padmasana or the lotus pose. They can sit in the sukhasana (comfortable pose) or siddhasana (perfected pose). You need not wait for practising pranayama till you get full mastery over the asana. Practise asana and side by side you can practise pranayama also. In course of time you will acquire perfection in both. Pranayama can also be practised by sitting erect in the chair.

In the *Bhagavad Gita* it is said: 'In a pure secret place, established in a fixed seat of his own, neither too high nor too low, with cloth, black antelope skin and kusa grass one over the other, there, making the mind one-pointed, with thought and the functions of the senses controlled he should practise yoga for the purification of the self, holding the body, head and neck erect, firm, gazing steadily at the tip of the nose without looking around.'

***Purification of Nadis**

Purification of nadis is important in the early stages of yoga and is necessary for the serious practice of pranayama. The practice of certain asanas removes the obstructions to the free flow of prana through the nadis, and paves the way for the practice of pranayama, while paschimottanasana and halasana, in particular, make the prana to flow

* See section on Kundalini

through the •sushumna nadi. If there are impurities in the nadis the ascent of •kundalini in the sushumna is seriously retarded.

The practice of •nadi suddhi (purification of the nadis) is a most effective method and brings about quick purification.

The Lungs

It will not be out of place here to mention a word on the lungs and their functions. The organs of respiration consist of two lungs and the air passages that lead to them. They are located in the upper thoracic cavity of the chest, one on each side of the median line. They are separated from each other by the heart, the greater blood vessels and the larger air-tubes. The lungs are spongy and porous and their tissues are very elastic. The substance of the lungs contains innumerable air-sacs which contain air. (After post-mortem, when they are placed in a basin of water, they float.) They are covered by a delicate serous membrane called the pleura which contains serous fluid to prevent friction of the lungs during the act of breathing. One wall of the pleura closely adheres to the lungs. The other wall is attached to the inner wall of the chest. Through this membrane the lungs are fixed to the wall of the chest. The right lung consists of three lobes. The left lung contains two lobes. Each lung consists of an apex and a base. The base is directed towards the diaphragm, the muscular dividing wall between chest and abdomen. The apex is situated above, near the root of the neck. It is the base that gets inflamed in pneumonia. The apex of the lung which does not get proper supply of oxygen gets affected by consumption. It affords favourable breeding ground for tubercle bacilli (T.B.). By the practice of *kapalabhati and *bhastrika pranayama and deep breathing exercises, these apices get a good supply of oxygen and thus tuberculosis is obviated. Pranayama develops the lungs.

The air-passage consists of the interior of the nose; pharynx (or throat); larynx (wind box or sounding box) which contains two vocal cords; trachea (or windpipe); right and left bronchii and the smaller bronchial tubes. When we breathe we draw in the air through the nose and, after it has passed through the pharynx and larynx, it passes into the trachea or windpipe, thence into the right and left bronchial tubes. These subdivide into innumerable smaller tubes called bronchioles, which terminate in minute subdivisions in the small air-sacs of

* See pages 192 and 223

• See section on Kundalini

the lungs (of which the lungs contain millions). The air-sacs of the lungs, when spread out over an unbroken surface, would cover an area of 140,000 square feet.

The air is drawn into the lungs by the action of the diaphragm. When it expands, the size of the chest and lungs is increased and the outside air rushes into the vacuum thus created. The chest and lungs contract when the diaphragm relaxes and the air is expelled from the lungs.

It is through the vocal cords that are located in the larynx that sound is produced. Larynx is the sounding box. When the vocal cords are affected by too much straining, as in singing and continuous lecturing, the voice becomes hoarse. In females these cords are shorter, hence they have a sweet, melodious voice.

The number of respirations per minute is 15. In pneumonia it is increased to 60, 70, 80 per minute. In asthma the bronchial tubes go into a spasm. They contract. Hence there is difficulty in breathing. Pranayama removes the spasm or constriction of these tubes.

A small membraneous flat cap covers the upper surface of the larynx. It is called the epiglottis. It prevents the food-particles or water from entering into the respiratory passage. It acts the part of a safety valve. When a small particle of food tries to enter the respiratory passage, cough comes in and the particle is thrown out.

Vital capacity is the capacity shown by the largest quantity of air a man can inhale after the deepest possible exhalation. The average number of breaths a man takes in one minute is fifteen.

A yogi measures the span of his life not by the number of years but by the number of his breaths.

Lungs purify the blood. The blood starts on its arterial journey, bright-red and rich, laden with life-giving qualities and properties. It returns by the venous route, poor, blue, laden with the waste matter of the system. Arteries are tubes or vessels that carry pure oxygenated blood from the heart towards the different parts of the body. Veins are vessels or tubes that carry back impure blood from the different parts of the body. The right side of the heart contains impure venous blood. From the right side of the heart the impure blood goes to the lungs for purification. It is distributed among the millions of tiny air-cells of the lungs. A breath of air is inhaled and the oxygen of the air comes in contact with the impure blood through the thin walls of the hair-like blood-vessels of the lungs, called pulmonary capillaries. The walls of the capillaries are very thin. They are like muslin cloth or a sieve. Blood exudes readily. Oxygen penetrates through the walls of these thin capillaries.

When the oxygen comes in contact with the tissues a form of combustion takes place. The blood takes up oxygen and releases carbonic-acid gas generated from the waste products and poisonous matter which has been gathered by the blood from all parts of the system. The purified blood is carried by the four pulmonary veins to the left auricle and thence to the left ventricle. From the ventricle it is pumped into the biggest artery, the aorta. From the aorta it passes into the different arteries of the body. It is estimated that in a day 35,000 pints of blood traverse the capillaries of the lungs for purification.

From the arteries the pure blood goes into the thin capillaries. From the capillaries the lymph of the blood exudes, bathes and nourishes the tissues of the body. Respiration takes place in the tissues. Tissues take up the oxygen and leave the carbon dioxide. The impurities are taken by the veins to the right side of the heart.

If the lungs are not developed properly they cannot perform the function of oxygenating the blood in an efficient manner. They will readily harbour the germs of consumption. You should try to possess a high lung power by the practice of pranayama or deep breathing exercises. Lungs which are endowed with a good capacity perform their functions satisfactorily under all conditions. They are proof against disease. In the vast majority of persons breathing is shallow and without rhythm. Lungs which have a good reserve capacity achieved by the practice of pranayama and deep breathing exercises will turn out extra work when there is an extra demand made upon them on account of lowered vitality from some cause or other.

Who is the Creator of this delicate structure? Are you feeling the invisible hand of God behind these organs? The structure of this body bespeaks undoubtedly of the omniscience of the Lord. The Indweller of our hearts supervises the working of the inner factory. Without His presence the heart cannot pump blood into the arteries and the lungs cannot carry out the process of purifying the blood. Pray. Pay your silent homage to Him. Remember Him at all times. Feel His presence in all the cells of the body.

Control of Breath

Control of breath is control of life itself. The more one masters the secret of breath-control, the more he can dominate his physical self. The practice of pranayama for a month destroys sins; practice for six months generates desire for wisdom; practice for one year gives Self-realisation. Proceed very gradually and step by step in the pranayama practice. Haste and hurry is never commended in the path of yoga.

The practice of pranayama exercises has an immediate good effect. You will find better concentration in all spiritual practices and study. By controlling the act of breathing you can efficiently control all the various motions in the body and the different nerve-currents that are running through the body. You can easily and quickly control and develop body, mind and soul through breath-control or the control of prana. It is through pranayama that you can control your circumstances and character and can consciously harmonize the individual life with the cosmic life.

The breath, directed by thought under the control of the will, is a vitalising, regenerating force which you can utilise consciously for self-development, for healing many incurable diseases in your system, for healing others and for other various useful purposes. It is within your easy reach at every moment of your life. Use it judiciously. Many yogis of yore, like Sri Jnanadeva, Trailinga Swami, Ramalinga Swami and others, utilised this breath, this force prana, in a variety of ways. You can also do so if you practise pranayama by prescribed breathing exercises.

Deep Breathing Exercises

Practise some deep breathing exercises for a few minutes daily in the fresh air of the early dawn. Deep breathing is only a variety of pranayama.

Each deep breath consists of a very full inhalation through the nose and a deep steady exhalation, also through the nose. Inhale slowly as much as you can. Exhale slowly as much as you can. During inhalation, observe the following rules:

1. Stand up. Place the hands on the hips; the elbows should be out and not forced backwards. Stand at ease.
2. Lengthen the chest upwards. Press the hip bones with the hands in a downward direction. A vacuum will be formed by this act and the air will rush in of its own accord.
3. Keep the nostrils wide open. Do not use the nose as a suction

pump. It should serve as a passive passage for both the inhaled and the exhaled air. Do not make any sound when you inhale and exhale. Remember that correct breathing is noiseless.
4. Stretch the whole upper part of the trunk.
5. Do not arch the upper chest into a cramped position. Keep the abdomen naturally relaxed.
6. Do not bend the head far backwards. Do not draw the abdomen inwards. Do not force the shoulders back. Lift the shoulders up.

During exhalation observe the following rules carefully:

1. Allow the ribs and the whole upper part of the trunk to sink down gradually.
2. Draw the abdomen upwards — slowly.
3. Do not bend the body too far forward. Arching of the chest should be avoided. Keep the head, neck and trunk in a straight line. Contract the chest. Do not breathe the air out through the mouth. Exhale very very slowly without producing any noise.
4. Expiration takes place by simply relaxing the inspiratory muscles. The chest falls down by its own weight, and expels the air out through the nose.
5. In the beginning do not retain the breath after inhalation. When the process of inhalation is over begin exhalation at once. When you have sufficiently advanced in your practice you can slowly retain the breath from five seconds to one minute, according to your strength and capacity.
6. When one round of three deep breaths is over you can take a little rest — 'respiratory pause' — by taking a few normal breaths. Then start the second round. During the pause, stand still in a comfortable position with the hands on the hips. The number of rounds can be fixed according to the capacity of the practitioner. Do 3 or 4 rounds and increase one round every week.
7. Standing erect, arms flowing open, chest wide, raise yourself gradually upon your toes, inhaling continuously and deeply all the time. Fill your chest with pure air. Then gradually exhale and slowly bring down your heels and your arms.

Pranayama in Hatha Yoga and Raja Yoga

The chief aim of pranayama is to unite the prana with the apana and take the united prana-apana slowly upwards toward the head. The effect or fruit of pranayama is the awakening of the sleeping kundalini.

A hatha yogi unites prana and apana through retention of breath (kumbhaka) and bandhas. He awakens the kundalini through the heat generated in retention of breath. He opens the *sushumna and takes the united prana-apana along the sushumna nadi. He takes sole refuge in pranayama. He always does kumbhaka, whereas a raja yogi does a little pranayama and a little kumbhaka to steady the mind and stop the vrittis. The raja yogi's chief aim is meditation through concentration of mind.

Pranayama is a great help — not only to hatha yogis, but also to raja yogis and vedantins — as it steadies the mind. A vedantic student who is in the habit of meditating on OM with feeling will actually think of Atman always, even while practising pranayama, and concentrate on the blissful Self. A raja yogi will concentrate on that special Purusha or Ishvara. A hatha yogi will concentrate on kundalini shakti in muladhara chakra and try to feel that the muladhara is pierced and kundalini is moving towards svadisthana.

Just as a goldsmith removes the impurities of gold by heating it in the hot furnace by strongly blowing the blow-pipe, so also the yoga student removes the impurities of the body and the senses by blowing his lungs, i.e. by practising pranayama.

Many have derived incalculable benefits through the practice of pranayama breathing exercises for a short period. Some people are unnecessarily alarmed, thinking there are dangers in the pranayama. There is absolutely no danger at all. The practice should be done in a systematic manner after having a thorough knowledge of the science and the technique.

Pranayama Exercises

Exercise No. 1: Sit in padmasana. Close your eyes. Concentrate on trikuti (the space between the two eyebrows). Close the right nostril with your right thumb. Inhale slowly through the left nostril as long as you can do it with comfort. Then exhale very very slowly through the same nostril. Do this twelve times. This is one round.

Then inhale through the right nostril by closing the left nostril with your right ring and little fingers and exhale very slowly through

---

* See section on Kundalini

the same nostril. Do twelve times. This is one round.

By closing one nostril the yogi helps the free full flow of breath in the other nostril.

Do not make any sound during inhalation and exhalation. Repeat your mantra during the practice. In the second week of practice do two rounds, in the third week three rounds. Take rest for two minutes when one round is over. If you take a few normal breaths when one round is over, that will give you sufficient rest and you will be fresh for the next round. There is no kumbhaka (retention) in this exercise. You can increase the number of rounds according to your strength and capacity.

Exercise No. 2: Inhale through both the nostrils slowly and gently. Do not retain the breath. Then exhale slowly. Do 12 times. This will constitute one round. You can do 2 or 3 rounds according to your capacity and strength and time at your disposal.

Exercise No. 3: Sit in your asana. Close the right nostril with your right thumb. Then inhale slowly through your left nostril; close the left nostril with your right ring and little fingers and open the right nostril by removing the right thumb. Exhale very slowly through the right nostril. Then draw the air through the right nostril as long as you can do it with comfort and exhale through the left nostril by removing the right ring and little fingers. There is no kumbhaka in this pranayama. Repeat the process 12 times. This will constitute one round.

Automatic Pranayama:

We all practise this pranayama daily unconsciously. When you are reading a sensational story book or solving a mathematical problem, your mind is very much absorbed in the subject matter. If you closely watch your breath on these occasions you will find that it has become very, very slow. When you see a tragic story being enacted in the theatre, when you hear very sad, striking news or some glad tidings, when you shed tears — whether of joy or sorrow — or burst into laughter, the breath is slackened; pranayama comes by itself. When you are deeply absorbed in doing japa or Brahma vichar (enquiry of Atman), concentration or meditation, pranayama comes by itself. The breath becomes slower and slower. Also in those yoga students who practise sirshasana, pranayama comes by itself. It is obvious from this that when the mind is deeply concentrated on any subject the respiration slows down or stops. Pranayama is being done automatically. Mind and prana are intimately connected. If you turn your attention to watch the breath on those occasions it will regain its normal state. Just as there is connection between wind and fire (light), so also there is connection between prana and mind.

Easy Comfortable Pranayama

Sit in lotus posture or other meditative pose in your meditation room before the picture of your chosen deity. Close the right nostril with the right thumb. Draw in the air very, very slowly through the left nostril. Then close the left nostril also with the little and ring fingers of the right hand. Retain the air as long as you comfortably can. (Stoppage of breath comes not through closing the nostrils but through stopping the lungs from operating.) Then exhale very, very slowly through the right nostril after removing the thumb. Now half the process is over. Then draw the air through the right nostril. Retain the air as before and exhale it very, very slowly through the left nostril. All these six processes constitute one pranayama. Do twenty in the morning and twenty in the evening. Gradually increase.

Have the mental attitude that all the divine qualities like mercy, love, forgiveness, peace and joy are entering into your system along with the inspired air, and that all undivine qualities like lust, anger, greed and pride are being thrown out along with the expired air.

You must adjust the inhalation, retention and exhalation so nicely that you do not experience the feeling of suffocation or discomfort at any stage of pranayama.

You should never feel the necessity of catching hold of a few normal breaths between any two successive rounds. The duration of inhalation, retention and exhalation must be properly adjusted. Exercise due care and attention and matters will turn out to be successful and easy in the end. Always inhale and exhale very, very slowly. Do not make the least sound. You must not unnecessarily prolong the period of exhalation, otherwise the next inhalation will be done in a hurried manner, and the rhythm will be disturbed. When this becomes effortless, maintain a ratio of inhalation, retention, exhalation of 1:4:2.

The External Kumbhaka: Draw the air through the left nostril till you count 3 OMs; throw it out through the right nostril immediately without retaining it, counting 6 OMs. Hold it outside till you count 12 OMs. Then draw the breath through the right; exhale it through the left and hold it outside as before, using the same units of OM for inhalation, exhalation and retention. Do six times in the morning and times in the evening. Gradually increase the number of rounds and the time of the kumbhaka. Do not strain or fatigue yourself.

There are three types of pranayama, viz. inferior, middle and superior (adhama, madhyama and uttama). The inferior pranayama consists of 12 *matras, the middle of 24, and the superior occupies a time of 36 matras. This is for inhalation. The ratio between inhalation, retention and exhalation is 1:4:2. If you inhale for a period of 12 matras you will have to make retention for a period of 48 matras. Then the time for exhalation will be for 24 matras. This is inferior pranayama. The same rule will apply to the other two varieties. First practise the inferior pranayama for a month. Then practise the middle for three months. Then take up the superior variety. That pranayama which produces perspiration is of the lowest type; that which produces tremor is of the middle type; that which produces levitation or rising of the body from the ground, is of the highest type.

If you want rapid progress in the practice, you must have four sittings — morning 4 a.m., afternoon 4 p.m., night 8 p.m., and at midnight 12 p.m., — and do 4 x 80 = 320 retentions. This pranayama exercise removes all diseases, purifies the nadis, steadies the mind in concentration, improves digestion, increases the digestive power, helps in maintaining brahmacharya and enables one to attain kevala kumbhaka (absolute retention) in due course of practice.

There is no danger in practising pranayama, asana, etc., if you are careful, if you use your commonsense. People are unnecessarily alarmed. There is danger in everything if you are careless. If you are careless in going down the staircase you will fall down and break your legs; if you are careless when you walk in the busy parts of a city you will be crushed by the motor cars; if you are careless when you purchase a ticket at the railway station you will lose your money-purse; if you are careless in dispensing mixtures you will kill the patients by giving a poison or a wrong medicine or administering a medicine in overdoses. Even so, when you practise pranayama you will have to be careful about your diet. You should avoid over-loading; you should take

---

* A matra corresponds to one second. Both the twinkling of an eye and the time occupied by one normal respiration are considered as one matra. The time taken in making three rounds of the knee with the palm of the hand — neither very quickly nor very slowly — snapping the fingers once, is called a matra.

light, easily digestible and nutritious food. You should be moderate in copulation. You should not go beyond your capacity in retaining the breath. You should first practise inhalation and exhalation only (without retention of breath) for one or two months. You should gradually increase the ratio of inhalation, retention and exhalation from 1:4:2 to 16:64:32. You should inhale very, very slowly. If these rules are observed there is no danger at all in the practice of pranayama.

Sivananda's Pranayama

Technique: Sit comfortably on a chair, sofa or easy-chair. Draw the air through both nostrils, as long as comfortable. Retain as long as comfortable. Repeat your mantra or OM while retaining the breath. Then exhale as long as comfortable. You need not observe any ratio between the inhalation, exhalation and retention; but let the inhalation and exhalation be deep and full.

Benefits: The benefits of this pranayama are incalculable. All the muscles are relaxed and all the nerves are toned. Rhythm and harmony are established in the entire being. The mind is calmed and circulation is promoted. An inexpressible peace and bliss come to reign within you.

You can do it in the morning while lying in bed. Your mind will become alert for commencing japa and meditation. You can do it when the mind is about to lose balance on account of the setting in of lust, anger or other evil thoughts; the mind will be filled with a great power that will prevent the evil thoughts from disturbing it. You can do it just before commencing your study; the mind will be concentrated easily and what you study will be indelibly impressed in your mind. You can do it during your office work; you will never be tired. When you return from the office you can practise this pranayama and you will be recharged with fresh energy.

The greatest advantage is that once you start doing it you will do it very often; and your mind can never find an excuse for not practising this very easy and comfortable pranayama, which has all the advantages of pranayama without its 'rules and regulations'. Do it from now without fail.

Pranayama While Walking

Walk with head up, shoulders back and chest expanded. Inhale slowly through both nostrils, counting OM mentally three times, one count for each step. Then retain the breath till you count twelve OMs. Then exhale slowly through both nostrils till you count six OMs. Take the respiratory pause or rest after one pranayama, counting twelve OMs. If you find it difficult to count OM with each step, count OM without having any concern with the steps.

Those who are very busy can practise the above pranayama during their morning and evening walks. It is like killing two birds with one stone. You will find it very pleasant to practise pranayama while walking in an open place, when a delightful gentle breeze is blowing. You will be invigorated quickly to a considerable degree. Practise, feel and realise the marked, beneficial influence of this kind of pranayama. Those who walk briskly, repeating OM mentally or verbally, practise natural pranayama without any effort.

Pranayama in Savasana

Lie down on the back, quite at ease, over a blanket. Keep the hands on the ground by the sides and the legs straight. The heels should be kept together, but the toes can remain a little apart. Relax all the muscles and the nerves. Those who are very weak can practise pranayama in this pose while lying on the ground or on a bedstead. Draw the breath in slowly without making any noise, through both nostrils. Retain the breath as long as you can do it with comfort. Then exhale slowly through both nostrils. Repeat the process twelve times in the morning and twelve times in the evening. Chant OM mentally during the practice. If you like you can practise in sukhasana (easy comfortable posture) also. This is a combined exercise of asana, pranayama, meditation and rest. It gives rest not only to the body but also for the mind. It gives relief, comfort and ease. This is very suitable for aged people.

Rhythmical Breathing

The breathing in men and women is very irregular. In exhalation the prana goes out 16 digits and in inhalation it comes in only 12 digits, thus losing 4 digits; but if you inhale for 16 digits as in exhalation, then you will have rhythmical breathing. Then kundalini will be roused. By the practice of rhythmical breathing you will enjoy real good rest. You can control the respiratory centre that is situated in medulla oblongata and other nerves also, because the centre of respiration has a sort of control effect on the nerves. Therefore breathing in and out in a measured manner will harmonise the whole system — the physical body, mind and sense organs — and will soothe the tired nerves. You will experience full repose and calmness. All the bubbling emotions will subside and the surging impulses will calm down. First inhale for 6 OMs and exhale for 6 OMs. Repeat 10 times. Gradually increase the number of rounds.

There is another variety or modification of rhythmic breathing: Inhale slowly through both nostrils for 4 OMs; retain the breath for eight OMs (internal kumbhaka); exhale slowly through both nostrils for four OMs; and retain the breath outside (external kumbhaka) for eight OMs.

Repeat the above process a number of times according to your strength and capacity. After some practice you can gradually increase the duration of inhalation and exhalation to eight OMs, and the period between breaths to sixteen OMs; but never try to increase the duration until you are sure that you have power and strength to do so. You must experience joy and pleasure in doing the same. You should not feel any undue strain. Pay considerable attention to keeping up the rhythm. Remember that the rhythm is more important than the length of the breath. You must feel the rhythm throughout the whole body. Practice will make you perfect. Patience and perseverance are needed.

Surya Bheda

Sit in padmasana or siddhasana. Close the eyes. Keep the left nostril closed with your right ring and little fingers. Slowly inhale without making any sound as long as you can do it comfortably through the right nostril. Then close the right nostril with your right thumb and retain the breath firmly pressing the chin against the chest (jalandhara bandha). Hold the breath till perspiration oozes from the tips of the nails and the roots of the hairs (hair follicles). (This point cannot be reached at the very outset. You will have to increase the period of kumbhaka gradually. This is the limit of the sphere of practice of surya bheda kumbhaka.) Then exhale very slowly, without making any sound, through the left nostril, keeping the right nostril closed with the thumb. Repeat OM mentally with feeling and meaning during inhalation, retention and exhalation. Exhale after purifying the skull by forcing the breath up.

This pranayama should be performed again and again, as it purifies the brain and destroys the intestinal worms and diseases arising from excess of wind (vayu). This removes the four kinds of evils caused by vayu and cures rheumatism. It also cures rhinitis, cephalagia and various sorts of neuralgia. The germs that are found in the frontal sinuses are removed. It destroys decay and death, awakens the kundalini shakti and increases the bodily fire.

Ujjayi

Sit in padmasana or siddhasana. Close the mouth. Inhale slowly through both the nostrils in a smooth, uniform manner till the breath fills the space from the throat to the heart. Retain the breath as long as you can do it comfortably and then exhale slowly through the left nostril by closing the right nostril with your right thumb. Expand the chest when you inhale. During inhalation a peculiar sound is produced owing to the partial closing of the glottis. The sound produced during inhalation should be of a mild and uniform pitch. It should be continuous also. This kumbhaka may be practised even when walking or standing. Instead of exhaling through the left nostril, you can exhale slowly through both nostrils.

This removes the heat in the head. The practitioner becomes very beautiful. The gastric fire is increased. It removes all the evils arising in the body and cures dropsy of the belly. It removes phlegm in the throat. Asthma, consumption and all sorts of pulmonary diseases are cured. All diseases that arise from deficient inhalation of oxygen, and diseases of the heart are cured. All works are accomplished by ujjayi pranayama. The practitioner is never attacked by diseases of phlegm, nerves, dyspepsia, dysentery, enlarged spleen, consumption, cough or fever. Perform ujjayi to destroy decay and death.

Sitkari

Fold the tongue so that the tip of the tongue might touch the upper palate and draw the air through the mouth with a hissing sound CCCCCCC (or Si, Si, Si, Si). Retain the breath as long as you can without the feeling of suffocation, and then exhale slowly through both nostrils. You can keep the two rows of teeth in contact and then inhale the air through the mouth as before.

The practice enhances the beauty of the practitioner and vigour of his body. It removes hunger, thirst, indolence and sleep. His strength will be just like that of Indra. He becomes the lord of yogis. He is able to do and undo things. He becomes invincible. No injury will affect him. When you are thirsty, practise this. You will be relieved of thirst.

Sitali

Protrude the tongue a little away from the lips. Fold the tongue like a tube. Draw the air through the mouth with the hissing sound Si. Retain the breath as long as you can with comfort. Then exhale slowly through both nostrils. Practise this daily again and again in the morning from 15 to 30 times. You can do this either in padmasana, siddhasana, vajrasana, or even when you stand or walk. This pranayama purifies the blood, quenches thirst and appeases hunger. It cools the system and destroys chronic dyspepsia, inflammation caused by various chronic diseases, fever, consumption, indigestion, bilious disorders, phlegm, the bad effects of poison, snake-bite etc. When you are caught up in a jungle or any place where you cannot get water, if you feel thirsty practise this pranayama. You will at once be relieved of thirst. He who practises this regularly will not be affected by the bite of serpents and scorpions. Sitali kumbhaka is an imitation of the respiration of a serpent. The practitioner gets the power of enduring the privation of air, water and food. He becomes proof against all sorts of inflammation and fever. Practise sitali in summer. This will purify your blood and cool the system too. Practise bhastrika in winter. This will cure asthma and consumption. Repeat OM or Rama mentally during the practice. Observe brahmacharya and diet-control. You will derive maximum benefits and will quickly purify the nadis or nerves.

Bhastrika

Bhastrika means 'bellows'. Rapid succession of forcible expulsion is a characteristic feature of bhastrika. Just as a blacksmith blows his bellows rapidly, so also you should move your breath rapidly.

Sit in padmasana. Keep the body, neck and head erect. Close the mouth. Next, inhale and exhale quickly ten times like the bellows of the blacksmith. Constantly dilate and contract. When you practise this pranayama a hissing sound is produced. The practitioner should start with rapid expulsions of breath following one another in rapid succession. When the required number of expulsions (say ten for a round) is finished, the final expulsion is followed by a deepest possible inhalation. The breath is suspended as long as it is comfortable. Then the deepest possible exhalation is done very very slowly. The end of this deep exhalation completes one round of bhastrika. Rest a while after one round is over, by taking a few normal breaths. This will give you relief and make you fit for starting the second round. Do three rounds daily in the morning. You can do another three rounds in the evening also. Busy people who find it difficult to do three rounds of bhastrika daily can do one round at least. This also will keep them quite fit.

Bhastrika is a powerful exercise. A combination of kapalabhati (see previous chapter) and ujjayi makes up bhastrika. Practise kapalabhati and ujjayi to start with. Then you will find it very easy to do bhastrika.

Some prolong the practice till they get tired. You will get perspiration profusely. If you experience any giddiness, stop the practice and take a few normal breaths. Continue the practice after the giddiness has vanished. Bhastrika can be done both in the morning and evening in winter. In summer do it in the morning only, during the cool hours.

Bhastrika relieves inflammation of the throat, increases gastric fire, removes diseases of the nose and chest and eradicates asthma, consumption, etc. It gives good appetite. It destroys phlegm which is the bolt or obstacle to the door at the mouth of the sushumna. It enables one to know the kundalini. It removes all diseases which arise from excess of wind, bile and phlegm. It gives warmth to the body. (When you do not have sufficient warm clothing in a cold region to protect yourself from cold, practise this pranayama and you will get sufficient warmth in the body quickly.) It purifies the nadis considerably. It is the most beneficial of all kumbhakas. Bhastrika kumbhaka should be specially practised, as it enables the prana to break through the three knots that are firmly located in the sushumna. It awakens the kundalini quickly. The practitioner will never suffer from any disease. He will always be healthy.

Let not bhastrika pranayama be over-violent. An intelligent moderation will ensure adherence to safety limits.

The number of exhalations or rounds is determined by the strength and capacity of the practitioner. You must not go to extremes. Some students do six rounds. Some do twelve also.

Repeat OM mentally with feeling and meaning throughout.

There are some varieties of bhastrika wherein one nostril only is used for breathing purposes, and in another variety the alternate nostrils are used for inhalation and exhalation.

Those who wish to do bhastrika for a long time in an intense manner should live on kitcherie, and take an enema or do basti in the morning before starting the practice.

Bhramari

Sit in padmasana or siddhasana. Inhale rapidly through both nostrils making sound of the bee (bhramari), and exhale rapidly through both nostrils, making the humming sound.

You can carry on the process till the body is bathed in perspiration. In the end inhale through both nostrils, retain the breath as long as you can do it comfortably and then exhale slowly through both nostrils. The joy which the practitioner gets in making this kumbhaka is unlimited and indescribable. In the beginning, heat of the body is increased as the circulation of blood is quickened. In the end the body-heat is decreased by perspiration. By success in this the yoga student gets success in samadhi.

Murchha

Sit in your asana and inhale. Retain the breath. Do jalandhara bandha by pressing the chin against the chest. Retain the breath till you expect fainting, and then exhale slowly. This is murchha kumbhaka as it makes the mind senseless and gives happiness. But this is not suitable for many.

Plavini

Practice of this pranayama demands skill on the part of the student. He who practises it can do jalastambha and float on water for any length of time. Mr. 'S', a yoga student, can float on water for twelve hours at a stretch. He who practises plavini kumbhaka can live on air and dispense with food for some days. The student actually drinks air like water, slowly, and sends it to the stomach. The stomach gets bloated a bit. If you tap the stomach when it is filled with air you will get a peculiar tympanic sound. Gradual practice is necessary. The help of one who is well versed in this pranayama is also necessary. The student can expel all the air from the stomach by gradual belching.

Kevala Kumbhaka

Kumbhaka is of two kinds viz. sahita and kevala. That which is coupled with inhalation and exhalation is termed sahita. That which is devoid of these, is called kevala (alone). When you get mastery in sahita, then you can attempt this kevala. When in due course of practice the kumbhaka subsists in many places without exhalation and inhalation and unconditioned by place, time and number — then that kumbhaka is called absolute and pure (kevala kumbhaka), the fourth form of 'regulation of breath'. Such powers as that of roaming about in space unseen follow this last form of pranayama. In *Vasishtha Samhita* it is said: 'When, after giving up inhalation and exhalation, one holds his breath with ease, it is absolute kumbhaka (kevala)'. In this pranayama the breath is suddenly stopped without inhalation and exhalation. The student can restrain his breath as long as he likes through this kumbhaka. He attains the state of raja yoga.

When kevala kumbhaka is attained by one, expiration and inspiration are dispensed with. There is nothing unattainable in the three worlds for him. In the commencement of his practice, he sweats. As a frog moves by leaps, so the yogi sitting in padmasana moves on the earth. With further increased practice he is able to rise from the ground. He levitates while seated in the lotus posture, and then arises in him the power to perform extraordinary feats. Any pain, small or great, does not affect the yogi. Then excretions and sleep are diminished; tears in the eye, salivary flow, sweat and bad smell in the mouth do not arise in him. With still further practice he acquires great strength, by which he attains bhuchara siddhi, which enables him to bring under his control all the creatures that tread the earth: tigers, elephants, wild bulls and even lions die by a blow given by the palm of this yogi. He becomes as beautiful as the god of love himself. By the preservation of the semen a good odour pervades the body of the yogi.

Through kevala kumbhaka the knowledge of kundalini arises. Kundalini is aroused and the sushumna is free from all sorts of obstacles. The yogi attains perfection in hatha yoga. This kumbhaka cures all diseases and promotes longevity. You can practise this kumbhaka three times a day. He who knows pranayama and kevala is the real yogi. What can he who has acquired success in kevala kumbhaka not accomplish in the three worlds?

Kumbhaka awakens kundalini shakti, steadies the mind, invigorates the different systems of the body and confers longevity on the practitioner. It augments the digestive 'fire' and gives good appetite. It produces a charming glow in the eyes and face. It eradicates various diseases of the lungs, stomach, kidneys, intestines and liver. Whenever you feel uneasy, depressed or dejected, practise pranayama.

Pranayama: Different Authorities

'Regulation of breath or the control of prana is the stoppage of inhalation and exhalation, which follows after securing that steadiness of posture or seat.'(*Yoga Sutras* II.49)

This is the definition of pranayama in the *Yoga Sutras of Patanjali*. You can take up the practice of pranayama after you have gained steadiness in your asana (seat). If you can sit for three hours in one asana, continuously at one stretch, you have gained mastery over the asana. If you are able to sit from half to one hour even, you can take up the practice of pranayama. You can hardly make any spiritual progress without the practice of pranayama.

Prana is vyashti (single) when the individual is concerned. The sum total of the cosmic prana is hiranyagarbha or samashti prana — just as one match-stick is vyashti while the whole match-box is samashti, and a single mango-tree is vyashti and while the whole mango grove is samashti.

The author of *Sivayoga Dipika* describes three kinds of pranayama: prakrita, vaikrita and kevala kumbhaka. 'If the prana is in the form of breath inhaled and exhaled, on account of its natural quality of going out and coming in, the pranayama is known as prakrita. If the prana is restrained by the threefold means of throwing out, taking in and stopping the breath in accordance with the rules prescribed in the scriptures, it is called vaikrita or artificial. But with great men who have risen above these two kinds of restraining breath, the sudden restraining of the vital currents directly (without inspiration and expiration) is kevala kumbhaka. Prakrita pranayama belongs to mantra yoga. Vaikrita belongs to laya yoga.'

In *Aparokshanubhuti* 118-120, Sri Sankaracarya writes:

> Pranayama is the control of all life-forces by realising naught but Brahman in all things as the mind, etc.
> The negation of the universe is the outgoing breath. The thought: 'I am Brahman' itself is called the incoming breath.
> The permanence of that thought thereafter is the restrained breath. This is the pranayama of the wise, while the pressing of the nose is only for the unknowing.

In the *Yoga Vasistha* (VI:1 25-26), Bhusunda says to Sri Vasistha:

> In the cool lotus of the heart within this visible tenement of flesh composed of the five elements, there are two vayus, viz., prana and apana, commingled in it. For those who tread smoothly and without any of the slightest efforts, the path of these two vayus will become the sun and the moon themselves in the heart-akasha (space), and will rove in the space and yet be animating and carrying their fleshy tabernacle. These vayus will go up and down to higher and lower states. They are of the same nature in the waking, dreaming and dreamless sleeping state, and permeate all throughout. I am moving in the direction of these two vayus and have rendered nil all my subtle desires in the waking state like unto those of the dreamless sleeping state. Divide a filament of the lotus-stalk into a thousand pieces and you will find these vayus more subtle than that. Hence it is difficult for me to talk about the nature of these vayus and their vibrations. Of these, prana does ceaselessly vibrate in this body with an upward motion both externally and internally, while apana having the same fluctuating tendency, vibrates both external and internal to the body, having a downward motion. It will be beneficial if the prana exhaled to the extent of 16 digits, is inhaled to the same extent. Only 12 digits are inhaled ordinarily. Those who have experienced the equalisation of prana in exhalation and inhalation will enjoy infinite bliss.
>
> Now hear about the characteristics of prana. The inhalation to the length of 12 digits of the prana which has been exhaled, is called (the internal) puraka (inhalation). It is also called the internal (puraka) when apana vayu re-enters the body from outside without any effort. When apana vayu ceases to manifest itself and prana gets absorbed in the heart, then the time occupied in such a state is internal kumbhaka. Yogis are able to experience all these. Then the prana in the space of the heart manifests itself externally (to the heart within) in diverse aspects without any affliction to the mind, then it is called (the external) rechaka (exhalation). When the externally fluctuating prana enters the nose and stops there at its tip, then it is called the external puraka. But when it is passing from the tip of the nose it goes down 12 digits, then also it is called the external puraka. When prana goes arrested without and apana within, then it is called the external kumbhaka. When the shining

apana vayu takes an upward bent within, then it is called the external rechaka. All these practices lead to liberation. Therefore they should ever be meditated upon. Those who have understood and practised well all the external and internal kumbhakas and others, will never be reborn.

The regular and systematic practice of pranayama as described by me is capable of yielding liberation. It should be practised both day and night. Those who follow these practices smoothly and control their minds by not letting them run in other directions, will in course of time attain nirvana.

Such practitioners will never thirst after material pleasures. They will ever be uniform in their practice — whether walking, standing, waking, dreaming or sleeping.

Prana, having flown out, will again be absorbed in the heart, having run back 12 digits. Similarly will apana be absorbed in the heart, having issued out of the heart and running back 12 digits to it. Apana, being the moon, will cool the whole body in its passage, but prana, being the sun, will generate heat in the system and cook or digest everything in it. Will pains arise in one who has reached that supreme state where the rays of apana (the moon) are drowned by prana (the sun)? Will rebirth arise in one who has reached that powerful seat when rays of prana, the sun, are devoured by apana, the moon? These will arrest at once the seven births (of they) who reach that neutral state where they find apana vayu consumed by prana, and vice versa. I eulogise that Chidatma, who is in that intermediate state where prana and apana are absorbed in one another. I meditate ceaselessly upon that Chidatma, who is in the space directly in front, at the end of my nose, where prana and apana both become extinct. Thus it is through this path of prana's control that I attained the supreme and immaculate reality, devoid of pains.

Importance and Benefits of Pranayama

There is no purificatory action greater than pranayama. Pranayama gives purity, and the light of knowledge shines. The karma of the yogi, which covers up the light and binds him to repeated births, becomes attenuated by the practice of pranayama, and is destroyed eventually.

Manu says: 'Let the defects be burnt up by pranayama.'

Patanjali says: 'By the practice of pranayama the mind becomes fit for concentration.' (*Yoga Sutras* II:53)

You will be able to concentrate the mind nicely after these defects of karma have been removed. The mind will be quite steady, like the flame in a windless place, as the disturbing energy has been removed. When the prana moves in the ether-principle, the breathing will be lessened. At this time it will be easy to stop the breath. The velocity of the mind will be slowly lessened by pranayama. It will induce dispassion.

Various siddhis are obtained by the advanced student in the practice of pranayama. If you can suspend one inch (or digit) of breath inside, you will obtain the powers of foretelling; if you can suspend two inches within, you will get the power of thought-reading; for suspending the breath for three inches, levitation; for four inches, psychometry, clairaudience, etc; for five inches, moving about unseen by anybody in the world; for six inches the power of 'kaya siddhi'; for seven inches, entering the body of another man; for eight inches, the power to remain always young; for nine inches, the power to make devas to work as your servants; for ten inches the powers of making the body very small or very large, and other siddhis; and for eleven inches you will attain oneness with Paramatma.

If you concentrate on the tip of the nose during kumbhaka, you will control prana. If you concentrate on the navel during kumbhaka all diseases will be cured. If you concentrate on the toe of the foot, you will get lightness of the body. Kumbhaka destroys sins and greyness of the hair and helps to get conquest over the mind. When through great practice the yogi can perform kumbhaka for a full three hours, then he can balance himself on his thumb. He undoubtedly attains all kinds of siddhis. Just as fire destroys the fuel, so also pranayama destroys the bundles of sins.

The pranayama practitioner becomes very handsome. The body becomes lean, strong and healthy and fat is reduced. There is lustre in the face, and the eyes sparkle like diamonds. His voice becomes sweet and melodious. The inner anahata sounds are distinctly heard. He is free from all sorts of diseases. The gastric fire is augmented and excreta becomes scanty. The student becomes so perfected in brahmacharya that his mind will not be shaken even if a celestial nymph tries to embrace him. His appetite becomes keen, nadis are purified and tossing of the mind is removed as the mind becomes one-pointed. Rajas and tamas are destroyed. The mind is prepared for concentration (dharana) and meditation (dhyana). Steady practice arouses inner spiritual light, happiness and peace of mind. Advanced students only will get all the other siddhis mentioned above.

The mind of a man can be made to transcend ordinary experience and exist on a plane higher than that of reason, known as super-conscious state of concentration, and get beyond the limit of concentration. He comes face to face with facts which ordinary consciousness cannot comprehend; this ought to be achieved by proper training and manipulation of the subtle forces of the body so as to cause them to give, as it were, an upward push to the mind into the higher regions. When the mind is so raised into the super-conscious state of perception, it begins to act from there and experiences higher facts, and higher knowledge. Such is the ultimate object of yoga, which can be achieved by the practice of pranayama. The control of vibratory prana means to a yogi the kindling of the fire of supreme knowledge, the realisation of the Self.

Pranic Healing

Those who practise pranayama can impart their prana in healing morbid diseases. They can also recharge themselves with prana in no time, by practising kumbhaka. Never think that you will be depleted of your prana by distributing it to others. The more you give, the more it will flow to you from the cosmic source (Hiranyagarbha). That is the law of nature. Do not become a niggard. If there is a rheumatic patient, gently massage his legs with your hands. Do kumbhaka when you massage, and imagine that the prana is flowing from your hands towards the leg of your patient. Connect yourself with Hiranyagarbha or the cosmic prana and imagine that the cosmic energy is flowing through your hands towards the legs of the patient. The patient will at once feel warmth, relief and strength. You can cure headache, intestinal colic or pain in any other portion or organ of the body, you can speak to the cells and give them orders: "O cells! Discharge your functions properly. I command you to do so." They will obey your orders. They too have got subconscious intelligence. Repeat OM when you pass your prana to others. Try a few cases. You will gain confidence and competence. You can cure scorpion-sting also. Gently massage the leg and bring the poison down.

You can have extraordinary power of concentration, strong will and a perfectly healthy and strong body by practising pranayama regularly. Pranayama is very helpful in relieving pain or discomfort in the body. You will have to direct the power of prana consciously to unhealthy parts of the body. For instance, suppose you have a sluggish liver. Sit on padmasana. Close your eyes. Inhale gently till you count OM three times. Then retain the breath till you count OM six times. Direct the prana to the region of the liver. Concentrate your mind there. Fix your attention on that area. Imagine that prana is interpenetrating the tissues and the cells of the lobes of the liver and doing its curative, regenerating and constructive work there. (Faith, imagination, attention and interest play a very important part in this.) Then exhale slowly. During exhalation imagine that the morbid impurities of the liver are thrown out. Repeat this process twelve times in the morning and twelve times in the evening. Sluggishness of liver will vanish in a few days. This is a drugless treatment.

You can take the prana to any part of the body during pranayama and cure any kind of disease, be it acute or chronic. Try once or twice in healing yourself. Your convictions will grow stronger. Why do you cry like the lady who is crying for ghee when she has butter in her hand, when you have a cheap, potent easily available remedy or agent at your command at all times? Use it judiciously. When you advance in your concentration and practice you can cure many diseases by mere touch. In the advanced stages many diseases are cured by mere will.

Distant Healing

This is known as 'absent healing' also. You can transmit your prana through space to your friend who is living at a distance. He should have a receptive mental attitude. You must feel yourself in direct relation and in sympathy with the man whom you heal with this distant healing method.

You can fix hours of appointment with him through correspondence. You can write to him: "Get ready at 4 a.m. Have a receptive mental attitude. Lie down in an easy chair. Close your eyes. I shall transmit my prana." Say mentally to the patient: "I am transmitting a supply of prana." Do kumbhaka when you send prana. Practise rhythmical breathing also. Have a mental image that the prana is leaving your mind when you exhale; it is passing through space and is entering the system of the patient. The prana travels unseen like the wireless (radio) waves and flashes like lightning across space. The prana that is coloured by the thoughts of the healer is projected outside. You can recharge yourself with prana by practising kumbhaka. This requires long, steady, regular practice.

Special Instructions

1. In the early morning, answer the call of nature and sit for the practice. Practise pranayama in a dry, well-ventilated room. Pranayama requires deep concentration and attention. It is always better to have the practice in a steady sitting posture. Do not keep anyone by your side, to avoid distraction of the mind.

2. Before you sit for pranayama practice, thoroughly clean the nostrils well. You can take a small quantity of fruit juice or a small cup of milk or coffee even before the practice. When you finish the practice take a cup of milk or light tiffin after ten minutes.

3. Spread a tiger-skin or deer-skin or a fourfold blanket. Over this spread a piece of white cloth. Then sit for the pranayama practice facing the north.

4. Have one sitting only in the morning during summer. If there is heat in the brain or head, apply amla oil or butter on the head before you take your bath. Take sugar candy dissolved in water. This will cool your whole system. Do sitali pranayama also. You will not be affected by the heat.

5. Strictly avoid too much talking, eating, sleeping, mixing with friends and exertion. 'Verily yoga is not for him who eats too much, who abstains to excess, is addicted to too much sleep, or even to wakefulness.' (*Bhagavad Gita* VI.16)

Take a little ghee with rice when you take your meals. This will lubricate the bowels and allow vayu to move downwards freely. 'Without observing moderation of diet, if one takes to the yoga practices he cannot obtain any benefit, but gets various diseases.' (*Gheranda Samhita* V:16)

6. Perfect celibacy for six months or one year will doubtlessly enable you to acquire rapid progress in the practice and in spiritual advancement. Do not talk with ladies. Do not laugh and joke with them. Shun their company entirely. Without brahmacharya and dietetic regulations if you practise yoga exercises you will not get maximum benefit in the spiritual practices. But, for ordinary health you can practise mild exercises.

7. Be regular and systematic in your practice. Never miss a day.

Stop the practice when you are ailing seriously. Some people twist the muscles of the face when they do kumbhaka (retention). It should be avoided. It is a symptom to indicate that they are going beyond their capacity. This must be strictly avoided. Such people cannot have a regulated inhalation and exhalation.

8. Obstacles in yoga are sleeping in daytime, late vigil at night, excess of urine and faeces, unwholesome food and laborious mental operation with prana. When one is attacked by any disease one says that the disease is due to the practice of yoga. This is a serious mistake.

9. Get up at 4 a.m. Meditate or do japa for half an hour. Then do asanas and mudras. Take rest for 15 minutes. Then do pranayama. Physical exercises can be conveniently combined with asanas. If you have sufficient time at your disposal you can do pranayama after finishing all the yoga exercises and meditation. Pranayama can also be performed as soon as you get up from bed just before japa and meditation. The mind gets one-pointed after the practice of pranayama. It will make your body light and you will enjoy meditation. You must have a routine according to your convenience and time.

10. First do japa and meditation. Then you can take to asanas and pranayama exercises. Then finish the course of practice by another short sitting in meditation.

11. Pranayama, though it concerns the breath, gives good exercise for the various internal organs and the whole body.

12. The general order of practice is: first of all asanas, then mudras, then pranayama and then meditation (dhyana). Since the early morning time is suitable for meditation, you can follow this order: japa, meditation, asanas, mudras and pranayama. This is a better way. You can follow the order which is suitable to you. After doing asanas, take rest for five minutes and then begin pranayama.

13. Some hatha yoga books interdict cold bath in the early morning. Probably the reason may be that one may catch cold or develop any complaint of the lungs, if he takes cold bath at 4 a.m., particularly in cold places like Kashmir, Mussoorie, Darjeeling, etc. There is no restriction in hot places. I am always in favour of morning cold baths before one starts the yoga practices, as it is refreshing and stimulating. It drives off drowsiness. It brings equilibrium of circulation of blood. There is a healthy flow of blood towards the brain.

14. Asanas and pranayama remove all sorts of diseases, improve health, energise digestion, invigorate the nerves, straighten the sushum-

na nadi, remove rajas and awaken kundalini. Practice of asanas and pranayama bestows good health and a steady mind.

15. The maintenance of the body is impossible without asanas or some kind of physical exercise or activities. Even an orthodox vedantin is an unconscious hatha yogi. He practises some kind of asana daily. He practises pranayama also unconsciously because during meditation pranayama comes by itself.

16. Whenever you feel uneasy, depressed or dejected, practise pranayama. You will be at once filled with new vigour, energy and strength. You will be elevated, renovated and filled with joy. Do this and try. Before you begin to write something — an essay, an article or a thesis — do pranayama first. You will bring out beautiful ideas and it will be an inspiring, powerful and original production.

17. Be regular in the practice. Regularity in the practice is very necessary if one wants to realise the maximum benefits of asanas and pranayama. Those who practise by fits and starts will not derive much benefit. Generally people practise for two months in the beginning with great enthusiasm and leave off the practice. This is a sad mistake. They always want a yoga teacher by their side. They have got the effeminate leaning mentality. They are lazy, torpid and slothful.

18. People do not want to remove mala (impurity) by selfless service, and tossing of the mind by yoga practices. They at once jump to awaken the kundalini and raise Brahmakara vritti. They will only break their legs. Those who attempt to awaken the kundalini by asanas and pranayama should have purity in thought, word and deed. They should have mental and physical brahmacharya. Then only they can enjoy the benefits of awakening the kundalini.

19. Sow the seed of spirituality in your young age. Do not waste veerya. Discipline the senses and mind. Do sadhana. When you become old, it will be difficult for you to do any rigid sadhana. Therefore be on the alert during your teens; you will see for yourself in a short time the particular benefits you derive from particular kinds of sadhana.

20. Everyone should select a course of a few exercises in asana, pranayama and meditation according to his temperament, capacity, convenience and requirement.

21. It is quite possible for a man to practise celibacy, albeit there are various sorts of temptations and distractions. A well-disciplined life, study of scriptures, satsang, japa, dhyana, pranayama, sattvic and

moderate diet, daily introspection and enquiry, self-analysis and self-correction, right conduct and practice of yama, niyama, physical and verbal tapas, will all pave a long way in the attainment of this end. People have irregular, unrighteous, immoderate, irreligious, undisciplined life. Hence they suffer and fail in the attainment of the goal of life. Just as the elephant throws sand on its own head, so also they themselves bring difficulties and troubles on their own heads on account of their foolishness.

22. Do not shake the body unnecessarily. By shaking the body often the mind also is disturbed. Do not scratch the body every now and then. The asana should be steady and firm as a rock when you do pranayama, japa and meditation.

23. You must find out for yourself according to your health and constitution what sort of dietetic regulation will suit and what particular pranayama will exactly help you. Then only can you safely proceed with your sadhana. First read all the instructions of the various exercises given in this book from the beginning to the end. Clearly understand the technique. If you have any doubts, just ask any yoga student to demonstrate and then practise it. This is the safest method. You should not select any one of the exercises at random and begin to practise it in a wrong way.

24. In all the exercises I have suggested the mantra 'OM' is the time-unit. You can have your guru mantra, Rama, Siva, Gayatri or mere number as the time-unit according to your inclination. Gayatri or OM is the best for pranayama.

In the beginning you must observe some time-unit for inhalation, retention and exhalation. The time-unit and the proper ratio come by themselves when you do them as long as you comfortably can. When you have advanced in the practice you need not count or keep any unit. You will be naturally established in the normal ratio through force of habit.

25. For some days in the beginning you must count the number and see how you progress. In the advanced stages, you need not distract the mind in counting. The lungs will tell you when the required number is finished.

26. Do not continue the pranayama when you are fatigued. There must be always joy and exhilaration of spirit during and after the practice. You should come out of the practice fully invigorated and refreshed. Do not bind yourself by too many rules.

27. Do not take a bath immediately after pranayama is over. Take some rest for half an hour. If you get perspiration during the practice, do not wipe it with a towel. Rub it with your hands. Do not expose the body to the chill draughts of air when you perspire.

28. Always inhale and exhale very slowly. Do not make any sound. In pranayamas like bhastrika, kapalabhati, sitali and sitkari, you can produce the lowest possible sound.

29. You should not expect the benefits after doing pranayama for two or three minutes only for a day or two. At least you must have fifteen minutes daily practice in the beginning regularly for days together. There will be no use if you jump from one exercise to another every day. You must have a particular exercise for your daily practice, which you should improve to a high degree. Other exercises, of course, you can have for occasional practice along with the daily exercise. You must have bhastrika, kapalabhati, and 'Easy Comfortable Pranayama' for your daily practice, and sitali and sitkari, etc. can be practised occasionally.

30. Inhalation is otherwise known as 'hisswasa' and exhalation is known as 'uchhwasa'. The mental process in kevala kumbhaka is called 'sunyaka' form of breath regulation. Steady, systematic practice and gradual increase of kumbhaka is known as 'abhyasa yoga'. Swallowing of air and living on this air alone is known as 'vayubhakshana'.

31. This is called kumbhaka (cessation of breath) when there is neither expiration nor inspiration and the body is motionless, remaining still in one state. 'Then he sees forms like the blind, hears sounds like the deaf, and sees the body like wood. This is the characteristic of one who has attained quiescence.'

32. Patanjali does not lay much stress on practice of different kinds of pranayama. He mentions: 'Exhale slowly, then inhale and retain the breath. You will get a steady and calm mind'. It is only the hatha yogis who developed pranayama as a science and have mentioned various exercises to suit different persons.

33. Some would take the order as exhaling, inhaling and retaining, others as inhaling, retaining and exhaling. The latter is much common. In Yajnavalkya, we find the different kinds of breath regulation mentioned in the order of inhalation (puraka), retention (kumbhaka) and exhalation (rechaka), whereas, in the Naradiya text we have them in the order of exhalation (rechaka), inhalation (puraka) and retention (kumbhaka). The two are to be regarded as optional.

34. A yogi should always avoid fear, anger, laziness, too much sleep or waking and too much food or fasting. If the above rule be well and strictly practised each day, spiritual wisdom will arise of itself in three months without doubt; in four months he sees the devas; in five months he becomes established in the direct knowledge of Brahman; and truly in six months he attains kaivalya at will. There is no doubt.

35. A neophyte should do inhalation and exhalation only, without any retention for some days. Take a long time to do inhalation. The proportion for inhalation and exhalation is 1:2.

36. Pranayama in its popular and preparatory form may be practised by everyone in any posture whatsoever, sitting or walking; and yet it is sure to show its benefits. But to those who practise it in accordance with the specific methods prescribed, fructification will be rapid.

37. Gradually increase the period of retention. Retain for four seconds in the first week, for eight seconds in the second week, for twelve seconds in the third week and so on, till you are able to retain the breath to your full capacity.

38. Commonsense should be used throughout your practice. If one kind of exercise is not agreeable to your system, change it after due consideration or consultation with your guru. This is commonsense. Where there is commonsense there is enjoyment, perfection and salvation.

39. You must nicely adjust the inhalation, retention and exhalation so that you should not experience the feeling of suffocation or discomfort at any stage of pranayama. You should never feel the necessity of catching a few normal breaths between any two successive rounds. The duration of inhalation, retention and exhalation must be properly adjusted. Exercise due care and attention. Matters will turn to be successful and easy.

40. You must not unnecessarily prolong the period of exhalation. If you do, the following inhalation will be done in hurried manner and the rhythm will be disturbed. You must so carefully regulate the kumbhaka that it is absolutely comfortable and you can perform not only one pranayama but also the full course or required rounds of pranayama. Experience and practice will make you alright. Practice makes one perfect. Be steady. Another important factor is that you must have efficient control over the lungs at the end of retention (kumbhaka) to enable you to do the exhalation smoothly and in proportion with the

inhalation.

41. Suryabheda and ujjayi produce heat. Sitkari and sitali are cooling. Bhastrika preserves normal temperature. Suryabheda destroys the excess of wind, ujjayi phlegm, sitkari and sitali bile, and bhastrika all the three.

42. Suryabheda and ujjayi must be practised during winter. Sitkari and sitali must be practised in summer. Bhastrika can be practised in all seasons. Those persons whose bodies are hot even in winter can practise sitali and sitkari during winter season.

43. The goal of life is Self-realisation. If you are really sincere and if you wish to have a quick, sure success, you must have a systematic routine for asana, pranayama, japa, meditation, study, etc. You must be very careful in keeping up brahmacharya. 'The effective means to control the mind are the attainment of spiritual knowledge, association with the wise, the entire abandonment of all vasanas and control of prana.' (*Muktikopanishad.*)

44. Some students who are studying vedantic books think that they are jnanis and they ignore asana, pranayama, etc. They also should practise these, till they are perfect in the preliminary qualifications of jnana yoga, e.g. tranquillity, control, renunciation, endurance, faith and concentration.

45. Do not hesitate. Do not be waiting to get a guru who will sit by your side and watch you daily for a long time. If you are sincere, regular and systematic and if you follow the rules and instructions of this book very carefully, there will be no trouble at all. You will undoubtedly get success. Slight errors may crop up in the beginning, it does not matter. Do not unnecessarily be alarmed. Do not give up the practice. You will yourself learn how to adjust. Commonsense, instinct and the shrill inner voice of the soul will help you in the path. Everything will come out smoothly in the end. Start the practice this very second in right earnest and become a real yogi.

The Aspirant's Daily Routine

Here is an ideal daily routine for whole-time aspirants. He who adheres to this routine will easily attain psychic powers within a year.

Get up at 4 a.m. Clean your teeth, hands, feet and face. Go into your room. All the time repeating your mantra, sit down on your mat. (The ideal seat has been described in the *Bhagavad Gita* as kusa-grass, deer skin and cloth placed one over the other.) Recite some hymns to the guru, meditate upon him and pray to him for success in your practice. Then commence the practice of asanas. Whenever you feel fatigued, do savasana (deep relaxation) for a few minutes. Conclude this practice with viparita karani. Once again seat yourself. Meditate upon your guru once again and commence the practice of pranayama, sitting on siddhasana or padmasana. Perform at least ten pranayamas to begin with (gradually increasing the number to eighty). After this, practise the kumbhakas, commencing with kevala kumbhaka by the right and then the left nadis. Then suryabheda, ujjayi, sitkari, sitali and bhastrika, etc. These should be followed by the mudras. After this, practise concentration; you will easily be able to hear the *anahata sounds now. At the conclusion of this practice, offer your practice to the Lord as an offering.

This is the routine, and all these should be done four times a day — in brahmamuhurtha (1½ hours before sunrise), at midday, in the evening and at midnight.

After the brahmamuhurtha practice is concluded, take a bath in lukewarm water and then engage yourself in your daily duties. After the midday practice, take a little rest and then take your meals. After this, engage yourself in the study of sacred books, or do japa. Commence your evening practice an hour and a half before sunset. (Viparita karani should not be practised either in the evening or after a meal.)

Padmasana and siddhasana are meant for japa and meditation. Vajrasana may suit some for this, and all will find it beneficial to practise for fifteen minutes after every meal.

---

* See section on Kundalini

General Order of Practice

Asana	Min. Duration	Max. Duration
Sirshasana:	10 mins	15 mins
Sarvangasana:	10 mins	15 mins
Halasana:	Repeat 3 or 4 times	
Matsyasana:	3 mins	4 mins
Paschimottanasana:	Repeat 4 or 5 times	
Bhujangasana:	Repeat 4 or 5 times	
Salabhasana:	Repeat 4 or 5 times	
Dhanurasana:	Repeat 4 or 5 times	
Ardhamatsyendrasana:	Repeat the asana twice both ways	
Mayurasana:	As long as possible	
Padahasthasana:	Repeat 3 to 4 times	
Trikonasana:	Twice	
Chakrasana:	Twice	
Savasana:	5 to 10 minutes	
Kapalabhati:	4 rounds	10 rounds
Pranayama:	20 rounds	40 rounds
Ujjayi:	10 rounds	20 rounds
Bhastrika:	5 rounds	10 rounds
Sitali:	10 rounds	20 rounds
Mahamudra:	6 rounds	12 rounds
Mahavedha:	6 rounds	12 rounds

Then, concentration and meditation.

Nauli:	6 times	10 times
Mula bandha:	6 times	10 times
Jalandhara bandha:	6 times	10 times
Uddiyana bandha:	6 times	10 times

Section III

Kundalini

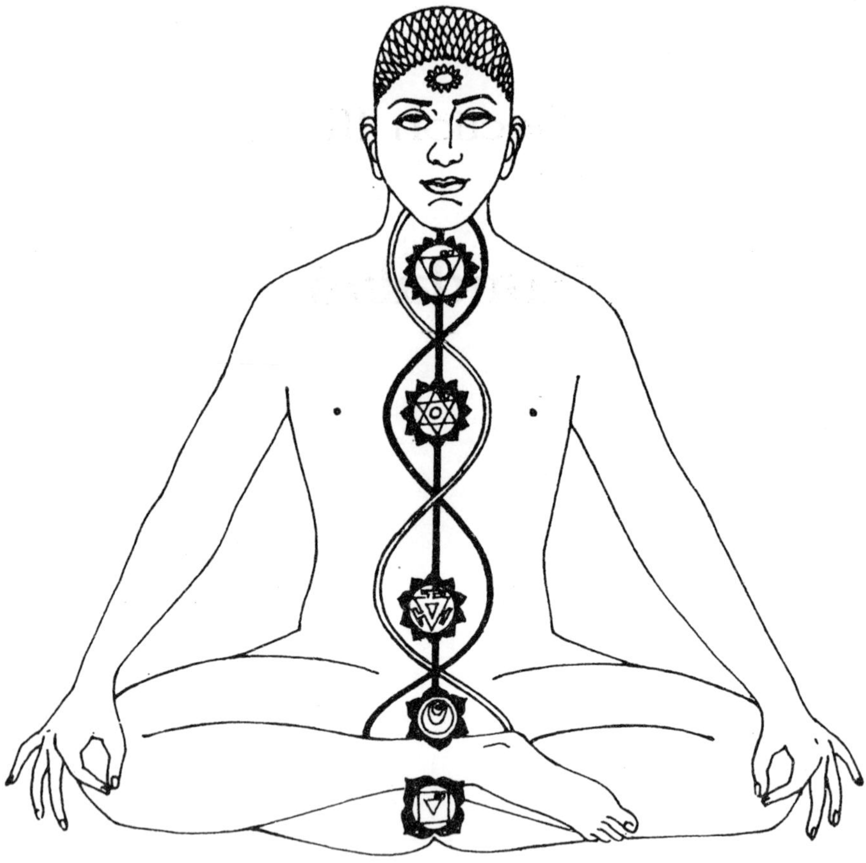

The chakras and ida, pingala and sushumna nadis

KUNDALINI

There are two main lines of yoga — dhyana (where meditation is the main discipline) and kundalini yoga — and there is a marked difference between the two. The first class of yoga is that in which samadhi is obtained by intellectual processes of meditation and the like, possibly with the aid of auxiliary processes of mantra, hatha yoga (other than the rousing of kundalini) and by detachment from the world; the second stands apart as that portion of hatha yoga in which, though intellectual processes are not neglected, the creative and sustaining shakti of the whole body is actually united with the Supreme Consciousness. The two forms of yoga differ in method and result.

Kundalini is so renowned that many seek to know Her. Having studied the theory of this yoga, one may ask: "Can one get on without it?" The answer is: "It depends upon what you are looking for." If you want to rouse kundalini shakti, to enjoy the bliss of union of Siva and shakti through Her, and to gain the accompanying powers (siddhis), it is obvious that this end can be achieved only by kundalini yoga. In that case there are some risks incurred. But if liberation is sought without desire for union through kundalini, then such yoga is not necesary; for liberation may be obtained by pure dhyana. Both are realisation; but whilst liberation is attainable by either method, there are other marked differences between the two. A dhyana yogi should not neglect his body, knowing that as he is both mind and matter, each reacts one upon the other. Neglect or mere mortification of the body is more apt to produce disordered imagination than a true spiritual experience. He is not concerned, however, with the body in the sense that the hatha yogi is. It is possible to be a successful dhyana yogi and yet to be weak in body, sick and short-lived.

Hatha yoga builds up its philosophy around kundalini, and the methods adopted are different from tantrik sadhana to which kundalini yoga actually belongs. Hatha yoga seeks to awaken kundalini through the discipline of the physical body, purification of nadis and controlling the prana. Through the asanas it tones up the entire nervous system and brings it under the conscious control of the yogi; through bandhas and mudras it controls the prana, regulates its movements and even blocks and seals it without allowing it to move; through kriyas it purifies the inner organs of the physical body; and, finally, through pranayama it brings the mind itself under the control of the yogi. The kundalini is made to go upwards to the sahasrara through these combined methods.

Before one studies kundalini yoga a knowledge of the nadis (ida, pingala and sushumna), chakras and kundalini is necessary.

Nadis

Nadis are astral tubes, made up of astral matter, that carry pranic currents. They can be seen by astral eyes only. They are not nerves. They arise from the kanda, which is the size and the shape of a bird's egg and lies above the genital organ and below the navel.

In the body of a human being the total number of nadis is 72,000. Of these the ten most important ones are ida, pingala, sushumna, gandhari, hastajihva, pusha, yasasvini, alambusha, kuhu and sankhini.

When the nadis have become purified through the practice of pranayama, lightness of the body, brilliance of complexion, increase of the digestive fire, leanness of the body and absence of restlessness are noticed.

Ida and Pingala

Ida and pingala nadis are situated on either side of the spinal column. Ida starts from the left testical, and pingala from the right. (Some take these tentatively as the right and left sympathetic cords, but they are really subtle tubes that carry prana.) The moon moves in the ida and the sun in the pingala. Ida is cooling, pingala is heating. The moon is of the nature of tamas and the sun is that of rajas. Ida flows through the left nostril and pingala through the right nostril. The breath flows through the left nostril for one hour and through the right nostril for one hour.

Ida and pingala meet with sushumna nadi at the muladhara chakra, and make a knot there. This meeting place is called brahma granthi. They meet again at the anahata and ajna chakras (see diagram).

Ida and pingala indicate time. Sushumna is the consumer of time. The yogi knows the time of his death. He takes his prana into sushumna, keeps it in brahmarandhra and defies time (death). [The famous yogi Sri Chang Dev of Maharashtra fought against death several times by taking the prana into sushumna. He was a contemporary of Sri Jnana Dev of Alandi, near Poona. It was he who had bhuta siddhi (control over wild animals) through his yogic practices. He came on the back of a tiger to see Sri Jnana Dev.]

Sushumna

The psychic nerve that is lodged in the hollow of the spinal column (brahma danda) is the chief nadi. It is called the sushumna nadi. It is the sustainer of the universe, the path of the universe and the path of salvation. Situated at the back of the anus, it is attached to the spinal column and extends to the brahmarandhra of the head, and is invisible and subtle. It runs along the length of the spinal cord or spinal column. The real work of a yogi begins when sushumna begins to function. A yogi tries his level best to make the prana run in the sushumna nadi (which is also known as the central brahma nadi). When prana moves in the sushumna, sit for meditation. You will have deep meditation.

Through the practice of pranayama the prana leaves the passages of ida and pingala and forces itself through the mouth of the sushumna and enters therein. Sushumna is the only passage through which, when the prana passes, the light of jnana is kindled. When the prana moves through the sushumna, the mind becomes steady. This steadiness of the mind is termed 'unmani avastha'. All the seeds of karma of the yogi are thereby burnt away.

If the coiled up energy, kundalini, passes up along the sushumna nadi and is taken up from chakra to chakra, the yogi gets different experiences, powers and bliss. When united with the pure mind, the sushumna nadi awakens one from his slumber of ignorance.

Chakras

Chakras are centres of spiritual energy. In other words, these are centres of prana-shakti manifested by prana-vayu in the living body, the presiding devatas of which are the names for the Universal Consciousness as It manifests in the form of these centres. They are also called padmas (lotuses) in Sanskrit. Located in the astral body, the chakras are not perceptible to the gross senses. Even if they were perceptible in the living body which they help to organise, they disappear with the disintegration of the organism at death. Only a clairvoyant can see them with his astral eyes. Tentatively, they correspond to certain plexuses in the physical body.

The chakras have corresponding centres in the spinal cord and the nerve-plexuses in the gross body. Each chakra has control and function over a particular centre in the gross body. (Some foolish doctors search for the chakras in the physical body. They cannot find them there. Since they cannot find any chakra in a dead body, they lose faith in yoga scriptures and kriyas.)

Subtle prana moves in the nervous system of the astral body, and gross prana moves in the nervous system of the gross physical body. The two are intimately connected and they act and react upon each other. The chakras are in the astral body even after the disintegration of the physical organism at death. According to one school of thought the chakras are formed during concentration and meditation only. This is not possible. The chakras should exist there in a subtle state, as the gross matter is the result of the subtle matter. Without that the gross body is impossible. (The meaning of this sentence should be taken to be that one can feel and understand the chakras during concentration and meditation only.)

Wherever there is an interlacing of several nerves, arteries and veins, that centre is called a plexus. (The physical gross plexuses — hepatic, cervical, brachial, coccygeal, lumbar, sacral, cardiac, epigastric, esophageal, pharyngeal, pulmonary, lingual, prostatic, etc.) Similarly there are plexuses or centres of subtle prana in the sushumna nadi. All the functions of the body — nervous, digestive, circulatory, respiratory, genito-urinary and all other systems of the body — are under the control of these centres in sushumna. They are subtle centres of vital energy and the centres of consciousness. These subtle centres of sushumna have their corresponding centres in the physical body. For example, anahata chakra, which is in the sushumna nadi, has its corresponding centre in the physical body at the heart (cardiac plexus).

At every chakra a particular element preponderates, and there is a presiding deity. In each one a certain animal is represented, which denotes that the centre has the qualities of that particular animal.

There are six important chakras: muladhara, svadhishthana, manipura, anahata, vishuddha and ajna; while sahasrara, situated at the crown of the head, is the chief chakra. Muladhara, svadhisthana, manipura, anahata and vishuddha are the centres of the five elements: earth, water, fire, air and ether, respectively. Ajna chakra represents the mind. The deities presiding over these mandalas also symbolically wield several weapons.

Petals on Chakras

Each chakra has a particular number of petals with a letter of the Sanskrit alphabet on each petal. The vibration that is produced at each petal is represented by the corresponding Sanskrit letter. The letters exist in the petals in a latent form and can be manifested, and the vibrations of the nadis felt, during concentration.

The number of petals of the lotuses varies. Muladhara, svadhishthana, manipura, anahata, vishuddha and ajna chakras have 4, 6, 10, 12, 16 and 2 petals respectively. All the 50 Sanskrit letters are on the 50 petals. The number of petals in each chakra is determined by the number and position of the yoga nadis around the chakra. I will make it still clearer. From each chakra a particular number of yoga nadis crop up. The chakra gives the appearance of a lotus with the nadis as its petals. The sound produced by the vibrations of the yoga nadis is represented by the corresponding Sanskrit letter. The chakras with their petals hang downwards when kundalini is at the muladhara chakra. When it is awakened, they turn upwards towards the crown of the head. They always face the side of kundalini.

Muladhara Chakra

Muladhara chakra is located at the base of the spinal column. It lies between the origin of the reproductory organ and the anus. It is just below the kanda (the source of all nadis) and the junction where ida, pingala and sushumna nadis meet. Two fingers above the anus, about two fingers below the genitals and four fingers in width, is the space where the muladhara chakra is situated. This is the suppport, as the other chakras are above this. Kundalini, which gives power and energy to all the chakras, lies at this chakra. Hence this, which is the support of all, is called muladhara chakra. The sacral plexus tentatively corresponds to this chakra.

From this chakra four important nadis emanate, giving the appearance of petals of a lotus. The subtle vibrations that are made by each nadi are represented by the Sanskrit letters: vam, sam, sham and sam. Here kundalini lies dormant. This chakra represents the earth element. The yellow square in the chakra is the symbol for the earth element. The bija mantra is 'lam', and the animal is the elephant. Brahma granthi or the knot of Brahma is in this chakra.

The wise yogi who concentrates and meditates on the muladhara chakra acquires the full knowledge of kundalini and the means to awaken it. When kundalini is awakened he gets the power to rise from the ground. He can control the breath, mind and semen. His prana enters the sushumna nadi. All his sins are destroyed. He acquires knowledge of the past, present and future. He enjoys natural bliss (sahaja ananda).

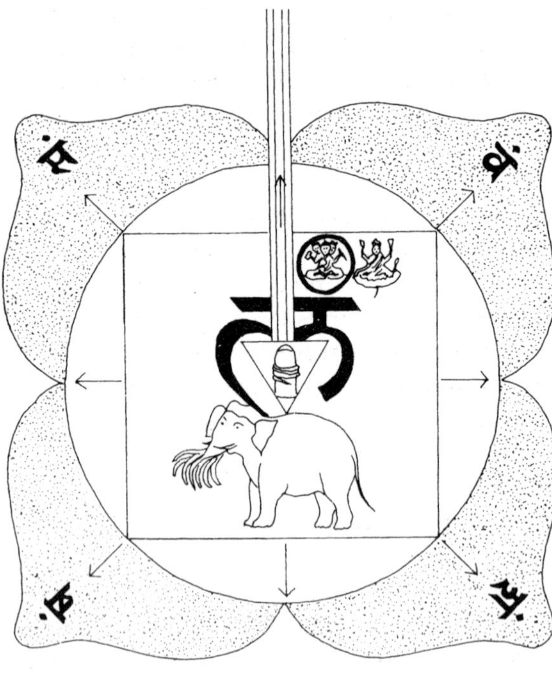

Muladhara Chakra

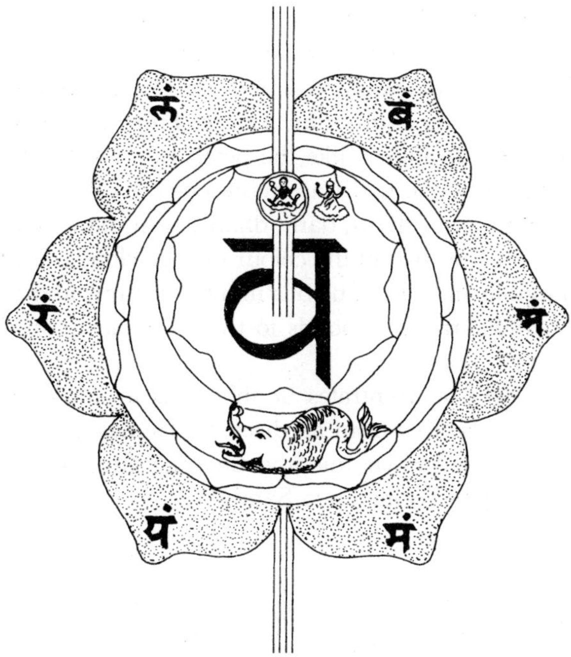

Svadhishthana Chakra

Svadhishthana Chakra.

Svadhishthana chakra is located within the sushumna nadi at the root of the reproductory organ. It has control over the lower abdomen, kidneys, etc. This chakra represents the water element. The animal is the alligator. Within this chakra there is a space like a crescent moon. The bija mantra is 'vam', and the colour of the chakra is pure blood-red. Its corresponding plexus is the prostate plexus. From this centre six yoga nadis emanate like the petals of a lotus. The vibrations that are produced by the nadis are represented by the Sanskrit letters: bam, bham, bam, yam, ram and lam.

He who concentrates at this chakra and meditates on the presiding devata has no fear of water. He has perfect control over the water element. He gets many psychic powers, intuitional knowledge and a perfect control over his senses. He has full knowledge of the astral entities. Lust, anger and greed and other impure qualities are completely annihilated. The yogi becomes the conqueror of death.

Manipura Chakra

Manipura is the third chakra from the muladhara. It is located within the sushumna nadi, in the region of navel. It has its corresponding centre in the physical body and has control over the liver, stomach, etc. It is a very important centre. From this chakra emanate ten yoga nadis which appear like the petals of a lotus. The vibrations that are produced by the nadis are represented by the Sanskrit letters: dam, dham, nam, tam, tham, dam, dham, nam, pam and pham. The chakra represents fire. It is of the colour of dark clouds. Within there is a space, triangular in form. The bija mantra is 'ram', and the animal is the ram. This chakra corresponds to the solar plexus in the physical body.

The yogi who concentrates at this chakra can acquire hidden treasures and will be free from all diseases. He has no fear at all from fire. 'Even if he is thrown into the burning fire, he remains alive without fear of death.' (Gheranda Samhita).

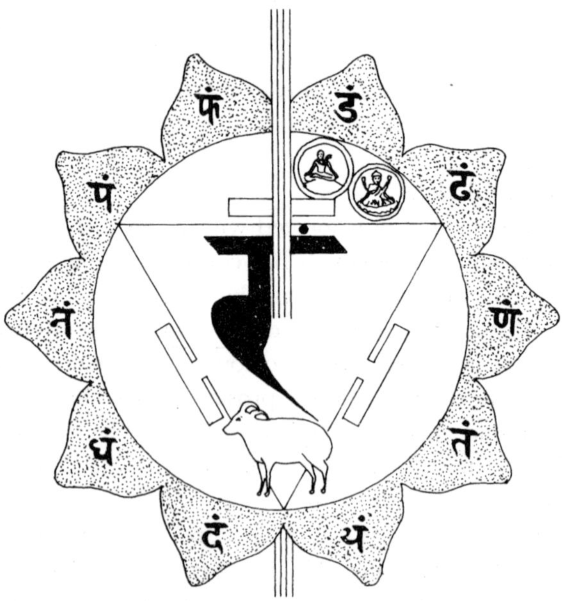

Manipura Chakra

Anahata Chakra

Anahata chakra is situated in the sushumna nadi. It corresponds to the cardiac plexus in the physical body and has control over the heart. The chakra is of deep red colour. Within it there is a hexagonal space of smokey or deep black colour. This chakra is the region of the air element. The animal is the black antelope. The sound that is produced by each nadi is represented by the following Sanskrit letters: kam, kham, gam, gham, gnam, cham, chham, jam, jham, jnam, tam and tham. 'Yam' is the bija mantra here. It is like the wish-fulfilling tree. Anahata sound is heard at this centre. You can very clearly hear this when you intently concentrate at this centre. When you do sirshasana for a long time, you can distinctly hear this sound. Vishnu granthi is in this chakra.

He who meditates on this chakra has full control over the air element. He gets the ability to fly in air, enter the body of another, etc. He gets cosmic love and all other pure divine qualities.

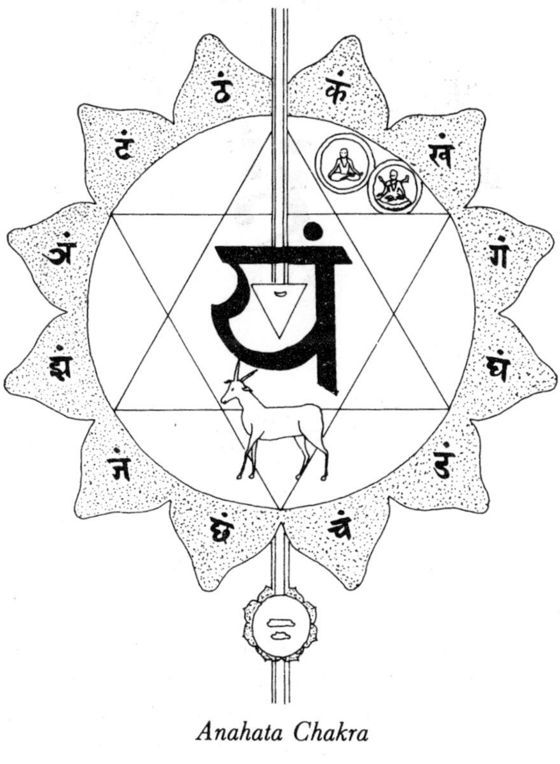

Anahata Chakra

Vishuddha Chakra

Vishuddha chakra is situated within the sushumna nadi at the base of the throat. It represents the ether element. It is of pure blue colour. From the centre emanate 16 yoga nadis which appear like the petals of a lotus. The vibrations that are produced by the nadis are represented by the 16 Sanskrit vowels. The animal is the elephant. The mandala is round in shape like the full-moon and is white in colour. The bija mantra is 'ham'. This chakra corresponds to the laryngeal plexus in the physical body.

He who practises concentration on this chakra will not perish. He attains the highest success and gets the full knowledge of the four *Vedas* by meditating on this chakra. He becomes a trikala jnani (one who knows the past, the present and the future).

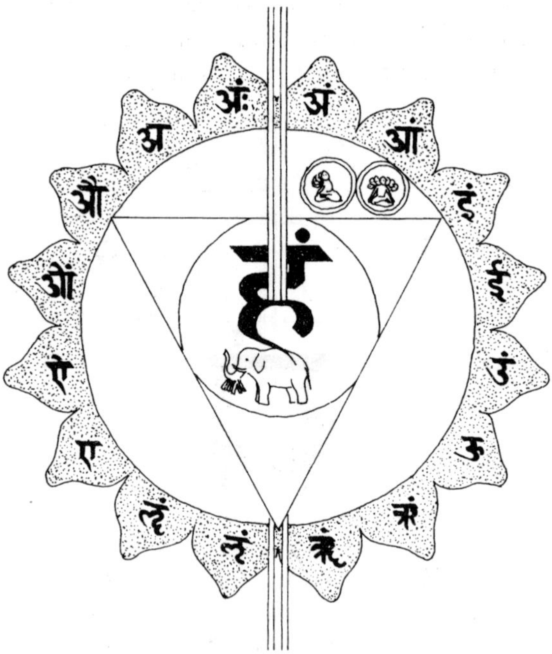

Vishuddha Chakra

Ajna Chakra

Ajna Chakra is situated within the sushumna nadi, and its corresponding centre in the physical body is at the space between the two eye-brows, which is known as trikuti. Pranava (OM) is the bija mantra for this chakra. This is the seat of the mind. There are two

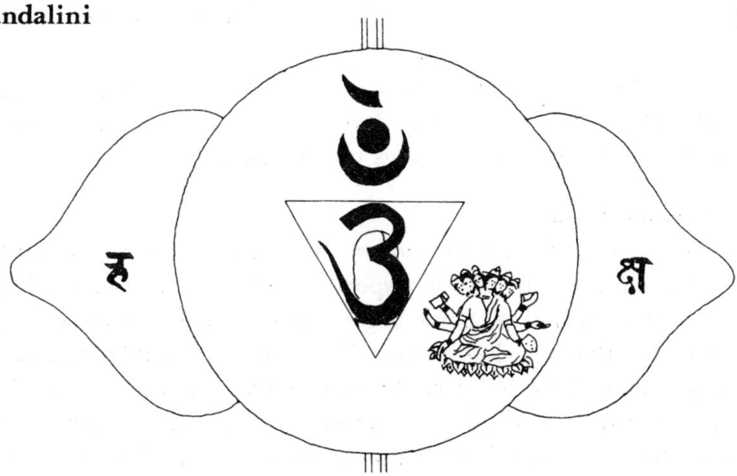

Ajna Chakra

petals (yoga nadis) on each side of the chakra and the vibrations of these nadis are represented by the Sanskrit letters ham and ksham. This is the Rudra granthi. The chakra is of pure white colour or like that of the full-moon. There is neither geometrical design nor animal. The corresponding centre in the physical body is at the cavernous plexus.

He who concentrates at this centre destroys all the karmas of the past lives. The benefits that are derived by meditation on this chakra cannot be described in words. The practitioner becomes a jivanmukta (liberated while living). He acquires all the 8 major and 32 minor siddhis. All yogis and jnanis, too, concentrate at this centre on the bija mantra OM. This is called bhrumadhya drishti (gazing at the space between the two eye-brows).

Sahasrara

The seventh chakra is known as sahasrara, and contains a thousand petals. It is located at the top of the head. The fontanelle that is located at the crown of the head is called the brahmarandhra, or hole of Brahman. It is very prominent in a new-born baby, when it is like a thin membrane. This changes to bone as the child grows. It corresponds to the sahasrara, and is the abode of the human soul. It bursts open in a fully developed yogi when his prana leaves the body through this hole at the time of his leaving the physical body. Yogis call it sukha-mandala, the space of happiness. Kundalini unites with Lord Siva here.

Just as electricity is stored in dynamos, so also the vital force or prana is stored in the chakras and the sushumna nadi. Prana plays a vital part in all psycho-physical processes. A detailed knowledge of nadis and chakras is necessary for a student who is treading the path of kundalini yoga. Only then can he have contemplation on these chakras. Meditation on these chakras brings psychic powers.

Chakra Concentration

A hatha yogi fixes his mind on the sushumna nadi, the middle path in the spinal canal, and on a specified centre, viz., the muladhara, manipura or ajna chakra. Some yogis ignore the lower chakras and fix their mind on the ajna chakra only. Their theory is that by controlling the ajna chakra all the lower chakras can be automatically controlled.

When you concentrate on a chakra, a threadlike connection is formed in the beginning between the mind and the chakra. The ascent along the sushumna from chakra to chakra is made gradually by patient efforts.

When the opening of the sushumna is shaken a bit, the kundalini shakti tries to enter the sushumna. Even this mere shaking of the opening of the sushumna causes a great deal of bliss. You become intoxicated. You will entirely forget the world. Great dispassion arises. You will become fearless. You will behold various visions, and witness the splendid inner light. You will get different siddhis, different types of bliss and different kinds of knowledge by controlling and operating on different chakras. For instance, if you have conquered the manipura chakra, you have already conquered fire. Fire will not burn you. [Panchadharana (five kinds of concentrations) will help you conquer the five elements. Learn them under a guru who is an adept yogi.]

What is Kundalini?

Kundalini shakti is the source for all occult powers. It is the coiled-up sleeping divine shakti that lies dormant in all beings. This mysterious kundalini lies face downwards at the mouth of the sushumna nadi. It has three and a half coils like a serpent. When it is awakened it makes a hissing sound like that of a serpent beaten with a stick, and proceeds to the other chakras through the brahma nadi (which is also called the chitra nadi) within sushumna. Hence kundalini is also called bhujangini or serpent power. The three coils represent the three gunas of prakriti – sattva, rajas and tamas — and the half represents the vikriti, the modification of prakriti.

If you are pure and free from all desires, kundalini will awaken by itself.

Need for a Guru

In olden days the aspirants were required to live with the guru for a number of years, so that the guru could study them thoroughly. The food during practice, what to practise and how, whether the students are qualified for the path of yoga, and the temperament of the aspirants and other important items have to be considered and judged by the guru. It is the guru who should decide whether the aspirants are of inferior, middling or superior type and fix different kinds of exercises. Sadhana differs according to the nature, capacity and qualifications of the aspirants. After understanding the theory of yoga, you will have to learn the practice from an experienced yogic guru.

For the practice of bhakti and vedanta you do not require a guru always by your side. After learning the scriptures from a guru for some time you will have to reflect and meditate alone in entire seclusion.

So long as there is the world, there are books on yoga and teachers also. You will have to search for them with faith, devotion and earnestness. You can get easy lessons from the guru and practise them at home also in the initial stages of practice. When you advance a bit, for advanced and difficult exercises you will have to stay with the guru. The personal contact with the guru has manifold advantages. You will be highly benefited by the spiritual magnetic aura of your guru.

In kundalini yoga you will have to break up the granthis (knots) and take the kundalini from chakra to chakra. These are all quite difficult processes. The method of uniting the apana and prana and sending it along the sushumna and breaking the granthis needs the help of a guru. You will have to sit at the guru's feet for a pretty long time. You will have to understand thoroughly the location of the nadis, chakras and the detailed technique of the several yogic kriyas.

Lay bare to your guru the secrets of your heart. The more you do the greater the sympathy and help you get from him. This sympathy means accession of strength to you in the struggle against sin and temptation.

'Learn thou this by discipleship, by investigation and by service. The wise, the seers of the essence of things will instruct thee in wisdom.' (*Bhagavad Gita*).

Some do meditation for some years independently. Later on they feel the necessity for a guru. They come across some obstacles or impediments, dangers, snares and pitfalls on the spiritual path. They may commit errors in sadhana also. It is very necessary to have a guru who has already trodden the path and reached the goal.

A guru is one who has full Self-illumination and who removes the veil of ignorance in deluded jivas. The number of realised souls may be less in this Kali Yuga when compared with the Satya Yuga, but they are always present to help the aspirants and they are always searching for the proper students.

Guru is Brahman Himself. Guru is Ishvara Himself. Guru is God. A word from him is a word from God. He need not teach. Even his mere presence or company is elevating, inspiring and soul-stirring. His very company itself is self-illumination, and living in his company is spiritual education. That which comes out of his lips is all *Vedas* or gospel-truth. His very life is an embodiment of *Vedas*.

The guru is your guide or spiritual preceptor, real father, mother, brother, relative and intimate friend. He is an embodiment of mercy and love. His tender smile radiates light, bliss, joy, knowledge and peace. He is a blessing to suffering humanity. Whatever he talks is upanishadic teaching. He knows the spiritual path, the pitfalls and snares on the way. He gives warning to the aspirants and removes obstacles on the path. He imparts spiritual strength to the students and showers his grace on their heads. He even takes their prarabdha (karma) on his own head. He is the ocean of mercy. All agonies, miseries, tribulations, taints of worldliness, etc., vanish in his presence.

A guru can awaken the kundalini of an aspirant through sight, touch, speech or mere thought. He can transmit spirituality to the student just as one gives an orange to another. When the guru gives a mantra to his disciples, he gives it with his own power and purity.

It is the guru who transmutes the little jiva-hood into great Brahman-hood. It is he who overhauls the old, wrong, vicious samskaras of the aspirants and awakens them to the attainment of the knowledge of Self. It is he who uplifts the jivas from the quagmire of body and worldly existence; removes the veil of ignorance, all doubts, infatuation and fear; awakens kundalini and opens the inner eye of intuition.

Mere study of books cannot make one a guru. Only one who has studied *Vedas* and who has direct knowledge of Atman can be considered a guru. If you can find peace in the presence of a mahatma and if your doubts are removed by his very presence you can take him as your guru.

The guru tests all the students in various ways. Some students misunderstand him and lose their faith in him. Hence, they are not benefited. Those who stand the tests boldly come out successful in the end. In days of yore the tests were very severe. Once Gorakhnath asked some of his students to climb up a tall tree and throw themselves head downwards on a very sharp trident. Many faithless students kept quiet, but one faithful student at once climbed up the tree with lightning speed and threw himself down. He was protected by the invisible hand of Gorakhnath. He had immediate Self-realisation. He had no attachment for his body. The other faithless students had strong attachment to their body and their own ignorance (avidya).

There is good deal of heated debate and controversy amongst many people on the matter of the necessity of a guru. Some of them assert with vehemence and force that a preceptor is not at all necessary for Self-realisation and spiritual advancement, and that one can have spiritual progress and Self-illumination through one's own efforts only. They quote various passages from scriptures and assign arguments and reasonings to support them. Others boldly assert with greater emphasis and force that no spiritual progress is possible for a man, however intelligent he may be, however hard he may attempt and struggle in the spiritual path, unless he gets the benign grace and direct guidance of a spiritual preceptor.

Now, open your eyes and watch carefully what is going on in this world in all walks of life. Even a cook needs a teacher. He serves under a senior cook for some years and obeys him implicitly. He pleases his teacher in all possible ways and learns all the techniques in cooking. He gets knowledge through the grace of his senior cook, his teacher. A junior lawyer wants the help and guidance of a senior advocate; students of mathematics and medicine need the help and guidance of a professor; a student of science, music and astronomy wants the guidance of a scientist and musician and an astronomer. When such is the case with ordinary secular knowledge, then what to speak of the inner spiritual path, wherein the student has to walk alone with closed eyes? When you are in a thick jungle and you come across several crossing footpaths you are in a dilemma. You do not know the directions and by which path you should go. You are bewildered. You want a guide here to direct you in the right path. It is universally admitted that an efficient teacher is needed in all branches of knowledge in this physical plane, and that physical, mental and moral culture and growth can only be had through the help and guidance of a capable master. This is a universal inexorable law of nature. Why do you deny then, friend, the application of this universally accepted law in the realm of spirituality?

Spiritual knowledge is handed down from a guru to his disciple. Study *Brihadaranyaka Upanishad*. You will have a comprehensive understanding. Gaudapadacharya imparted Self-knowledge to his disciple Govindacharya; Govindacharya to his disciple Sankaracharya; Sankaracharya to his disciple Gorakhnath; Gorakhnath to Nivrittinath; Nivrittinath to Jnana Dev. Totapuri imparted knowledge to Ramakrishna; Ramakrishna to Vivekananda. It was Ashtavakra who moulded the life of Rajah Janaka. It was Gorakhnath who shaped the spiritual destiny of Rajah Bhartrihari. It was Lord Krishna who made Arjuna and Uddhava establish themselves in the spiritual path when their minds were in an unsettled condition.

The student and the teacher should live together as father and devoted son with extreme sincerity and devotion. The aspirant should have an eager, receptive attitude to imbibe the teachings of the master. Then only will he be spiritually benefited; otherwise there is not the least hope of spiritual life for the aspirant, or complete regeneration of his old nature.

It is a great pity that the present system of education in India is not favourable to the spiritual growth of seekers. The minds of the students are saturated with materialistic poison. Aspirants of the present day have not got any idea of the true relationship of guru and a disciple. It is not like the relationship of a student and teacher or professor in schools and colleges. Spiritual relationship is entirely different. It involves dedication. It is very sacred. It is purely divine.

The Time

It is stated in *Gheranda Samhita* that yogic practices should not be commenced in winter, summer and rainy seasons, but only in spring and autumn. This depends upon the temperature of the particular place and the strength of the individual. Generally cool hours are best suited. In hot places you should not practise during the day. Early morning hours are suitable. You should completely avoid practices in summer in those places where the temperature is hot even in winter. If you live in cool places you can practise even during the day.

As instructed in the previous lessons you should not practise when the stomach is loaded. Generally yogic practices should be done only after a bath. A bath is not beneficial immediately after the practices. You should not sit for yogic practices when your mind is restless or when you are worried.

The Age

Young boys under 18 years of age whose bodies are very tender should not have too much practice. They have a very tender body which cannot stand the exertion of yogic exercises. Further, a youth's mind will be wandering and unsettled, and so in youth one cannot concentrate well. Yoga exercises require intense and deep concentration. In old age when all vitality is sapped by unnecessary worry, anxieties, troubles and other worldly problems, one cannot do any spiritual practice. Yoga requires full vitality, energy, power and strength. Therefore the best period for practices is from 20 to 40 years of age. Those who are strong and healthy can take to yogic practices even after the age of 50.

The Awakening of Kundalini

One should become perfectly desireless and should be full of vairagya before attempting to awaken kundalini. It can be awakened only when a man rises above lust, anger, greed, infatuation and other impurities. Kundalini can be awakened through rising above desires of the senses. The yogi who has got a pure heart and a mind free from passions and desires will be benefited by awakening kundalini. If a man with a lot of impurities in the mind awakens the shakti by sheer force through asanas, pranayamas and mudras, he will break his legs and stumble down. He will not be able to ascend the yogic ladder. This is the chief reason for people going out of the way or getting some bodily infirmities. There is nothing wrong in the yoga. People must have purity first; then a thorough knowledge of the sadhana, a proper guide, and a steady, gradual practice. When kundalini is awakened there are many temptations on the way, and an aspirant without purity will not have the strength to resist.

Kundalini can be awakened by pranayama, asanas and mudras by hatha yogis; by concentration and training of the mind by raja yogis; by devotion and perfect self-surrender by bhaktas; by analytical will by the jnanis; by mantras by the tantrikas; and by the grace of the guru through touch, sight or mere thought. Rousing of kundalini and its union with Siva at the sahasrara chakra effect the state of samadhi and liberation. No samadhi is possible without awakening the kundalini.

For a selected few, any one of the above methods is quite sufficient to awaken the kundalini. Many will have to combine different methods. This is according to the aspirant's growth and position in the spiritual path. The guru will find out his real position and will prescribe a proper method that will successfully awaken the kundalini in a short period. This is something like the doctor prescribing a proper medicine to a patient to cure a particular disease. One kind of medicine will not cure the diseases of different patients. So also, one kind of sadhana may not suit all.

You will have to take the kundalini up to sahasrara chakra through some special exercises such as maha bheda, shakti chalana, etc. As soon as kundalini is awakened, it pierces the muladhara chakra. It should be taken to sahasrara through the other chakras. When kundalini is at one chakra intense heat is felt there, and when it leaves that centre for another chakra the former chakra becomes very cold and appears lifeless.

Freedom from lust, anger, likes and dislikes and possession of balance of mind, cosmic love, astral vision, supreme fearlessness, desirelessness, siddhis, divine intoxication and spiritual bliss are the signs to denote the awakening of kundalini. When it is at rest a man has full consciousness of the world and its surroundings; when it is awakened he is dead to the world. He has no body-consciousness. When kundalini travels from chakra to chakra, layer after layer of the mind becomes opened and the yogi acquires psychic powers. He gets control over the five elements. When it reaches the sahasrara chakra he is in the chid-akasa (knowledge-space).

Problems on the Path

There are many persons nowadays who, foolishly imagining that they have attained purity, commit errors in selecting some methods and neglect many important items of sadhana. They are poor, self-deluded souls. Self-assertive aspirants, too, will select some exercise of their own fancy in an irregular manner and leave all the exercises when they get some serious troubles.

Awakening of the kundalini shakti, its union with Siva, enjoying the nectar and other functions of kundalini yoga that are described in the yoga scriptures are misrepresented and taken in a literal sense by many. They think that they are Siva and ladies are Shakti and that mere sexual union is the aim of kundalini yoga. After having some wrong interpretation of the yogic texts, they begin to offer flowers and worship their wives with lustful propensities. The term 'divine intoxication that is derived by drinking the nectar' is also misrepresented. They take a lot of wine and other intoxicating drinks and imagine they have enjoyed the Divine ecstasy. It is mere ignorance. They are utterly wrong. This sort of worship and union is not at all kundalini yoga. They divert their concentration on sexual centres and ruin themselves.

Some foolish young boys practise one or two asanas, mudras and a little pranayama, too, for a few days, in any way they like, and imagine that the kundalini has gone up to their neck. They pose as big yogis. They are pitiable, self-deluded souls.

It is easy to awaken the kundalini, but it is very difficult to take it to sahasrara chakra through the different chakras. It demands a great deal of patience, perseverance, purity and steady practice. The yogi who has taken it to sahasrara chakra is the real master of all forces. Generally yogic students stop their sadhana halfway on account of false satisfaction. They imagine that they have reached the goal when they get some mystic experiences and psychic powers. They desire to demonstrate such powers to the public to get reputation and fame and to earn some money. This is a sad mistake. Full realisation alone can give final liberation, perfect peace and highest bliss.

Before awakening the kundalini, you must have purity of body, purification of nadis, purity of mind and purity of intellect.

The following asanas, mudras and bandhas are useful for concentration, meditation and awakening kundalini:

Padmasana
Siddhasana
Sukhasana
Sirshasana
Sarvangasana
Matsyasana
Paschimottanasana
Mayurasana
Ardha Matsyendrasana

Vajrasana
Urdhva
Padmasana
Mula bandha
Jalandhara bandha
Uddiyana bandha
Maha mudra
Maha bandha
Maha vedha
Yoga mudra
Viparita karani mudra
Kechari mudra
Vajroli mudra
Shakti chalana mudra
Yoni mudra

Kundalini Yoga

The first step in kundalini yoga is the purification of the nadis. When sushumna is pure, then only will kundalini pass through it. Purification of the nadis is done by the practice of pranayama. One should practise control of breath with concentration of the mind. The yogi opens the mouth of sushumna nadi through pranayama, bandhas and mudras and thereby kundalini is awakened and passes upwards along the sushumna nadi. Then the kundalini passes along the six chakras and eventually gets united with Lord Siva seated on the sahasrara or thousand petal lotus at the crown of the heat. Nirvikalpa samadhi ensues and the yogi gets liberation and all the divine powers.

The awakened kundalini that is taken up to manipura chakra may drop down again to muladhara. It has to be raised up again with effort. One should become perfectly desireless and should be full of dispassion before he attempts to awaken kundalini. Kundalini is like a thread, and is resplendent. When it travels from chakra to chakra, layer after layer of the mind becomes open and the yogi acquires various siddhis (psychic powers).

The rousing of kundalini shakti is attended by intense heat. You should apply butter or amalaka oil to the head, and eat butter and sugar-candy. You should not be unnecessarily alarmed by the heat and other symptoms. They will pass off soon. Be brave, courageous and cheerful. You will now develop clairvoyance, and your inner eye will be opened.

As soon as kundalini is awakened you will lose your body-consciousness. You will not get any experience like fainting. You will experience higher consciousness of higher realms, new visions and new joy. (Rousing of kundalini does not necessarily bring about, in all cases, trance with all accompanying events — such as unconsciousness of the body, its coldness, etc.)

You will experiences a particular ananda (bliss) at each centre also, and a great upward pull on the anus and the lower end of the spine. Sometimes you will feel a great tingling sensation at the lower end of the spine. You will feel as though some great change in your system will happen soon. In dream you will feel that you are trying to come out of your body. You will feel great pressure at the end of the spine.

When you meditate with closed eyes you will see, in your body, two luminous strings in which luminous lotuses are placed at intervals. The strings pass through the image of your ishtam seated in one of these lotuses in the region of the heart. Continue your meditation. You will feel that your anus and a spot in the top of the head are connected by these strings. You may feel that you will lose your physical consciousness. Be not afraid. Be bold and courageous. You will have rare spiritual experiences. You will have cosmic vision. Do not open your eyes now. You will come back to normal consciousness.

Pure emotions will rise in your heart. You will begin to love every creature, to feel that the whole world is nothing but pure consciousness. The tables, chairs, men, women and other things will all appear to contain this consciousness, just as vessels contain their contents. You will feel that all things are made of this consciousness. This rare experience will give you great bliss. You will feel that the Lord is sporting in all things as this pure consciousness and you will actually lose the sense of material nature of things around you.

You will have sakara realisation and bhava samadhi at the anahata chakra. You will experience nirvikalpa samadhi at sahasrara.

May you all attain the exalted state of nirvikalpa samadhi through regular and constant meditation. That yogi in whom the kundalini has been awakened and taken upwards to the top of the head (sahasrara chakra), is the real King of kings or Emperor of emperors. He has all divine wealth and glory. All psychic powers roll under his feet. He can command nature, he can command the elements. His glory is indescribable.

Need for Purification

Aspirants cry for inner spiritual experiences. They cry for the awakening of kundalini and samadhi. When the experiences actually begin to manifest, they tremble with fear and stop their sadhana. The receptacle is not pure or strong enough to receive the divine light. When they are about to go above body-consciousness during meditation they are terribly frightened. They open their eyes to find out whether they have their bodies or not. When the breath stops during deep meditation and when it tries to move towards sahasrara, they are alarmed. They open their eyes to see whether the breath moves in the nostrils or not and then the meditation is broken.

Be not troubled. Be not anxious about the awakening of kundalini. Direct your full energy and attention to purifying the mind, and to getting rid of various sorts of impurities of the mind — subtle egoism, subtle attachments and ties, subtle cravings, subtle hidden personal desires and ambitions, etc. This is most important. You will not be benefited much, even if the kundalini is awakened, if subtle desires, etc., remain in the chitta. Beware of hidden under-currents of desires. Purify your mind. Destroy desires and cravings. Do the right method of sadhana.

Two yoga students approached yogi Kaka Bhusunda to learn yoga. The master said: "O dear students, wait in my ashram for twelve years. Practise restraint, moral discipline, asana and pranayama. Later on I shall put you in samadhi. I shall teach you the secrets of awakening the kundalini and taking it to sahasrara." One student was very impatient. He practised some yoga kriyas for some time. He then worried the teacher daily to show him the way to enter into samadhi. The teacher kept quiet for a long time. The student left the ashram. The other student was very patient and sensible. He strictly adhered to the instructions of his guru. He never spoke a word to the guru. Twelve years passed. The guru thought: "The student is ready now. His nadis are purified. He is sattvic. He possesses all the divine virtues. He is fit now for higher initiation." He asked the student to sit in front of him, and through his pure thought made the student's kundalini shakti pass into sushumna nadi. The student enjoyed the bliss of nirvikalpa state.

The grace of the guru alone is the passport for the yoga student to enter the realms of divine bliss. The grace of the guru can descend only on that student who is exerting himself. The guru showers his grace in exchange for the hard-earned merit achieved by the disciple. Considerable patience, faith in the guru and rigid practice are necessary if one desires to achieve the highest goal of yoga. The other student missed the goal on account of his impatience.

O impatient aspirants, be patient. You will get everything when the time comes. Do not bother much about awakening kundalini. Let it awaken by itself spontaneously. Premature awakening is not desirable. Do your sadhana and tapas systematically and regularly. Just as the gardener who waters the trees daily gets the fruits when the time comes, so also you will enjoy the fruits of your sadhana when the time comes. Do proper sadhana. Kundalini will take care of itself.

Pranayama for Purification of Nadis

The vayu cannot enter the nadis if they are full of impurities. Therefore, first of all they should be purified and then pranayama should be practised. The nadis are purified by two processes, viz. nirmanu and samanu. The nirmanu is done by physical cleansing of the shat-kriyas (see page no. 187). The samanu is done by a mental process with bija mantras, as follows:

1. Sit in padmasana. Meditate on the bija for air *yam* which is of smokey colour. Inhale through the left nostril. Repeat *yam* 16 times. Retain the breath till you repeat this bija 64 times. Then exhale through the nostrils very, very slowly till you repeat *yam* 32 times.
2. The navel is the seat of the fire principle. Meditate on this, then draw the breath through the right nostril repeating the fire bija *ram* 16 times. Retain the breath till you count *ram* 64 times. Then exhale slowly through the left nostril till you repeat *ram* mentally 32 times.
3. Fix the gaze at the tip of the nose. Inhale through the left nostril repeating the bija *tham* 16 times. Retain the breath till you repeat it 64 times. Imagine that the nectar that flows from the moon runs through all the vessels of the body and purifies them. Then exhale slowly through the right nostril, till you repeat the bija *lam* 32 times.

The nadis are purified nicely by the practice of the above three kinds of pranayama, sitting firmly in your usual posture.

Pranayama for Purification of the Sushumna

Having become firm in the posture and having preserved perfect self-control, in order to clear away the impurities of the sushumna the yogi should sit in padmasana; and having inhaled the air through the left nostril he should retain it as long as he can and then exhale through the right. Then drawing it again through the right and having retained it, he should exhale it through the left. Then he should draw it through the same nostril by which he exhaled it before, retain it and exhale. To those who practise according to these rules through the right and left nostrils, the nadis become purified within three months. He should practise retention of breath at sunrise, at midday, at sunset and at midnight, slowly, 80 times a day, for 4 weeks. All the pranas are unified during kumbhaka or retention of breath. The yogi offers the oblations of the senses into the prana fire. (Senses merged in the state of kumbhaka are considered as oblations.)

In the early stage, perspiration is produced; in the middle stage a tremor of the body; and in the last stage, levitation in the air. These results ensue out of the repression of the breath, while sitting in the lotus posture.

When perspiration rises with effort, one should rub it into his body well. By this the body becomes firm and light. In the early course of the practice, food with milk and ghee is excellent. One sticking to this rule becomes firm in his practice and gets no burning sensation in the body. As lions, elephants and tigers are gradually tamed, so also the breath, when rigidly managed, comes under control.

So long as the prana does not enter the sushumna, so long as the mind is not free from lust, anger, greed and jealousy, so long as the semen is not steadfast and is not moving upward to the sahasrara as ojas (through sublimation), it is hypocrisy if one says "I meditate for six hours. I enter into samadhi. I have attained God-realisation or Self-realisation." The words of such a man are no better than the words of a big fool! Do not believe him a bit. Do not sit in his company. Shun him ruthlessly.

By the practice of pranayama the purification of the nadis, brightening of the gastric fire, hearing spiritual sounds distinctly and good health result. When the nerve centres have been purified through the regular practice of pranayama, the air easily forces its way up through the mouth of the sushumna, which is in the middle. It is after such entry that the yogi becomes dead to the world, being in that state called samadhi. Drawing up the apana and forcing down the prana from the throat, the yogi, free from old age, becomes like a youth of sixteen.

Anahata Sounds (Nada)

Anahata sounds are the mystic sounds heard by the yogi during his meditation. It is a sign of the purification of nadis. Some students can clearly hear the sounds through either ear and some by both the ears. There are loud as well as subtle sounds. From the loud one will have to contemplate on the subtle and from the subtle to the subtler. Beginners can hear the sound only when the ears are closed. Advanced students can concentrate on the anahata sound even without closing the ears. Anahata sounds proceed from the anahata centre of the sushumna nadi.

Technique: Sit in your usual asana, with closed eyes. Close the ears with the thumbs. Hear and minutely observe the internal sound through the ears. The sound that you hear from within will make you deaf to all external sounds. In the beginning of your practice you will hear many loud sounds. Later on they are heard in a mild way. The mind having at first concentrated itself on any one sound fixes firmly to that and is absorbed in it. The mind, becoming insensible to the external impressions, becomes one with the sound, as milk with water, and then becomes rapidly absorbed in the inner sound.

Nada that is heard through the ears is of ten kinds. The first is the sound *chini* (like the pronunciation of the word); the second is *chinichini*; the third is the sound of a bell; the fourth is that of a conch; the fifth is that of a lute; the sixth is the sound of cymbals; the seventh is the tune of a flute; the eighth is the voice of a drum (bheri); the ninth is the sound of a double-drum (mridanga); and the tenth is the sound of thunder.

You cannot expect the sound immediately after you close your ears. You should concentrate and keep your mind one-pointed. The particular sound that you hear today you may not hear every day. But you will hear any one of the ten anahata sounds.

The description given above is laya (absorption) through nada, anahata sound. In the same manner, laya can be effected by concentration at the tip of the nose and at the space between the two eyebrows (brumadhya drishti), meditation on soham mantra and mahavakyas, and other methods also.

Experiences on Awakening of Kundalini

During meditation you will behold divine visions, experience divine smells, divine tastes, divine touch and hear divine anahata sounds. You will receive instructions from God. These indicate that the kundalini shakti has been awakened. When there is throbbing in muladhara, when hair stands on end, when uddiyana, jalandhara and mulabandha come involuntarily, know that kundalini has awakened.

When the breath stops without any effort, when kevala kumbhaka comes by itself without any exertion, know that kundalini shakti has become active. When you feel the currents of prana rising up to the sahasrara, when you experience bliss, when you repeat OM automatically, when there are no thoughts of the world in the mind, know that kundalini shakti has awakened.

When in your meditation the eyes become fixed on the space between the eyebrows, when the sambhavi mudra operates, know that kundalini has become active. When you feel vibrations of prana in different parts inside your body, when you experience jerks like the shocks of electricity, know that kundalini has become active. During meditation when you feel that there is no body, when your eyelids become closed and do not open in spite of your exertion, when electric-like currents flow up and down the nerves, know that kundalini has awakened.

When you meditate, when you get inspiration and insight, when nature unfolds its secrets to you, all doubts disappear and you understand clearly the meaning of the vedic texts, know that kundalini has become active. When your body becomes light like air, when you have a balanced mind in perturbed conditions, when you possess inexhaustable energy for work, know that kundalini has become active.

When you get divine intoxication, when you develop power of oration, know that kundalini has awakened. When you involuntarily perform difficult asanas or yoga postures without the least pain or fatigue, know that kundalini has become active. When you compose beautiful sublime hymns and poetry involuntarily, know that kundalini has become active.

That aspirant who has firm faith in yoga scriptures, who is courageous, devotional, humble, generous, merciful, pure and dispassionate, can easily awaken kundalini and attain success in samadhi. He should also be equipped with right conduct and self-restraint; he should constantly engage himself in the service of his guru and be free from lust, anger, attachment, greed and vanity.

If you awaken kundalini forcibly by violent methods when your heart is impure and when desires lurk in your mind, you will come across temptations of various sorts, when you move from plane to plane. You will have a downfall. You will have no strength of will to resist these temptations.

Kundalini, the sustaining power, is the basis on which the whole edifice of the science of yoga has been built. The kundalini shakti is both cosmic and individual. The cosmic is called maha kundalini and the individual one the kundalini.

Sadhana, dhriti, sthirata, dhairya, laghava, pratyaksha and nirvikalpa samadhi are the seven stages of kundalini yoga.

Eight Major Siddhis

An accomplished yogi in the path of kundalini yoga is in possession of eight major siddhis: anima, mahima, laghima, garima, Prapti, prakamya, vasitvam and ishitvam.

1. *Anima*: The yogi can become as minute as he pleases.
2. *Mahima*: This is the opposite of anima. He can become as big as he likes. He can make his body assume a very large size. He can fill up the whole universe.
3. *Laghima*: He can make his body as light as cotton or feather. The body is rendered light by plavini pranayama. The yogi produces a diminution of his specific gravity by swallowing large draughts of air. He travels in the sky with the help of this siddhi. He can travel thousands of miles in a minute.
4. *Garima*: This is the opposite of laghima. In this the yogi acquires an increase of specific gravity. He can make the body as heavy as a mountain.
5. *Prapti:* The yogi standing on the earth can touch the highest things. He can touch the sun or the moon or the sky. Through this siddhi the yogi attains his desired objects and super-natural powers. He acquires the power of predicting future events and the powers of clairvoyance, clairaudience, telepathy, thought-reading, etc. He can understand the languages of the beasts and birds. He

can understand unknown languages also. He can cure all diseases.
6. *Prakamya*: The yogi can dive into the water and can come out at any time he likes. (The late Trilinga Swami of Benares used to live for six months underneath the Ganges.) It is also the process by which a yogi makes himself invisible sometimes. By some writers it is defined to be the power of entering the body of another. (Sri Sankara entered the body of Rajah Amaruka of Benares. Tirumular in Southern India entered the body of a shepherd. Rajah Vikramaditya also did this.) It is also the power of keeping a youth-like appearance for any length of time. (Rajah Yayati had this power.)
7. *Vashitvam*: This is the power of taming wild animals and bringing them under control. It is the power of mesmerising persons by the exercise of will and of making them obedient to one's own wishes and orders. It is the restraint of passions and emotions. It is the power to bring men, women and the elements under subjection.
8. *Ishitvam*: This is the attainment of divine power. The yogi who has this power can restore life to the dead. (Kabir, Tulsi Das, Akalkot Swami and others had this power of bringing the dead back to life.)

Minor Siddhis

The yogi acquires the following minor siddhis also:

1. Freedom from hunger and thirst.
2. Freedom from the effects of heat and cold.
3. Freedom from raga-dvesha (likes and dislikes).
4. Clairvoyance.
5. Clairaudience.
6. Control of mind.
7. The yogi can take any form he likes.
8. He can enter into another body, can animate a dead body and enter into it by transferring his soul.
9. He can have death at his will.
10. He can play with the devas after seeing them.
11. He can get whatever he likes.
12. He has knowledge of past, present and future.

13. He is beyond the pairs of opposites.
14. Whatever he predicts will come to pass.
15. He can turn base metal into gold.
16. He can take as many bodies as he likes to exhaust all his karmas in one life.
17. He has the jumping power of a frog.
18. He becomes the lord of desire, destroys sorrows and diseases.
19. He gets knowledge of his past life.
20. He gets knowledge of the cluster of stars and planets.
21. He gets the power of perceiving the siddhas.
22. He gets mastery of the elements (bhuta jaya) and mastery of prana (prana jaya).
23. He can move to any place he likes.
24. He gets omnipotence and omniscience.
25. He rises in the air and leaves the ground.
26. He can point out the place where a hidden treasure lies.

The Gradational Ascent of the Mind

Purity of mind leads to perfection in yoga. Regulate your conduct when you deal with others. Have no feeling of jealousy towards others. Be compassionate. Do not hate sinners. Be kind to all. Success in yoga will be rapid if you put your maximum energy into your yoga practice. You must have a keen longing for liberation and intense dispassion also. You must be sincere and earnest. Intense and constant meditation is necessary for entering into samadhi.

The mind of a worldly man with base desires and passions moves in the muladhara and svadhisthana chakras or centres (situated near the anus and the reproductive organ, respectively).

If one's mind becomes purified it rises to the manipura chakra (the centre in the navel) and experiences some power and joy.

If the mind becomes more purified, it rises to the anahata chakra (the centre in the heart) experiences bliss and visualises the effulgent form of the ishta devata or the tutelary deity.

When the mind gets highly purified, when meditation and devotion become intense and profound, the mind rises to vishuddha chakra (the centre in the throat) and experiences more and more powers and bliss. Even when the mind has reached this centre there is a possibility for it to come down to the lower centres.

When the mind reaches the ajna chakra (the centre between the two eyebrows) he attains samadhi and realises the supreme Self, or Brahman. There is a slight sense of separateness between the devotee and Brahman.

If he reaches the spiritual centre in the brain, the sahasrara chakra, the thousand-petalled lotus, the yogi attains nirvikalpa samadhi or super-conscious state. He becomes one with the non-dual Brahman. All sense of separateness dissolves. This is the highest plane of consciousness or supreme asamprajnata samadhi. Here kundalini unites with Siva.

The yogi may come down to the centre in the throat to give instructions to the students and do good to the others (lokasangraha).

Section IV

Swara Yoga

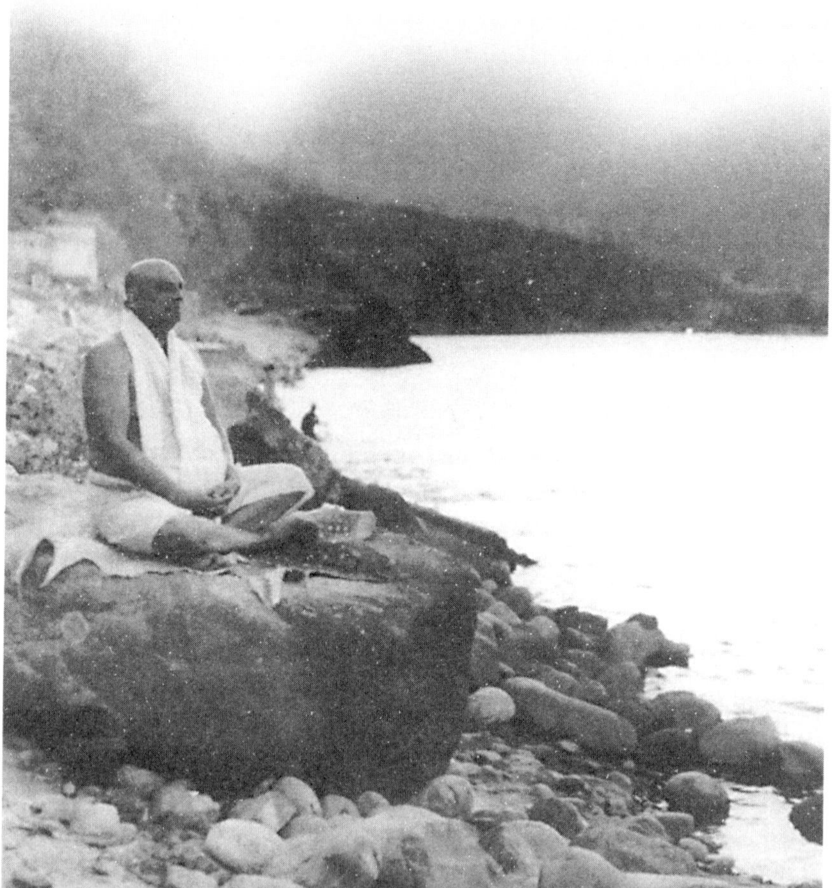

Meditating on the Ganges bank

SWARA YOGA

The sane leading of a healthy life of longevity and peace that shall bless us with immortality, depends upon the nature of the flow of breath through the three nadis, and the rhythm and ease with which it flows.

Ida or chandra nadi (the moon) is determined by the flow of breath through the left nostril. Pingala or surya nadi (the sun) is determined by a flow in the right nostril.

These two nadis function alternately. The change of flow from one nostril to the other is called vishuvat. The time when this change occurs is highly inauspicious.

When, during the change of flow, there is an obstruction in the new channel, naturally there will be a forcible expulsion of the obstructing matter and the clearance of the passage, generally resulting in a mild or heavy sneezing. (That is why sneezing is considered as an ill-omen.)

When the breath changes its flow from one nostril to the other in quick succession with every breath, it is said to be in sushumna and is considered to be inauspicious for any act. This state of flow is also called vishuvat, which means destroyer of all actions. It denotes tossing of the mind, restlessness, haste, non-fixity and hesitation of the mind, and a defective posture of the body as well. In this state one is advised to take rest and recover the balance of mind. No act should be done at this time because it denotes that the mind is not steady or firm in its motive and that there is doubt and hesitation. Hasty actions always make one repent afterwards.

There is a second variety of sushumna and it is cognised by the flow of breath simultaneously through both the nostrils. It is further characterized by the evenness of flow without any jerk and by a concentration of the mind on any one of the six chakras.

During this sushumna it is the best opportunity to concentrate and meditate upon the Lord, there being a natural tendency of the mind as such to be calm and fixed. There should be no other undertaking.

It is very difficult to maintain a constant flow of breath through sushumna, and therefore even the short and insignificant duration for which the sushumna flows should be utilised to give the maximum good.

Swara Vijnana

Each of the two nadis, ida and pingala, function alternately for a period of 2½ ghatikas (one hour) at a stretch, beginning from sunrise. Thus, in the course of twenty four hours the breath flows twelve times in ida and twelve time in pingala. This indicates the normal functioning of the breath and the nadis, and good health as well.

Generally, sushumna does not function when a man is engaged in actions, either mental or physical. Only when the mind gets concentrated and controlled with all its vrittis subsided, the sushumna (flow of breath simultaneously from both the nostrils) functions. If, on the other hand, the other variety of sushumna (fluctuation of the flow at rapid speed and with jerk) functions during the waking state of a man or when the mind is not in a meditative mood, it denotes certain disturbances in the normal flow of breath.

Changing the Flow

The auspicious and inauspicious flows are mentioned above, so that each individual can regulate and direct the flow of breath along a particular channel at a particular time to bless his undertakings with success. A knowledge of the various means of changing the direction of flow, therefore, is essential. There are various means of changing the course of breath from one nostril to the other, a few of which are mentioned below:

1. Plug the nostril (any one) with a light cotton pad. The breath will flow through the other nostril.
2. You can close the nostril through which the breath flows with your thumb. This will divert the flow through the other nostril.

3. When the breath flows through the left nostril, place the left palm on the ground (while sitting on the ground in sukhasana or padmasana) and press the left elbow on the left side just underneath the ribs, applying a little pressure. Slightly incline your body towards the left side. The flow of breath will change from left to right. The same should be done on the right side with the right elbow if you wish to change the flow from right to left.
4. You can use a yoga danda (a small staff of about one cubit in length with a 'U' shaped piece fixed horizontally at the top). Place the portion of the arm just below the armpit in the U-shaped groove. Apply slight pressure and bend a little on that side. The flow will be diverted to the other side. The same can also be done with the help of a long staff while walking or standing.
5. The mind also can be trained to control the flow. Just as you can control the bodily muscles by a mere thought of the mind, the flow can be changed from one nostril to the other.
6. If you are lying on your left side, the flow will be through the right nostril and vice versa.

You shall have to change the flow as and when necessary, according to your requirements.

Changing the flow to sushumna is slightly difficult and maintaining it there is still more difficult.

The following methods will help one in changing the flow from either of the nadis to sushumna:

1. Lie flat on your back on the ground, without using a pillow. Concentrate on the tip of the nose or on the space between the two eye-brows. Sushumna will function.
2. Sit erect in sukhasana, padmasana or siddhasana. Do a few rounds of bhastrika pranayama. Concentrate as above. The flow will be through sushumna.
3. Concentration on any one of the six chakras will also help a flow in sushumna.

It is the steadiness of the vertical posture in which the spinal column will be in a straight line, and the intensity of the concentration and fixity of thought, that goes to ensure a flow of breath in sushumna. That alone will help maintain the flow. If any one of the above three concentrations gets disturbed, the breath will be diverted along the right or left nostril.

Use of the Nadis

During the flow of ida nadi, strength, vitality and good digestion are ensured. During the flow of pingala nadi, digestion takes place but poisons are formed in the system. Sushumna leads to final beatitude.

While sleeping on the left side, the pingala nadi functions and the mind sleeps well because ida nadi is given rest. If ida nadi flows while sleeping, it will be a disturbed sleep, maybe with much dreaming. Therefore you should always sleep on your left side allowing the pingala nadi to function. Thus two things are had — sound sleep and ideal digestion leading to health and strength and vitality.

You can keep your consciousness awake while allowing the senses and the lower mind to sleep if you go to sleep on your right side. This should be attempted only when you are freed from the tossing of the mind and desires, and are sure that no dream will occur.

In all your external activities which are calculated to do good — individual and universal, see that they are started while the pingala nadi functions. The following are some of the good acts that can be begun during a flow in ida. Entering new mode or walk of life, starting scriptural studies, travelling, meeting friends, relations and elders; erecting buildings and temples; cultivation; taking new appointments; marriage; wearing new clothes and jewellery; and preparing nourishing medicines. Ida nadi should function while study of mantra sastra relating to rajasic or tamasic deity is started. While eating and taking bath also, ida nadi should function.

In short, acts of lasting good should be started while breath flows through ida and all acts that are either transitory or temporary in their nature should be performed while pingala nadi functions.

Sushumna should always be reserved for spiritual good, for concentration and meditation and for doing kumbhak (retention of breath).

Let the breath flow through ida, the left nostril, throughout the whole day from sunrise to sunset, and through pingala, the right nostril, throughout the night from sunset to sunrise.

This is the practice of swara sadhana. He who practises thus is verily a great yogi. Practise this now. Wake up to drink the nectar of immortality. Shake off your habitual sloth, indolence, inertia and all aspects of tamas. Leave off your idle talk, gossiping and the obnoxious habit of criticising others. Do something practical.

Section V

Brahmacharya

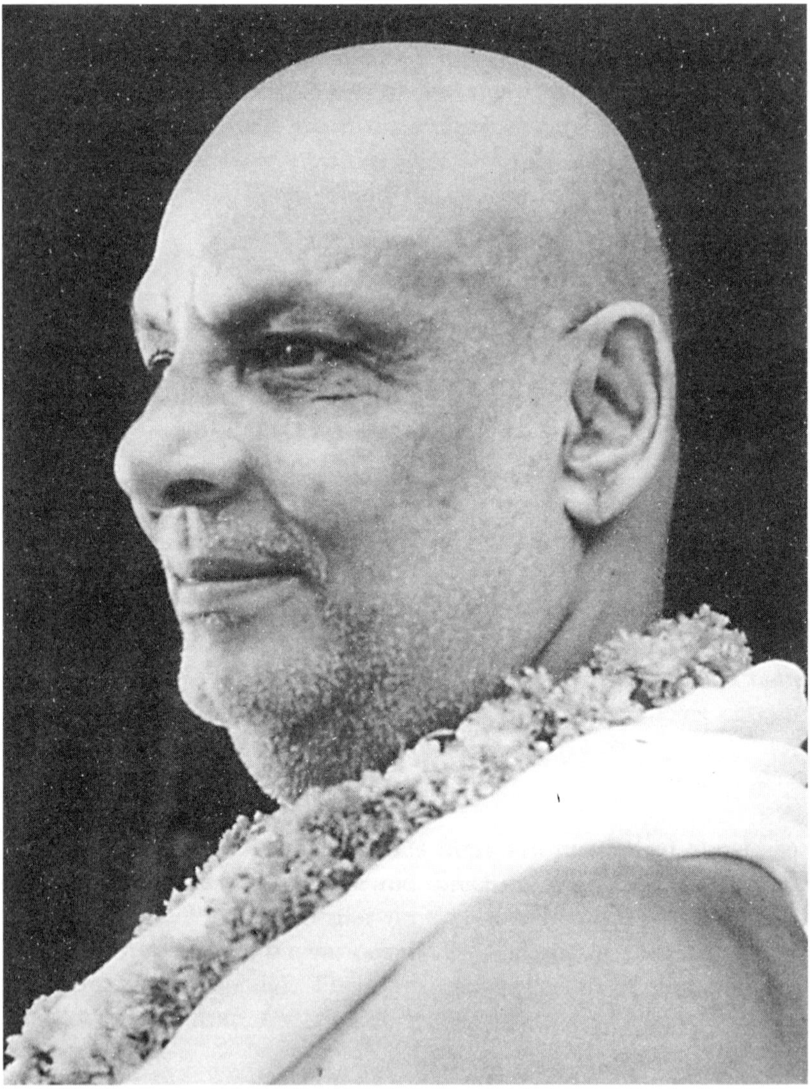

Energy filled him and overflowed to all

BRAHMACHARYA

Brahmacharya

The word 'brahmacharya' has several meanings. The literal meaning is 'movement towards God'; or, where the mind moves in God. It is the conduct by which you attain Brahman or God, it is life in the Absolute, it is purity in thought, word and deed.

A brahmachari (or one whose mind always moves in God) is a master of the three worlds. He can turn out immense mental, physical and intellectual work. He has a magnetic aura around his face. He can influence people by speaking a few words, or even by his very presence. When there is purity the rays of the mind are not dissipated, and focussing of the mind becomes easy. Concentration and purity go together. Although a sage talks a few words only, a deep impression is produced on the minds of the hearers. This is due to his spiritual force which is conserved by the preservation of semen and its transmutation. All the spiritual leaders have been true brahmacharis. Jesus, Sankara, Jnana Deva and Samartha Ram Das were all brahmacharis.

Brahmacharya is the bright light that shines in the house of the human body. It is the fully blossomed flower of life around which the bees (of strength, patience, knowledge, purity and firmness) wander about humming hither and thither. In other words, he who observes brahmacharya will be endowed with the above qualities. Scriptures declare emphatically: "By the practice of brahmacharya, longevity, glory, strength, vigour, knowledge, undying fame, virtues and devotion to Truth increases."

Brahmacharya is the basis for attaining immortality. It is the substratum for a life of peace in the Atman or pure spirit. It is the firm support for one who is established in the direct knowledge of Brahman, which is eagerly longed for by sages, aspirants and yoga students. Even rishis and devas are at the feet of a genuine and established brahmachari. With this power only, one has to open the sushumna (the important psychic nerve current that passes through the spinal column) to allow the kundalini to pass through.

The yogi gets perfection by attaining brahmacharya. It helps him in achieving divine knowledge and other siddhis or psychic powers — anima (atomic size), manima (colossal size), garima (excessive bulk), laghima (extreme lightness), prapti (attainment of desire), prakamya (unhampered will), isitva (lordliness) and vasittva (control over everything), and the nine riddhis which are inferior to siddhis.

The limited meaning of the word 'brahmacharya' is celibacy or continence.

Celibacy

The term 'celibacy' is from the latin 'calebs', and signifies the state of living unmarried. It also includes character-building or right moulding of character. It is of vital importance. It is the gateway to liberation or eternal bliss, it bestows super-human strength and supreme bliss, and it is the basis for morality. Absolute celibacy is the sine-qua-non of divine life or spiritual higher life. The door to nirvana or perfection is complete celibacy.

Celibacy means control of not only the reproductive organ but also the control of all senses, in thought, word, and deed. Mere control of animal passion alone will not constitute celibacy. That is incomplete. You must control all the organs — the ears that want to hear lustful stories, the eye that wants to see objects that excite passion, the tongue that wants to taste exciting objects. The door to nirvana or perfection is complete celibacy. It is the master-key to open the realms of elysian bliss. The avenue to the abode of supreme peace begins from celibacy.

Celibacy is of two kinds: viz, physical and mental. Physical celibacy is the control of body; mental celibacy is the control of evil thoughts. He who is free from lustful thoughts even in his dreams, is a veritable god on this earth. He is worthy of the world's adoration. In mental celibacy no bad thoughts will enter the mind. It is a little more difficult than the physical but through sincere exertion you can be well established in it. You must keep the ideal always before you. Then you will realize it soon. There is no doubt of this.

The special virtues of endurance and bravery are intimately connected with the cultivation of chastity. Strict abstinence is not merely from sexual intercourse but also from auto-erotic manifestations, from masturbation, from homosexual acts and from all sexual perverse practices. Self-indulgence is not a safe-guard against involuntary dreams. There must be a permanent abstention from indulgence in erotic imagination and voluptuous reverie.

The following are the eight kinds of breaks, so to say, in the current of the practice of unbroken celibacy. You must avoid these with great care, sincere exertion and vigilant circumspection:

1. Looking at the opposite sex.
2. Desire to touch, embrace or be near a person of the opposite sex.
3. Amorous sport (playing with him or her).
4. Praising his or her qualities to your friends.
5. Conversing with him or her in private.
6. Lustful thought of a man or woman.
7. Strong determination to have intercourse with a man or woman.
8. Sexual enjoyment.

Though the first seven kinds do not cause actual loss of semen, yet the semen is separated from the blood and it tries to escape when opportunity arises, either in dreams or in other ways. In the first seven kinds man enjoys mentally.

A real brahmachari should ruthlessly avoid the above. Only one who is free from all of them can be called a true celibate. A break in any one of these vows is a break of celibacy. This point should be very well borne in mind.

Pure air, pure water, wholesome food, physical exercises, out-door games, walking with a brisk step, rowing, swimming, light games (like tennis etc.) all contribute to the maintenance of good health, strength and a high standard of vitality. There are indeed many ways to gain health and strength and these ways are doubtless indispensable, but celibacy is the most important of all. Without it all your exercises are nothing. It is the master-key for opening the realms of health and happiness. It is the corner-stone of the edifice of bliss and unalloyed felicity, it is the only specific thing that keeps up true manliness.

Yama is the first step of raja yoga. It is the practice of ahimsa, satyam, asteyam, brahmacharya and aparigraha (non-killing, truthfulness, non-stealing, celibacy and non-receiving of gifts.). In jnana yogis, dama (self-control) is the foundation for the student.

Benefits of Celibacy

The *Siva Samhita* says:

> Death is hastened by letting out semen from the body; life is saved and prolonged by preserving it in the body. Therefore semen must be preserved very carefully... There is no doubt that people are born and live a healthy life by preserving semen, and die prematurely for want of semen by letting it out of the body; knowing this the yogi should always preserve semen and lead a life of strict celibacy.

Celibacy is a potent weapon for waging war against the internal devils of lust, anger, greed etc. It contributes to perennial joy, uninterrupted and undecaying bliss. It gives tremendous energy, clear brain, gigantic will-power, bold understanding, retentive memory and good power of enquiry. Through celibacy alone you can have physical, mental and spiritual advancement in life.

Celibacy is the basis for the attainment of perfection of body. For this, complete celibacy must be observed. This is of paramount importance. By the practice of yoga the semen becomes transmuted into ojas shakti. The yogi will have a perfect body. There will be charm and grace in his movements. He can live as long as he likes. That is the reason why Lord Krishna says to Arjuna: "Therefore, become a yogi, O Arjuna."

Those who practise celibacy generally complain that they get mental fatigue owing to continence. This is only a deception of the mind. You sometimes get a pseudo-hunger, whereas when you actually sit for dinner you have no real appetite and do not take any food. So also there is a false mental fatigue. If you observe celibacy you will have immense mental strength. You will not be able to feel it always, but you will manifest it when the occasion arises in the same way as a wrestler manifests his physical strength in the arena, though he feels as a normal man in ordinary times.

Practice of celibacy immensely augments one's mental energy and mental strength. Mental strength is far superior to physical strength. Look at Mahatma Gandhi. Physically he was weak, but mark his tremendous mental strength. He had acquired this by constant and careful practice of non-violence, truthfulness and celibacy. He influenced the world through this power alone. The intellect becomes sharp and clear by continence. Strength and fortitude are obtained.

He who practises celibacy will tide over a crisis of any disease very easily. If it takes a month for an ordinary man for recovery, this man will be completely alright in a week. Practice of celibacy gives strength, (inner) good health, peace of mind and long life. It invigorates the mind and nerves, it helps to conserve physical and mental energy, it augments strength, vigour and vitality, and it gives power to face all the difficulties in the daily battle of life. A perfect celibate can move the world and command nature and the five elements as Jnana Dev did.

Awaken your hidden faculties, potential energies of all descriptions through celibacy. Attain God-consciousness quickly and get over the miseries of this mundane life with its concomitant evils of birth, death and sorrow.

Celibacy and Longevity

It is on the mere attainment of establishment of good conduct that you may be able to attain full age and eternal happiness. You can attain full age even if you are devoid of all other qualities, by the establishment of good conduct only. Good conduct is character-building. You must have a good character, otherwise you will lose your vital energy and thereby attain premature death. Scriptures declare that the full life of a man is one hundred years. This you can attain only by remaining established in celibacy.

You have to remember one thing more! The secrets of longevity are based chiefly upon discretion in the choice of food and drink, temperance, sobriety, chastity and a hopeful optimistic outlook on life; and so gluttons, drunkards, the idle, the dissipated or the lazy cannot hope to attain full age. There are instances of men who have attained longevity and intellectual powers despite their loose immoral ways. Obviously this is due to their karma. But they would have been still more powerful and brilliant had they possessed a good character and continence as well.

Blessed is he who has taken the vow of celibacy till the end of life.

Twice blessed is he who is sincerely struggling to destroy lust and attain perfect purity. Thrice blessed is he who has completely rooted out lust and has attained Self-realisation. Glory be to such exalted souls! They are veritable gods on earth. May their blessings be upon you all.

Need for Celibacy

A goldsmith converts impure gold into pure gold by adding acids and burning it several times in the crucible. Even so you will have to purify your impure mind and body by constant sadhana. A man used the words 'Sala badmash', in anger against a stranger when he was crossing the Ganges in a boat. The stranger became furious, caught hold of the neck of the man and threw him into the Ganges. How mentally weak that stranger was, though he was physically strong! A little sound, a single word, upset his mind and threw him out of balance. He became a slave of anger. Had he possessed continence, discrimination and self enquiry he would not have done this rash, brutal action. He who is established in celibacy can control anger and move the whole world.

Celibacy is the sum and substance of yoga. Through ignorance this is forgotten. It is the supreme yoga which Lord Krishna emphasises repeatedly in the *Bhagavad Gita*. In Chapter VI: 14, it is very clearly stated that the vow of celibacy is necessary for meditation. In Chapter XVII: 14, He says that it is one of the requisites for the austerity of the body.

Lambichus states that the gods do not hear him who invokes them if he is impure from sexual connections. In Islam strict continence is required on the pilgrimage to Mecca. It is required for the Hebrew congregation during the Theophany at Sinai and before entering the temple. Ancient India, Egypt and Greece enforced the rule that the worshipper must abstain from intercourse with the opposite sex during and before worship. In Christianity continence was required as a preparation for both baptism and the eucharist. The highest type of Christian was a celibate. Christian teachers praised celibacy, and marriage came to be in their eyes only a secondary good for those who were unable to observe continence. The bishops of the Greek Church are always celibates, being chosen from the monks.

Throughout the folklore runs the idea that second sight and the vision of the super-natural are especially, if not solely, the privilege of celibates. A tribe on the Rio Negro enjoined celibacy upon their shamans because they believed that medicine will prove ineffectual if adminstered by a married man.

Man has degraded himself to a great degree by becoming a puppet of passion. Also, he has become an imitative machine. He has lost his power of discrimination. He has sunk into the most abject form of slavery. What a lamentable plight indeed. If he wishes to regain his lost divine state and glory his whole being must be transformed; his sex-desire must be completely transmuted by entertaining sublime, divine thoughts and practice of regular meditation. Transmutation of sex-desire is a potent, efficacious and satisfactory way for realising eternal bliss.

Celibacy is the very foundation of yoga. Just as a house that is built on a rotten foundation will surely fall down, so also will you fall down from your meditation if you have not laid down the foundation properly. You may meditate for a period of twelve years and yet you will have no success in samadhi if you have not destroyed the subtle lust or the craving seed that lingers in the innermost recesses of your heart. You will have to carefully search out this dire enemy — lust — that lies hidden in various corners of the mind. You can detect its presence only if you are vigilant. Intense self-examination is very necessary. Just as powerful enemies can be conquered only if you attack them from all sides, so also you can keep the powerful senses under control only if you check them from all sides, from within and from without, from above and from beneath.

The vow of celibacy will give you sure protection against temptation. It is a strong weapon to attack lust. If you do not take a vow of celibacy the mind will tempt you at any moment. You will have no strength to resist temptations and you will become a sure victim. He who is weak and effeminate is afraid of taking the vow. He brings in various excuses and says: "Why should I be bound by a vow? My will is strong and powerful. I can resist any sort of temptation. I am doing meditation on God. I am practising will-culture." He repents in the long run. He has no control over the senses. Only that man in whom the subtle desire for the object of pleasure lurks in the corner of his mind brings in such excuses. You must understand rightly and have discrimination and dispassion, then only your renunciation will be lasting and permanent. If renunciation is not the outcome of discrimination and dispassion the mind will simply be waiting for an opportunity to get back the object that has been renounced.

The future well-being of India rest entirely on celibacy and celibacy alone. It is the duty of sannyasins and yogins to train students in celibacy, to teach asana and pranayama and disseminate the knowledge of Atman far and wide. They can do a lot in improving the situation, as they are whole-timed men. They should come out of their caves and huts for the upliftment of the world. It is 'All this is Brahman' now for them.

The duty of the parents, guardians, teachers and professors is, therefore, to lead a life of celibacy themselves and to train youngsters in brahmacharya also. Training of youths means nation-building.

Nowadays children beget children. Early marriages have wrought physical degeneration. Man with his boasted intellect has to learn lessons from birds and animals. Lions, elephants and other powerful animals have better self-control than men. Lions cohabit only once in a year. After conception the female animals will never allow the male animals to approach them till the young ones are weaned and they themselves become healthy and strong. Only man violates the laws of nature and consequently suffers from innumerable diseases. He has degenerated to a far lower level than animals in this respect. Food, sleep, fear, copulation are common to both animals and men. That which differentiates man from animals is the power of enquiry. If he does not possess these higher faculties he is also an animal only.

Eminent doctors of the West say that various kinds of disease arise from loss of semen, particularly in young age. There are boils in the body, acne or eruptions on the face, blue lines around the eye, absence of beard, sunken eyes, pale face with anaemia (poverty of blood), loss of memory, loss of eye-sight, short sightedness, discharge of semen along with urine, enlargement of testes, pain in the testes, debility, drowsiness, laziness, gloominess, palpitation of heart, difficulty of breathing, phthisis, pain in the back, loins, head and joints, etc; weak kidneys, passing urine in sleep, fickle-mindedness, lack of thinking power, bad dreams, wet dreams, restlessness of mind etc.

Have you realised, my dear friends, the importance of celibacy? Have you recognisd the true significance and glory of celibacy? How can you expect to be strong and healthy if the energy that is acquired through various means with great difficulty and at a great price, is wasted daily? It is impossible to be strong and healthy unless men and women and boys and girls try their level best to keep up the vow of celibacy. If our mother-land wants to rise high in the scale of nations her children, both male and female, should study this important subject in all its bearings, understand its supreme importance and observe this great vow strictly.

Virya — The Vital Fluid

According to ayurveda, semen (virya) comes out of the marrow that lies concealed inside the bones. It is found in a subtle state in all the cells of the body. Out of food is manufactured chyle. Out of chyle comes blood. Out of blood comes flesh. Out of flesh comes fat. Out of fat comes bone. Out of bone comes marrow. Out of marrow comes semen. These are the seven dhatus (elements) that support this life and body. Mark here how precious is semen. It is the essence of essences. One drop of semen comes from forty drops of blood.

Just as sugar is all-pervading in the sugar-cane, and butter in milk, so also semen pervades the whole body. Just as butter-milk is thin after the butter is removed, so also semen is thinned by its wastage. The more the wastage of semen, the more is the weakness. In yoga scriptures it is said: 'Falling of semen brings death; preservation of semen gives life.' Semen is the real vitality in man. It is the hidden treasure for man. It imparts spiritual brilliance to the face and strength to the intellect. It is the essence of life, thought, intelligence and consciousness.

The cells of the testes have been endowed with the peculiar property of secreting semen from the blood. Just as bees collect honey in the honeycomb drop by drop, so also the cells of the testes collect the semen drop by drop from the blood. Then this fluid is taken by the two ducts or tubes to the vesiculae seminalis. Under excitement it is thrown out by special ducts (called ejaculatory ducts) into the urethra, where it is mixed with the prostatic fluid. (For a detailed description and function of all these internal sexual organs, refer to any anatomy book. This knowledge is necessary. I will pass on to the most important portion — sadhana or practical methods to preserve this vital fluid.)

Semen nourishes the physical body, heart and intellect. Only that man who uses the physical body, heart and intellect can have perfect brahmacharya. A wrestler who uses his physical body only but keeps the intellect and heart undeveloped cannot expect to have full brahmacharya. He can have brahmacharya of the body only but not of the mind and heart. The semen that belongs to the heart and mind will certainly flow out. If an aspirant does only japa and meditation, if he does not develop the heart and if he does not practise physical exercise, he will have only mental brahmacharya. That portion of the semen which goes to nourish the heart and body will flow out. But an advanced yogi who dives deep in meditation will have full brahmacharya even if he does not take physical exercise.

A tree draws the essence from the earth. It is circulated throughout the tree through its twigs, branches, leaves, flowers and fruits. The shining colour and life in the leaves, flowers, etc. is due to this essence. Similarly the semen that is manufactured by the cells of the testes gives colour and vitality to this body and different organs.

One of the students of Dhanvantari approached his teacher after finishing his full course of ayurveda and asked him: "O Bhagavan! Kindly let me know the secret of health now." Dhanvantari replied: "Seminal energy is verily Atman. The secret of health lies in the preservation of this vital force. He who wastes this energy cannot have physical, mental, moral and spiritual development."

If the spermatic secretion in men is continuous it must either be expelled or reabsorbed. As a result of the most patient and persevering scientific investigations it has been established that whenever the semen is conserved and thereby reabsorbed into the system, it goes towards enriching the blood and strengthening the brain. Dr. Dio Louis thought that the conservation of this element is essential to the strength of body, vigour of mind and keenness of intellect. Another writer, Dr. E.P. Miller, writes: "All waste of spermatic secretions, whether voluntary or involuntary, is a direct wastage of the life-force. It is almost universally conceded that the choicest element of the blood enters into the composition of the spermatic secretion. If these conclusions are correct, then it follows that a chaste life is essential to man's well-being."

Just as the oil flows through a wick and burns with glowing light, so also the semen flows up by the practice of yoga sadhana and is converted into spiritual energy. This nourishes the brain cells.

For protecting the semen, it is essential to wear always a strip of cloth (dark-red coloured) over the private parts; for then there will be no night emission and growth of testicles. It is befitting for a celibate to wear always wooden sandals as thereby the semen will be conserved, eyes will be benefited, life prolonged and holiness and lustre will increase.

When the vital fluid is once lost it can never be recouped in your lifetime by your taking any amount of almonds, nerve tonics, milk, cream or cheese.

The vital energy, the seminal energy which supports your life, which is the prana of pranas, which shines in your sparkling eyes, which beams in your shining cheeks, is a great treasure for you. Remember this point well. Grasp fully the importance and value of this vital essence of life. Seminal energy is all-power, all-wealth. It is God in motion. It is God's manifestation. The *Bhagavad Gita* says: "I am the seed or vitality in men."

If the seminal energy is transmuted into spiritual energy by pure thoughts it is called sex-sublimation in Western psychology. Just as chemical substance is sublimated or purified, so also the sexual energy is purified and changed into divine energy by spiritual sadhana, by entertaining sublime, soul-elevating thoughts of self or Atman. In yoga he is called urdhvaretas or one in whom the seminal energy has flowed upwards into the brain as ojas shakti. There is no possibility of semen going downwards by sexual excitement. This process is extremely difficult. It demands constant and protracted sadhana and perfect discipline. That yogi who has achieved perfect sublimation has perfect control over lust. There is no fear of his downfall. He is perfectly safe. This stage is a very high stage. A microscopic minority only like Sri Sankaracharya, Sri Dattatreya and Jnana Dev of Alandi attained this sublime exalted state.

Mind and Virya

Mind, prana and virya (seminal energy) are one. They are under one connection or circuit. If the mind is controlled, prana and virya are automatically controlled. He who suspends or restrains the prana, restrains also the working of the mind and the movement of virya. Again if the virya is controlled and if it is made to flow upwards into the brain by pure thoughts and the practice of viparita karani mudra, etc., mind and prana are automatically controlled.

There is intimate connection between the mind and senses. Mind operates and gains experiences of this world through the five organs of perception. It enjoys through them. It extracts the work through the five organs of action. Control of the sense organs, therefore, is really control of the mind. The practice of yama, niyama, dama, sama, pratyahara, etc., aims at controlling the senses and the mind indirectly.

Mind enjoys through sound, touch, sight, taste and smell in conjunction with the five sense organs. It derives highest pleasure through touch. Sexual pleasure is the chief form of pleasure for the mind. Everybody runs after it and dies in it. Then comes the taste for nice food and drink. Sight enjoys pleasure from form or beauty. Hearing derives pleasure from music. The organ of smell is not as troublesome as the tongue. If the tongue is controlled, all other organs are automatically controlled.

An aspirant complains, "As I continue meditation, layer after layer of impurities are arising from the subconscious mind. Sometimes they are so strong and formidable that I am bewildered as to how to check them. I am not perfectly established in truth and brahmacharya. The old habits of speaking lies and lust are still lurking in me. Lust is troubling me vigorously. The very idea of a woman agitates my mind. My mind is so sensitive that I am not able to hear or think of them. As soon as the thought comes in the mind, the meditation and also the peace of the whole day is spoiled. I advise my mind, coax it, frighten it, but it is of no avail. My mind revolts. I do not know how to control this passion. Irritability, egoism, anger, greed, hatred, attachment, etc, are still lurking in me. As far as I have analysed the mind, lust is my chief enemy and it is a very strong one too. I request you to be kind enough to advise me as to how to get rid of the same."

The mind will again and again try to do some mischief inwardly. It is very diplomatic. It is very difficult to find out its ways and secret underground operation. It demands a subtle intellect and carefully repeated introspection and vigilant watchfulness. Whenever the mental image of a woman crops up in your mind with evil thoughts, repeat mentally 'OM' and do mental prostration. Gradually old evil thoughts will go.

He who has controlled the mind has also controlled the prana. The mind is set in motion or rendered active by two things — viz. the vibration of prana and vasanas (subtle desires). If one of these things dies, the other also dies by itself. When the mind is absorbed, then the prana is restrained. Where the prana is fixed, there the mind also is absorbed. When the mind and prana are not restrained, all the sense organs keep actively engaged in their respective functions.

The average man has no control at all over his mind. The mind runs riot in all directions. It does havoc, it sways him, it is in a state of constant agitation and commotion, surging with emotions and bubbling with impulses. It is being impressed at all times with the images or pictures of a thousand objects clamouring for his attention through the five senses. Each sense organ drags the mind to its

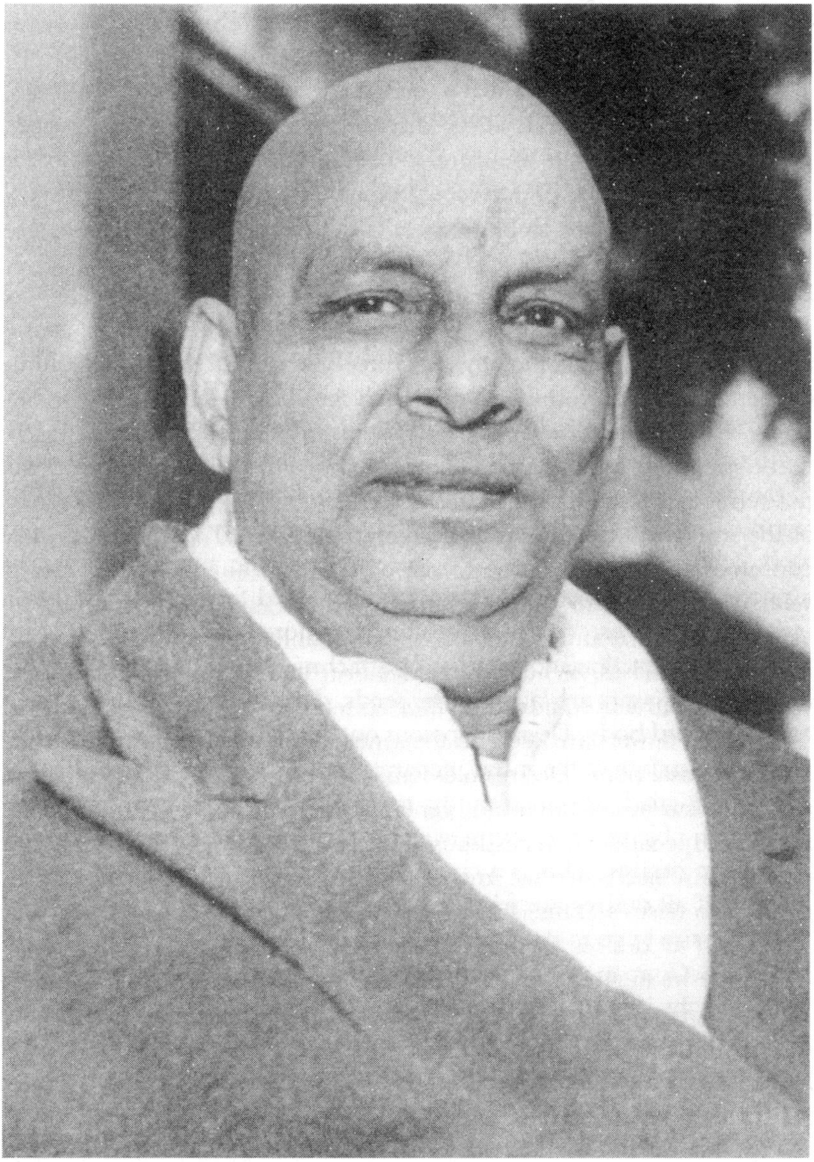

particular object of enjoyment for its own gratification. The ear drags the mind whenever it hears good music. The tongue propels the mind to run to coffee hotels and tea stalls. The control of all the senses is absolutely necessary for keeping up perfect celibacy.

There is not a moment's rest for the mind. Cares, worries, anxieties, fears of various sorts, diseases, abuses, hatred, lust, anger, etc. torment and agitate the mind constantly from within. He who has control over thoughts, impulses, emotions, moods, instincts, senses etc. is the real Emperor of emperors. He is the happiest man.

Destroy Vasanas (Subtle Desires)

Vasana (subtle desire) is a wave in the mind-lake. It causes attraction, attachment for objects, and bondage. If there is no subtle desire in the mind you will not be attracted by a woman.

Desire is the cause for the restlessness of mind. As soon as a desire manifests, there is an immediate sensual over-flowing. The mind will not retrace its steps till it gets the object and enjoys it. The restlessness of the mind will continue till the object is obtained and enjoyed. The common run of men cannot resist or suppress any desires, owing to weak will. A desire may be suppressed for the time being by an aspirant, but it manifests again with redoubled force when a suitable opportunity arises. When all desires are thoroughly eradicated there will not be attraction, admiration or attachment for any object outside.

Just as flowers are latent in the seeds, desires are latent in the mind and the causal body. Desires blossom out like flowers one by one, come out to the surface of the mind, generate thoughts and excitement in the mind and goad one incessantly to strive to possess and enjoy the particular objects of enjoyment. Desires cause actions and actions strengthen desires. This is a circle. On the advent of direct knowledge of the Self all desires are fried up entirely.

A desire to go to the theatre or cinema is impure. A desire to read *Bhagavad Gita*, to do spiritual sadhana, is pure. Increase the pure desire; all the impure ones will die by themselves. A keen desire to have Self-realisation will destroy all kinds of desires. It is a valuable asset for you in the path of Self-realisation.

Whenever a desire arises in the mind, consult always with your power of discrimination. It will at once tell you that the desire is attended with pain and that it is only a vain temptation set up by this mischievous mind. It will advise you to renounce the desire immediately and to do spiritual sadhana. Discrimination will guide you to take the help of will and drive the desire away immediately. For an aspirant on the path of jnana yoga discrimination and will are two potent weapons to destroy evil temptations and passion.

When desire is eradicated, will-power increases. If you have controlled five desires it will be very easy for you to control the sixth, as you gain additional power. You can actually feel this.

This attack is from inside. There should be attack from outside also. It is done through restraint of the senses. You must not allow the sense-vibrations to enter from outside into the mind through the avenue of the sense organs. Control of mind alone is not sufficient. The senses must be rendered calm by the practice of restraint. Desire for enjoying a woman for instance, should be destroyed by crushing the sexual desire within as soon as it arises in the mind. When you move about in the bazaar the organ of sight must be withdrawn by the practice of restraint when it runs with sexual desire towards a woman.

A strong counter-desire for liberation will decidedly help you in the destruction of worldly desires, subtle desires and cravings. Give up all desires through one strong desire for God-realisation. Give up also the desire for God-realisation, in the long run. This process is like removing a thorn by another thorn and throwing both the thorns away eventually when the business is over. The method is quite simple.

In the vast majority of persons the sexual craving is very intense. In some, the sexual desire occasionally comes but passes off quickly. There is mere agitation of a simple nature in the mind. By proper method of spiritual sadhana this also can be completely eradicated.

Cravings are the real seeds for taking birth. These cravings give rise to actions. The wheel of worldly existence is kept up by these cravings. The cravings induce excitement of the mind and you become very passionate. Sage Valmiki says in *Yoga Vasishtha*: "You can drink the whole ocean; you can swallow fire; you can carry the whole Himalayas in the palm of the hand, but it is very difficult to destroy desires." For a man of determination, patience and perseverance with burning dispassion and discrimination, the work is nothing. It can be done in the twinkling of an eye. Nip the cravings in their buds. Root them out through proper sadhana. Search all the roots of cravings by digging deep in the mind, and burn them beyond resurrection.

Imagination emanates from the bed of memories, innate tendencies and desires. Then comes attachment. Along with imagination, emotion and impulse (which exist side by side) manifest themselves. Then comes sexual irritation — craving and burning sensation in the mind and throughout the body. Cupid carries a flowery bow equipped with the arrows of fascination, suppression, intoxication, attraction and burning. If you destroy fascination at the very outset you will not have burning. The irritation and burning in the mind percolates into the physical body just as water inside the pot percolates into the surface of the pot. If you are vigilant you can drive off the bad imagination itself in the very beginning and avert the impending danger. Even if you allow the thief (imagination) to enter the first gate, keep a careful watch at the second gate when the sexual irritation manifests. You can easily stop the strong sexual impulses from being transmitted to the organ itself. Draw the sex-energy up towards the brain through hatha yoga methods and pranayama. Divert the mind. Chant 'Om' or any other mantra with concentration. Pray. Meditate.

If you still find it difficult to control the mind, immediately seek satsang (the company of wise people) and do not remain alone. When the strong impulse manifests suddenly and is transmitted to the organ you forget everything and become blind. You will become a prey to lust. Later on you will repent.

The glory of satsang (association with wise saints, yogis, sannyasins and mahatmas) is immeasurable. The glory and power of satsang is described in various ways in the *Bhagavatam, Ramayana* and other scriptures. Sankara says: "One gets dispassion by association with wise people. The state of freedom from delusion is induced by developing dispassion. By acquiring freedom from delusion, the mind becomes quite steady. When the mind is absorbed, one gets liberation."

Even a moment's company with wise people is quite sufficient to overhaul the old vicious tendencies of worldly-minded people. The magnetic aura, the spiritual vibrations and the powerful thought-currents of developed adepts produce a tremendous influence on the minds of worldly people. The personal contact of mahatmas is a blessing in reality for a worldly person. Service of saints purifies the mind. Satsang elevates the mind to a magnanimous height. Just as a single match-stick burns huge bundles of cotton in a few seconds, so also the company of saints burns all ignorance, all thoughts and impressions of passion and evil actions within a short time.

If you cannot get satsang in your own place, you can visit places of pilgrimage like Rishikesh, Varanasi, Nasik, Prayag, Haridwar, etc.

Study of books written by realised persons is also tantamount to satsang. The only potent specific for inducing burning dispassion and desire for liberation is satsang.

Passion is the instinctive urge for externalisation, self-preservation and self-multiplication. It is the diversifying power which is directly opposite to the force that moves towards the integration of being.

Control over passions constitutes the essence of truth. Self-denial or refraining from greed and indulgence is truth. Truth is eternal life and existence. Untruth is change, decay and death.

Self-control is the holding in check of the instinctive urges that try to drag the individual away from truth. Self-control is a universal rule which applies to all men and all women, at all places and at all times. It is the very key to beatitude. Indulgence in objects is the effect of the failure of the individual to discriminate the truth from untruth. Desire to have contact with and enjoy external things is the outcome of the ignorance of the truth which is God.

Be careful in destroying passion. Even Brahma the Creator does not know the exact seat of passion. In the *Bhagavad Gita* you will find that senses, mind and lower buddhi are seats of passion. The vital sheath is another seat. Desire is all-pervading in the body, mind and senses. Every cell, every atom, every molecule, every electron, is surcharged with passion. There are undercurrents, crosscurrents and intercurrents in the mighty ocean of passion wherein the crocodiles of cravings are swimming. You must completely destroy the passion in all places.

Intense musing on the objects of senses does more harm to the inner spiritual life than actual sense-gratification. If the mind is not rendered pure by sadhana, mere mortification of the external senses will not produce the desired effect. Although the external senses are mortified their internal counter-parts, which are still energetic and vigorous, take revenge upon the mind and produce intense mental disturbance and wild imagination.

How to Overcome Lust

It is easy to tame a tiger, or a lion or an elephant; it is easy to play with a cobra; it is easy to walk over fire; it is easy to uproot the Himalayas; it is easy to get victory in the battlefield — but it is difficult to eradicate lust. However, you need not despair, even a bit. Have faith in God, in His name and in His grace. Mere human effort alone will not suffice. Lust cannot be completely uprooted from the mind except by the grace of the Lord. You are bound to succeed if you have faith in Him. Then you can destroy lust in the twinkling of an eye. The Lord makes a dumb man to speak and a lame man to ascend a steep hill. Divine grace is needed. God helps those who help themselves. If you do total self-surrender, Mother Nature herself does the sadhana.

A passionate bachelor is ever-thinking: "When can I live with a young wife?" A dispassionate householder in whom discrimination has dawned is ever thinking: "When can I disentangle myself from the clutches of my wife and retire into forests for contemplation on Atman?" You must think over the difference.

You have no lustful look when you see your mother and sister although they are beautiful, well-dressed and decorated with ornaments and flowers. You look at them with affection and pure love. There are no lustful ideas. You will have to develop such a pure attitude when you look at other women also. Looking at a woman with a lustful heart is tantamount to sexual enjoyment. That is the reason why Lord Jesus says "If you look at a woman with a lustful heart you have already committed adultery in your heart."

When you are in the company of the opposite sex try to identify yourself with the sexless, all-pervading soul. Constantly make the endeavour. The sex-idea will gradually vanish and with it the attraction and lust also. Do not try to run away from the opposite sex. Try to see the Self in all forms and remember that the Atman is sexless. Mental repetition of this formula will give you strength.

For a scientist, a man or woman is a mass of electrons; for a tiger, an object of prey; for a passionate man or woman, an object of enjoyment; for a man of discrimination and dispassion, a combination of flesh, bone, urine, faecal matter, pus, perspiration, blood, phlegm, etc; for a full-blown jnani, 'All is Brahman only'. Names and forms are all mental creations only, even as a rope might be imagined to be a snake.

You should try to get discrimination between the real self and the unreal, impure body. You should hammer the mind, and point out to the mind about the defects of a sexual life — viz: loss of energy, enervation of senses, disease, birth and death, attachment and various sorts of miseries, etc.; and about the components of the body, viz., flesh, bone, excreta, urine, pus, phlegm, etc. You should always think of the ever pure immortal Atman and the glory of the spiritual life, the attainment of immortality, eternal bliss and supreme peace. Gradually the mind will be weaned from looking at the opposite sex, however attractive he or she might be. The mind will shudder to look at him or her with an evil thought. Ladies also should undergo the above practices to get themselves established in purity.

If you clearly understand the serious damages that come through an impure life and if you determine to attain the goal of life by leading a pure life, you must keep your mind busily engaged in divine thoughts, concentration, meditation, study of religious books and service of humanity, or do some gardening and other useful work, and avoid evil company, visiting cinemas and picture houses.

You may be able to stop copulation for months and years but there should not be any sexual craving or attraction for the opposite sex. Evil thoughts should not arise when you look at the opposite sex, or when you are in their company. If you succeed in this direction, then you are established in perfect brahmacharya. You have crossed the danger zone. There is no harm in looking at the opposite sex but you must have a chaste look. When you look at a young person you can think within yourself, "Prostrations unto Thee, O Mother. Thou are an image of the manifestation of Mother Kali. Do not tempt me. Do not allure me. I have understood now the secret of maya and her creation. Who has created these forms? There is an omnipotent, all-pervading and all-merciful Creator behind these names and forms. This is all decaying, false beauty. The Creator or God is Beauty of beauties. He is the fountainhead of beauty. Let me realise this Beauty of beauties by meditation."

You will have to cultivate feelings of devotion, admiration and awe when you look at an alluring form, by remembering the Creator of this form. Then you will not be tempted. If you are a student of vedanta think and feel: "Everything is Self only. The names and forms are illusory. They have no independent existence apart from Self."

Self-realisation alone can completely destroy or burn the sexual desire and the tendencies in-toto. There is neither sex nor sexual desire in Brahman. Brahman is eternally pure. By constant thinking on that sexless Atman you will be established in brahmacharya. This is the most powerful and effective method. This is the best kind of sadhana for those who know the right technique of enquiry. For others, yoga practices, meditation etc., will attenuate or thin out the sexual desire to a very great extent. "The objects of the senses turn away from the abstinent man leaving the longing behind; but this longing also turns away after he attains Self-realisation." (*Bhagavad Gita* Chapter II: 59.)

Only advanced students on the path of jnana yoga can rely on the method of Brahma vichara (enquiry of Brahman) alone for the destruction of lust. For the vast majority of persons a combined method is very congenial and healthy. When the enemies are very powerful, a combined method is used for their destruction. So also in the destruction of this powerful enemy — passion — a combined method is absolutely necessary.

Asanas, mudras, etc., can act powerfully on the physical body. Have a cold hip bath. This is the physical method. Pranayama will act on the pranamaya kosha (the vital sheath). This is the vital method. Fasting, pratyahara (withdrawal of senses), control of senses, vow of silence, dietetic discipline, etc. will purify the senses. Japa (repetition of Lord's name), dhyana (meditation), svadhyaya (study of scriptures), satsang (association of holy men), vichara (enquiry) etc. will purify the mind. Do not think of women. Do not look at women. Avert the sexual thoughts by sublime divine thoughts. This is the mental method. A healthy combination of physical, vital and mental methods is an indispensable requisite.

Brahmacharya or purity can be attained only through constant striving. It cannot be achieved in a day or a week. Your most powerful friend is the name of the Lord. It will destroy lust from its very root. So always recite and sing Ram, Ram, Ram. Self-control must be your ideal. Self-control gives you immense inner spiritual strength. Therefore, practise self-control.

You must not have false contentment, you must not be puffed up with pride for your little achievement in celibacy. If you are put to the test you will fail hopelessly. You must be ever-conscious of your shortcomings and must constantly strive to get rid of them. The greatest effort is necessary. Then only will you have sanguine success in this direction.

Fasting and Celibacy

Fasting controls passion. It calms the emotions. It controls the senses also. Fasting is a great tapas. It purifies the mind. It destroys a great multitude of sins.

A glutton can never dream of becoming a brahmachari. Control of tongue is a sine-qua-non if you want to control lust. The tongue must be controlled first. Then it will be easy to control the passion.

There is an intimate connection between the tongue and the organ of generation. The tongue is an organ of knowledge. It is born of the pure portion of the water-element. The organ of generation is an organ of action. It is born of the active, dynamic portion of the water-element. They are sister organs as their source is the same. If the tongue is stimulated with stimulating food, at once the reproductive organ also gets excited. There should be selection and restriction in diet. Food must be simple, bland, spiceless, non-irritating and non-stimulating. Moderation in food is very necessary. Stuffing the stomach is highly deleterious. Fruits are highly beneficial. You should take food only when you are really hungry. When you fast do not allow the mind to think of delicious dishes, otherwise you will not derive much benefit. Dietetic restrictions and fasting are very useful auxilliaries in controlling the carnal mind and in the attainment of celibacy. You should not ignore or make light of them on any account. Young, robust brahmacharis should observe fasting whenever passion troubles them.

You must not labour under the delusion that you have eradicated lust completely by adjusting the diet a bit, by practising pranayama and by doing a little japa, and then think that you have nothing more to do. Temptation may overcome you at any moment. Eternal vigilance and rigorous sadhana are very essential. You cannot attain perfect brahmacharya by limited effort.

Celibacy in Active Life

The ignorant man is an instrument in the hands of his tendencies and karmas. He slowly gains strength by understanding his real essential nature, by doing spiritual sadhana and by removing the desires and egoism.

This world is nothing but sex and ego. Ego is the chief thing. It is the basis. The sex is hanging on to the ego. If the ego is destroyed by enquiry of 'Who am I?' the sex-idea takes to its heels by itself. Man, master of his destiny, has lost his divine glory and has become a slave in the hands of sex and ego on account of ignorance. Sex and ego are the products of nescience. The dawn of knowledge of Self annihilates these two enemies of Atman, the two dacoits who are plundering the little helpless, ignorant, false jiva, the illusory 'I'.

The practice of celibacy is not attended with any danger or any disease or any undesirable results, such as the various sorts of complex which are wrongly attributed by the western psychologists, who have no practical knowledge of the subject. They have the wrong, ill-founded idea that the ungratified sex energy assumes the forms of various complexes in disguise, such as touch-phobia etc. This complex is due to some other causes. It is a morbid state of mind due to excessive jealousy, hatred, anger, worry and depression brought about by various causes.

On the contrary, even a little self-restraint or a little practice of continence is an ideal 'pick-me-up'. It gives inner strength and peace of mind. It invigorates the mind and nerves. It helps to conserve physical and mental energy. It augments memory, will-force and brain-power. It bestows tremendous strength, vigour and vitality. It renovates the system or constitution, rebuilds the cells and tissues, energises digestion and gives you power to face the difficulties in the daily battle of life.

Sex-sublimation is within your reach if you wish to attain it. The path is quite clear, straight and smooth, if you understand it and if you apply yourself with patience, perseverance, determination and strong will, if you practise discipline of the senses, right conduct, right thinking, right action, regular meditation, assertion, auto-suggestion and enquiry of 'Who am I?' Atman is formless. Feel this. Can there be any trace of lust or impurity in the eternal pure Atman?

Morality is a relative term. A man who observes celibacy for one year but who occasionally visits a woman once in two or three years is more moral than the passionate man who cohabits daily with his married wife. A man who constantly dwells on sexual thoughts is the most immoral person. But, the ignorant foolish worldly persons judge the standard of morality from their own view-point and look to the external conditions only, not to the internal mental state.

When you cannot control the lustful thoughts, at least control the physical body. Do vigorous sadhana. A time will come when you will be absolutely free from vicious thoughts. This is a hard struggle for you; but you will have to do it anyhow, my friend, if you want eternal peace and immortal life.

If you are weak, take a vow of celibacy for a month and then extend it to three months. You will gain some strength. You will be able to prolong the period to six months. Gradually you will be able to extend the vow to one or two or three years. Sleep separately and do vigorous japa, kirtan and meditation daily. You will hate lust now. You will experience freedom and indescribable joy. Your partner in life should also do japa, kirtan and meditation daily.

Repression or suppression of sexual desires will not help very much. It will again manifest with redoubled force when the suitable opportunity arises, when your will becomes weak, when dispassion wanes, when there is a slackening in meditation or sadhana, when you become weak owing to an attack of any disease. The sexual energy must be transmuted into spiritual energy (ojas shakti) by the practice of japa, prayer, meditation, study of religious books, pranayama, asanas, etc. You must develop devotion and burning desire for liberation. You must constantly meditate on the pure, immortal, sexless, bodiless, desireless Atman. Then only the sexual desire will be annihilated.

Celibacy for Woman

In olden days there were brahmacharinis in India. They did not wish to lead a life devoted to householder's duties. They served rishis and sages in hermitages and enquired into the nature of Brahman.

Sulabha was a very learned lady. She was born in a royal family. A celibate, she was instructed in the religion of emancipation and observed the practice of asceticism. She was firm in the practices that belong to that mode of life and was firm and steady in her vows. Never uttering a word without reflecting on its propriety, she led the life of sannyasini. She appeared before Janaka in his court and had a great discussion with him on the science of the Self.

Gargi was also a celibate. She also was a highly cultured lady and had a lengthy discussion with Yajnavalkya on the science of the Self. The dialogue between them comes in the *Brihadaranyaka Upanishad*.

In Europe also there are many women who are celibate and who entirely dedicate their lives to a life of severe austerity, prayer and meditation. They have their own hermitages. In India even at the present moment there are educated women who are leading the life of celibates. They do not wish to marry. This is due to the force of good tendencies of previous birth. They are giving education to the girls in schools. They give free tuition privately to poor girls and train them in sewing and other household works. They study religious books and practise meditation in the morning and evening. They keep a daily spiritual diary. They conduct satsang classes and kirtan among women. They train them in the practice of asanas and pranayama. They give discourses on *Bhagavad Gita* and *Upanishads*. They deliver lectures on religious subjects in English, Sanskrit and Hindi. During Christmas, Easter holidays and other important occasions they hold religious conferences for ladies on a grand scale, for mass spiritual awakening. Sometimes they visit villages and distribute medicines freely to the poor. They are equipped with the knowledge of first-aid, homeopathy, allopathy and biochemic systems of medicine. They are trained in nursing the sick.

Such girls and women are really a blessing to India. They lead a life of purity and self-sacrifice. They enjoy bliss, prosperity and renown here and will also attain the immortal abode of supreme peace hereafter.

The world is in dire need of such ideal women. I wish that the world abounded with such glorious women. I do not condemn women. I do not oppose giving them education and freedom. I have the highest veneration for women, I adore them as devis (goddesses), but I am not in favour of such freedom for women as will ruin them. I am in favour of such education and culture as will make them immortal and glorious; that will make them ideal women, ideal wives like Sulabha, Mira, Savitri and Damayanti.

Women should not do anything that can bring dishonour or infamy on them and their family and a blot on their character. Without character a man or a woman is considered as dead while living. They should be very careful and cautious when they move in society. They should avoid too much talking, too much mixing, guff and giggling. They should always walk in a dignified manner and not with the swinging of the hips. They should never look at man with a flirting gesture. Clothes should not be too tight or revealing.

Loose life is not perfect freedom. Some women of India have ruined themselves by taking advantage of this false freedom. What is there in a woman's life if her purity is lost? She is only a living corpse if there is no purity, although she is rolling in wealth and moves in high circles in society. Promiscuous mixing will lead to disastrous results. Even rishis and yogis who are clad in rags, who live in seclusion, will be pulled down by the dark forces of nature if they are careless. Then what to speak of women who daily eat dainties and sweetmeats, who are clad in perfumed velvet and silk with lace borders, who are given to too much mixing, who do not lead a life of self-control, who have no religious training and discipline and who have no idea of inner life and the religion of emancipation.

Celibacy for Householders

It is quite possible for a man to practise celibacy while remaining in the world, albeit there are various sorts of temptations and distractions. Many have achieved this in times of yore. There are many at the present moment also. A well-disciplined life, study of religious scriptures, satsang (association with the holy men), japa, meditation, pranayama, pure and moderate diet, daily introspection and enquiry, self-analysis and self-correction, right conduct, practice of ethics and moral disciplines, physical, verbal and mental tapas (austerity) in accordance with the teachings of the seventeenth chapter of the *Bhagavad Gita* — all these will pave a long way in the attainment of this end. People lead an irregular, unrighteous, immoderate, irreligious and undisciplined life; hence they suffer and fail in the attainment of the goal of life. Just as the elephant throws sand on its own head, so also the people themselves bring troubles and tribulations on their own heads on account of their foolishness.

If a man leads a life of celibacy even in the householder's life and has copulation occasionally for the sake of progeny only, he can bring forth healthy, intelligent, strong, beautiful self-sacrificing children. The ascetics and savants of ancient India, when married, used to follow this excellent rule very carefully for the same purpose and also to teach by practice and precept how to lead a life of a brahmachari even as a householder.

You will have to train your wife also in the study of *Bhagavad Gita, Upanishads, Bhagavatam* and Ramayana and in fasting, diet regulation etc.

As soon as a son is born to you, your wife becomes your mother because you are yourself born as the son. Change the mental attitude. Serve her as a World Mother. Start spiritual practice. Destroy passion. Every morning as soon as you get up from bed, touch her feet and prostrate before your wife, taking her for World Mother. Do not feel ashamed. This practice will remove the idea of 'wife' from your mind. If you cannot do prostration physically, at least do it mentally.

Thirsty aspirants who are treading the path of Self-realisation, who are householders above fifty years of age, should give up contact with their partners in life, even very occasionally. They should observe perfect physical brahmacharya if they want realisation in this very birth.

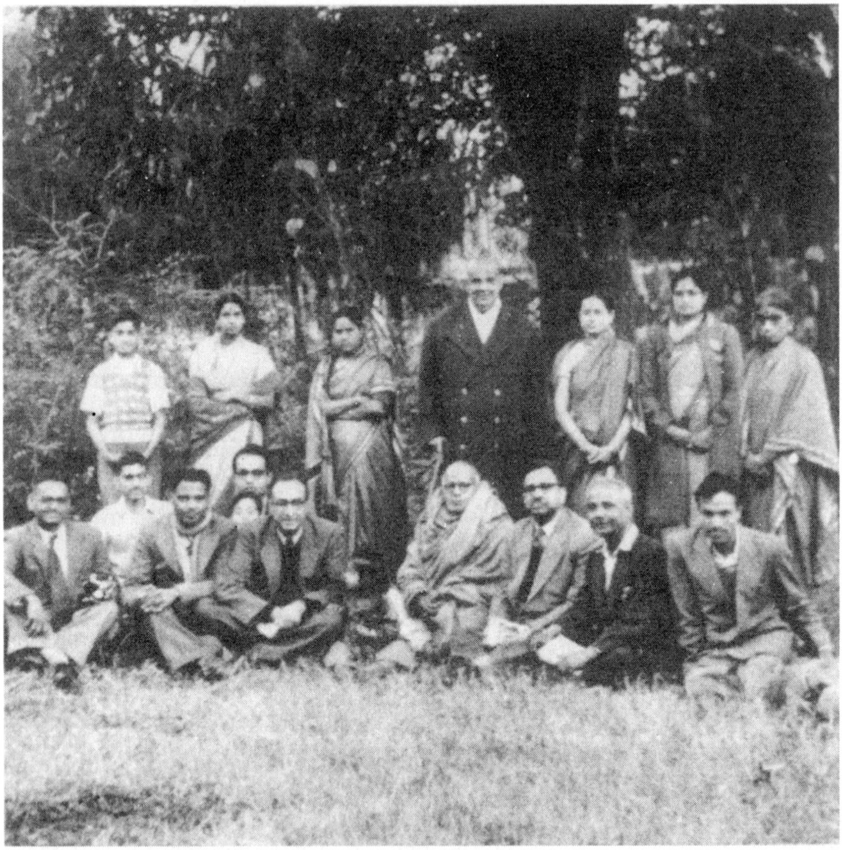

Swami Sivananda with a group of householder devotees

The Stage of Studentship

'Brahmacharya' is the term used for the first of the four stages of life according to the Hindu tradition, viz: brahmacharya or the stage of the student; grihastha or the household life; vanaprastha or the stage of a hermit; and sannyasa or the life of renunciation.

Each order has its own duties. In none of these stages must a man grasp at the special duties of the other three. At the present moment it is difficult to maintain or observe the exact details of the ancient rules, as the conditions have changed very much.

A brahmachari should study religious books till he reaches the age of twenty-five. If he has taken the vow of life-long celibacy to become a life-long brahmachari he need not enter the stage of a householder. He can devote his whole life to spiritual pursuits. He should have real lasting dispassion and discrimination. Then only will he be really benefited.

If he does not want life-long brahmacharya, after finishing his studies the student enters the order of the householder, when he is ready to take on the duties and responsibilities of the householder's life.

Of all the stages of life, that of the householder is the highest, as it verily supports the other three. Herein he can help the brahmachari, the vanaprasthi and the sannyasin. (If one leads a well regulated household life, there is no need for sannyasa. Many sannyasins are failures in their household life and therefore they had to take to sannyas.) Living in this world with all its responsibilities, he lives a religious life.

So, remaining as a householder, one should help the sannyasins and the poor, and nurse the sick. These are the virtues that householders should practise. One-tenth of income should be set apart for helping the poor. Thus one can grow in spirituality and attain God-realisation in one's own house.

Eknath and Guru Nanak were householders. Lord Rama and Lord Krishna were householders. Therefore, marriage is no hindrance to spirituality and God-realisation. You must live a life of detachment, prayerfulness, worshipfulness, meditation, realisation, aspiration and renunciation. You should not think that when you retire you will come to Hardwar and do sadhana. You must start your quest for God-realisation even now. When you are young the mind is very pliable. Good habits can be easily formed. A little meditation, a little japa, a little pranayama, a little asana — all these will help you to attain God-realisation.

The householder's life is the field for developing various virtues such as mercy, love, generosity, patience, tolerance, purity, prudence and right judgement. The central teaching of the *Bhagavad Gita* and *Yoga Vasistha* is that Self-realisation should be attained in and through the world.

If a householder visits his wife only occasionally for bringing progeny to keep up the line and not for sensual gratification he will be styled a brahmachari.

After he has finished the stage of a householder and after fixing up his son in a proper position, he can become a vanaprastha, either alone or with his wife. He should not remain in the house till the end of life. He will be having various anxieties and attachment for children if he remains in the house. If a vanaprastha wants to take sannyasa, he can do so. Vanaprastha is only a preparatory step to sannyasa.

The glory and freedom of a sannyasin can hardly be described. A sannyasin only can cut off all sorts of attachments. Otherwise some sort of subtle connection will always remain. When once one takes sannyasa, he becomes a dead man to the family members. Otherwise they always think of getting something from him. The subtle attachment in the mind still remains in both parties. This is quite sufficient to bring one back to the wheel of birth and death.

Rules for Brahmacharis

'Brahmacharya' is also the name given to the stage which precedes sannyasa in ashrams in India.

A brahmachari should avoid looking at the opposite sex with lustful eyes. He should not play, cut jokes or converse with them. He should avoid sexual intercourse without fail. If he breaks any of the above rules he violates the vow of brahmacharya.

When you walk along the road, do not look hither and thither like a monkey. Look at the tip of your toes and walk gently with a grave attitude or look at the ground and walk. This is a great help in maintaining brahmacharya. You can look at the tip of the nose also.

Bring the image of your chosen deity in your mind if the thought of the opposite sex crops up. Repeat your mantra vigorously. If sexual feelings arise in your mind when you look at the mating of animals and birds or at the bare body of the opposite sex, it indicates that lust is still lurking in your mind. Some people are so passionate and weak that even the thought or sight or touch of them causes discharge. Pitiable is their lot.

You should have the attitude that women are manifestations of the World Mother. You should adore them. Otherwise you will begin to hate women and will not develop cosmic love. This practice is for one who is beginning the practice of the feeling that everything is Self (Atma bhav). The above mental picture is kept up to annihilate lust. It is a mental discipline. Cosmic love is a great unifying force. Therefore cultivate cosmic love through selfless service, loving every creature on this earth.

The cultivation of this attitude that all women are your mothers and sisters is very difficult. You may fail to develop it one hundred and one times. It does not matter. Stick to your practice tenaciously. You are bound to succeed eventually. You will have to destroy the old mind and build a new mind. Nevertheless you will have to do it if you want to attain immortality and eternal bliss. You will surely succeed if you are fiery in your resolve and if you have iron determination. It will gradually manifest by constant practice. You will be soon established in that attitude.

After you are perfectly moulded and well established in celibacy you can test your strength by moving with the opposite sex, very cautiously, for some time. If your mind is very pure then, there is no sex-idea; if the mind ceases to act through the practice of renunciation of desires, serenity and self control, remember you have gained real spiritual strength. You are safe now. You should not stop your sadhana thinking that you are a master over the senses. If you stop it, you will have a hopeless fall. Even if you are a jivanmukta and dynamic yogi, you should be very careful when you move with worldly persons.

When the impurities emerge from the subconscious mind and come to the surface of the conscious mind with formidable force, don't try to resist them. Repeat your mantra.

Passion will subside by protracted japa and meditation on Atman. Do not try to run away from ladies. Then maya will chase you terribly. Try to see the Self in all forms.

You must understand the psychological working of the sex-impulse. When there are itches on the body, mere scratching of it is a pleasure. Sex-impulse is only a nervous itching. The satisfaction of this impulse begets a delusive pleasure but it has a disastrous effect on the spiritual well-being of the person.

You must segregate yourself for some time and live in a place full of invigorating air of health, peace and joy. Live with spiritually advanced men and stop reading all books except those that are directly spiritual. Put an end to going to exciting cinemas and films if you have got that habit. Do not read those journals which excite your lower instincts. Do not converse with those who are eager to convey irritating news and disturb your mental poise.

Lack of spiritual sadhana is the main cause for all sexual attractions. Mere theoretical abstention from sensuality will not bring you good results. You must mercilessly cut off all formalities in social life and lead a pious life freed from the business of bodily existence. Leniency to internal lower tendencies will land you in the region of suffering. Excuse will be of no use in this respect. You must be sincere in your purpose for the sublime life of spirituality. Half-heartedness will leave you in your old state of misery.

If you suffer from spermatorrhoea, observe the rules of right living. Remember God always. Fast for a day, taking only diluted juice of lemon or orange. For one week live on fruits only. For the next week take only milk and fruits before nightfall. Then have your usual midday meal. Take enema until you resume your usual meals. Reduce your sleep. Sleep on your left side. Do not sleep on the back or on the stomach. Get up at 4 a.m. and engage yourself in spiritual sadhana. Scrupulously avoid anything that may excite passion. Complete cure may take at least one to six months, according to the intensity of the disease. If the disease is of long standing the cure may take a long time, as nature's processes are slow (but sure). Whenever you are haunted by sensual thoughts, you should try to replace them by holy thoughts about your favourite deity.

One should not mind if the discharge of semen is very occasional. In case of constipation the use of an enema is most essential. The use of laxatives is not of much benefit as it creates heat in the body. Answer calls of nature before going to bed. Always wear a kowpeen or suspension bandage or trunks.

The following rules are applicable equally to those suffering from night losses and spermatorrhoea as to those who are victims of habits resulting in loss of vitality:

1. Do not be alone. Be in the company of others.
2. Do vigorous japa and kirtan.

3. Chant OM very loudly several times.
4. Run fast for some distance.
5. Enquire "In whom does this desire arise?" Do not identify yourself with the body and mind.
6. Assert your higher nature. You are the Soul or Atman. The mind is your servant. Stand as a witness to the actions of the mind.
7. Pray to God. Chant elevating hymns.
8. Feel the presence of God within you.
9. Engage yourself in the study of some elevating religious work. This will give you strength and prevent you from a fall.
10. Give up bad company, loose talk, drama, cinema and novels. Do not mix freely with the members of the opposite sex. When this is found absolutely necessary in the course of the daily duties of life, mentally address them as 'Mother', look at their feet and speak the minimum words with pure attitude.
11. Minimise your needs. Do not look into the mirror frequently. Lead a disciplined rigorous life.
12. Do not ride too much on a bicycle.
13. Root out love of leisure and ease. Overcome laziness and always be engaged in some useful work. Let your mind be always busy with study of spiritual literature or active work along some good lines. Let there not be time enough for idle pleasure.
14. Let the work you do be a source of joy to you. Find pleasure in your work. Let it not be done under compulsion. The mind turns away from such work and takes recourse to other objects for seeking pleasure. You should work spontaneously and happily so that there may not be any occasion for the mind to resort to unhealthy practices. Work for the sake of the Lord. Then all work becomes interesting. Take to hard physical labour, but do not exhaust yourself. Do the work as a hobby. Then you can do your work without anxiety or worry.
15. Do asanas (specially sirshasana, sarvangasana and siddhasana); practise deep-breathing and bhastrika pranayama; take long walks; take part in sports.
16. Always take a cold water bath. Do not use scents or fancy clothings. Do not attend dance or music parties. Do not sing. You may take part in some chanting without showing your musical talents.
17. Give up smoking, intoxicating drinks and non-vegetarian food.

18. Give up tea, coffee, chillies, excess of salt and excess of sugar. Have occasional fasts (once a week). Do not drink even water on that day. Do not drink milk without mixing ginger in it.
19. Avoid dainty dishes, sauces, savouries and pastries.
20. Do not look at the mating of animals, birds etc.

This weakness will pass away. Do not be anxious, worried or depressed over it. Worry will only weaken you more. Learn lessons from the past and be benefited therefrom. Do not brood over the past and be weakened. Change your angle of vision. Practise enquiry. Meditate on the advantages of celibacy.

You are the child of the Lord of the universe. Bliss is within you. There is not an iota of pleasure in sense-objects. Dissociate yourself from the body; identify yourself with the Lord. If your mind is pure and healthy, your body too will be pure and healthy. Therefore forget the past and take to a new, better life of virtue and spirituality, love of God and aspiration for the higher divine life. Develop a taste for divine life. Do more sadhana with greater intensity. You will be a completely changed and blessed person.

Section VI

Concentration and Meditation

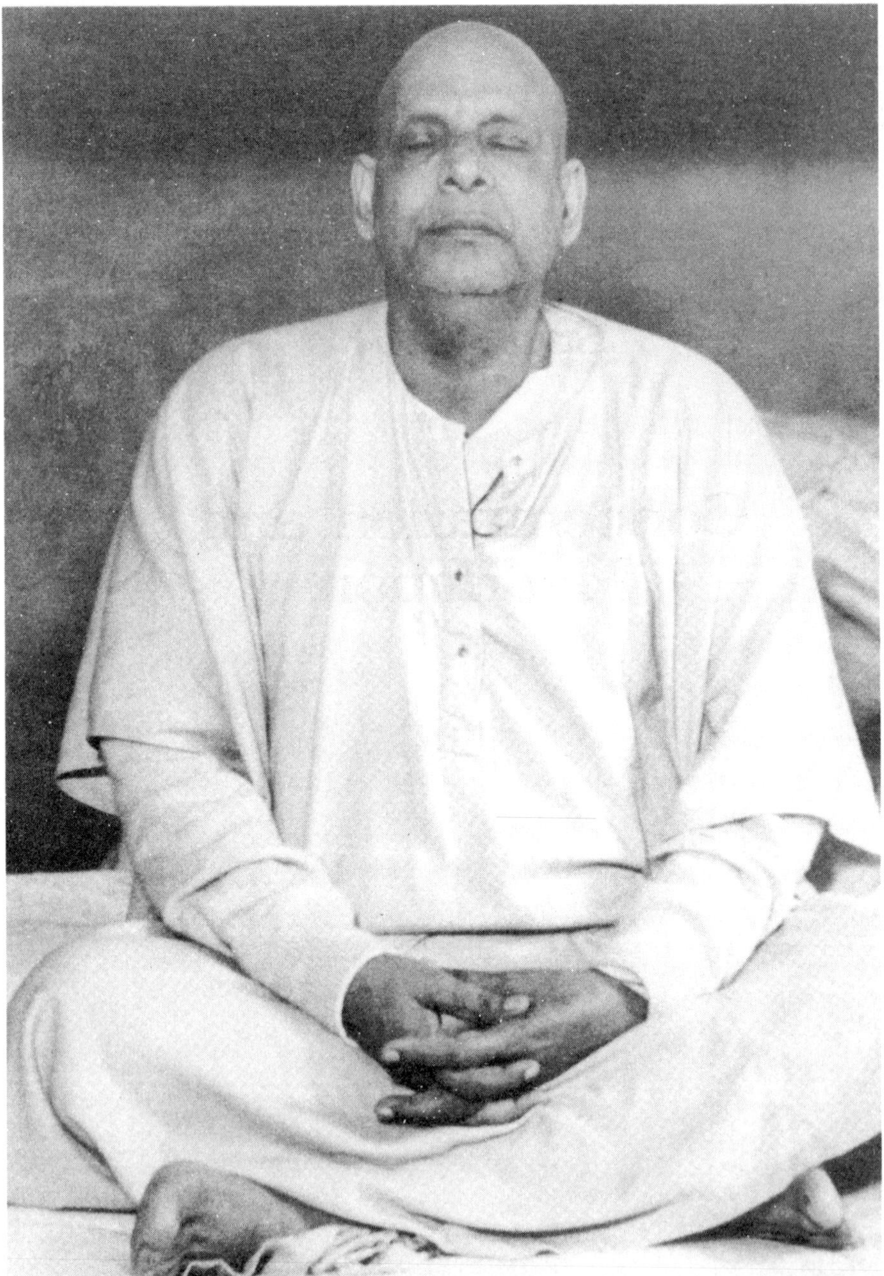

In meditation

DHARANA, DHYANA, SAMADHI

Concentration or dharana is centering the mind on one single thought. Hatha yogis concentrate their mind on the six chakras. Concentration is a great necessity for all aspirants.

During concentration the various rays of the mind are collected and focussed on the object of concentration. There will be no tossing of the mind. One idea occupies the mind, and the whole energy of the mind is concentrated on that one idea. The senses become still and do not function.

When there is deep concentration there is no consciousness of the body and surroundings. There is no concentration without something to rest the mind upon. The mind should be trained to concentrate on gross objects in the beginning; and later on, you can successfully concentrate on subtle objects and abstract ideas.

Concentration is purely a mental process which needs an inward turning of the mind. It is not a muscular exercise. There should be no undue strain on the brain. You should not fight and wrestle with the mind. When you concentrate avoid tension anywhere in the body or mind. Think gently of the object in a continuous manner. Do not allow the mind to wander away

The practice of concentration and the practice of pranayama are interdependent. If you practise pranayama you will get concentration. Natural pranayama follows the practice of concentration. A hatha yogi practises pranayama and then controls the mind. He rises upwards from below. A raja yogi practises concentration and thus controls his prana. He comes downwards from above. They both meet on a common platform in the end.

There are different practices according to the different capacities, tastes and temperaments. To some, the practice of pranayama will be easy to start with; to others, the practice of concentration will be easier.

Those who practise concentration off and on will have a steady mind only occasionally. Sometimes the mind will begin to wander and will be quite unfit for application. You must have a mind that will obey you at all times sincerely and carry out all your commands in the best possible manner at any time. Steady and systematic practice will make the mind very obedient and faithful.

Chakra Concentration

A hatha yogi fixes his mind on the sushumna nadi, the middle path in the spinal canal, and on a specified centre — the muladhara, manipura or ajna chakra. Some yogis ignore the lower chakras and fix their mind on the ajna chakra only. Their theory is that by controlling the ajna chakra all the lower chakras can be automatically controlled.

When you concentrate on a chakra, a threadlike connection is formed in the beginning between the mind and the chakra. The ascent along the sushumna from chakra to chakra is made gradually by patient efforts.

When the opening of the sushumna is shaken a bit, the kundalini shakti tries to enter the sushumna. Even this mere shaking of the opening of the sushumna causes a great deal of bliss. You become intoxicated and entirely forget the world. Great dispassion arises. You will become fearless. You will behold various visions, and witness the splendid inner light. You will get different siddhis, different types of bliss and different kinds of knowledge by controlling and operating on different chakras. For instance if you have conquered the manipura chakra you have already conquered fire. Fire will not burn you.

Pancha Dharana (Five Concentrations)

Practice of these five concentrations should be learnt under a guru who is an adept yogi.

There are five elements: earth (prithvi), water (apas), fire (agni), air (vayu) and space (akasha). To the body of the five elements, there is the five-fold dharana.

Prithvi dharana: From the feet to the knees is said to be the region of the earth. It is four-sided in shape, yellow in colour and has the sanskrit letter *la* along the region of earth i.e. from the feet to the knees. Contemplating upon this, one should concentrate there for a period of two hours daily. He then attains mastery over the earth. Death does not trouble him since he has obtained mastery over the 'earth' element.

Ambhasi dharana: The region of water is said to extend from the knees to the anus. Apas is semi-lunar in shape and white in colour. It has the letter *va* for its seed-letter. Carrying up the breath with the letter *va* along the region of water, one should contemplate on Lord Narayana, having four arms, a crowned head and dressed in orange-colour clothes. Practising concentration there daily for a period of two hours, one is freed from all sins. Then one has no fear from water.

Agneyi dharana: From the anus to the heart is said to be the region of fire. Agni is triangular in shape, red in colour and has the letter *ra* for its seed-letter. Raising the breath with the letter *ra* along the region of fire, one should contemplate on Rudra, who has three eyes, who grants all wishes and who is of the colour of the midday sun. Practising concentration there daily for a period of two hours, he is not burnt by fire even though his body enters into the fire-pit.

Vayavya dharana: From the heart to the middle of the eyebrows is said to be the region of air. It is black in colour and shines with the letter *ya*. Carrying the breath along the region of air, one should contemplate on Ishvara, the omniscient. The yogi does not meet his death through air.

Akasha dharana: From the centre of the eyebrows to the top of the head is said to be the region of space. It is circular in shape, smokey in colour and shines with the letter *ha*. Raising the breath along the region of akasha one should contemplate on Sadasiva. By practising this concentration one obtains the power of levitation. The yogi gets all the siddhis.

Concentration on Solar Plexus

The solar plexus is often called the abdominal brain. It is an important centre of the nerves, connected with the sympathetic nervous system. It is located in the epigastric region, behind the pit of the stomach on either side of the spinal column. It has control of the main internal organs of man and plays an important part in the control of emotions and of various bodily functions. It plays a much more important part than is generally recognised, being one of the most vital parts of the body. It is composed of white and grey brain matter. Yogis refer to it as the storehouse of prana, or the powerhouse. (Men have been instantly killed by a severe blow over the solar plexus.) The solar plexus is literally the sun of the nervous system. When the sun is shining harmoniously, the whole of the physical system is harmonious. It radiates strength and energy to all parts of the body. Thoughts and prana, when directed towards the centre through pranayama, will stimulate and awaken the 'sunshine' latent therein.

Technique: Sit erect in padmasana or siddhasana. Close your eyes. Draw the air slowly through the left nostril, as long as you can do so with comfort. Keep the right one closed with your right thumb. Repeat OM mentally. Then retain the breath. Have the attention well directed towards the solar plexus. Concentrate your mind there. Do not make any undue strain of the mind or undue effort of any kind. Consciously direct the prana to the region of the solar plexus through the retained breath. Imagine: "I am breathing in prana, happiness, joy, strength, vigour, love." Then slowly exhale through the right nostril. Then inhale through the right nostril, retain it as before and exhale through the left. Repeat the process 12 times in the morning. Fear, depression, weakness and all other undesirable emotions which stand in the way of spiritual advancement will vanish. You will become more and more confident of success in Self-realisation.

Dhyana (Meditation)

The practice of concentration leads to meditation. Meditation is the flow of continuous thought on one idea. When persisted in it brings about the experience of super-consciousness, or samadhi.

Every human being has within himself various tremendous powers, potentialities, capacities and latent faculties. He must awaken these dormant powers and faculties by the practice of yoga and meditation, then only can he change his environment and influence others, and enter into the superconscious state of samadhi.

During medtation the mind becomes calm, serene and steady. The various rays of the mind are collected and focussed on the object of meditation. There will be no tossing of the mind. The whole energy of the mind is concentrated on that one idea.

Considerable changes take place in the mind, brain and nervous system by the practice of meditation. New nerve currents, vibrations and cells are all formed. The whole mind and nervous system are remodelled.

Meditation eventually leads to samadhi or superconscious state, wherein the yogi gets divine knowledge of his real nature. When he is established in samadhi he is liberated. He shines as a jivanmukta, a beaconlight for the world. Glory to the jivanmuktas; may you all shine as jivanmuktas here and now!

Various kinds of lights manifest during meditation owing to deep concentration. In the beginning a bright white light, the size of a pin's point, will appear in the forehead at the space between the two eyebrows, (which corresponds tentatively to the ajna chakra).

At times you will see some lustrous forms of devatas or some other physical forms. You will see your favourite deity or your guru. Siddhas, rishis and others give their darshan to encourage you. You can see beautiful gardens, palatial buildings, rivers, mountains and golden temples —sceneries so lovely and picturesque as cannot be adequately described.

Samadhi

Samadhi is of two kinds: jada samadhi and chaitanya samadhi. A hatha yogi through the practice of kechari mudra can shut himself up in a box and remain underneath the ground for months and years. There is no higher supernatural knowledge in this kind of samadhi. This is jada samadhi. In chaitanya samadhi there is perfect 'awareness'. The yogi comes down with new super-sensuous wisdom.

Nirvikalpa is the state of super-consciousness. There are no imaginations of any sort in this condition. This is the goal of life. All the mental activities and the functions of the intellect and the senses cease entirely. The aspirant rests in Atman. There is no distinction between subject and object. The world and the pairs of opposites vanish completely. This is a state beyond all relativity. The aspirant gets knowledge of Self, supreme peace and infinite, indescribable bliss. (This is also called yogarudha state, or the state of one who is established in yoga.)

*For detailed information on meditation and samadhi, see **Raja Yoga: The Yoga System of Patanjali**. Vol.IV in this series.

APPENDIX

Human Body: The Primal Source of all Attainments

1. The body of all beings, from Brahma down to the least inanimate particle, is composed of earth, water, fire, air and ether. They are ensouled by Atman.
2. The human body, which is the primal source of all attainments, is a strong boat, so hard to secure yet within easy reach, so cheap when once attained.
3. Having obtained a human body which is the gateway for liberation, he who attaches himself too much to worldly life is to be regarded as one who has fallen down from a high state.
4. This human body is a prison! Having entered it, you should struggle hard to get out of it.
5. The wise man does not even wish for human existence, for connection with the body causes selfish distractions and delusion.
6. Identification with the body or attachment to the body is the cause for fear.
7. Life is a voyage in the infinite ocean of time where scenes are perpetually changing.
8. Do not love or hate your body and senses. Be indifferent towards the body, senses and all objects. Never be disgusted with life. Be disgusted with worldliness.
9. Action, emotion and intelligence are the three horses that are linked to the body-chariot.
10. Keep this body in proper condition. Make better use of it. A sound and healthy body will help you in your daily spiritual practices. With

perfect and radiant health you can achieve the highest success in your life.

11. Whenever the physical body becomes unfit for further evolution on account of sickness or old age, the Lord destroys the body and thus enables the jiva to assume a new healthy body for his further growth or quick evolution.

12. This body-consciousness remains till one gets knowledge of the Self and consequent emancipation.

Yogic Recipes:

1. Meditation and study	Padmasana, siddhasana, svastikasana or sukhasana.
2. Sex sublimation, syphillis, spermatorrhoea, pyorrhoea, gonorrhoea, sterility, awakening of kundalini, bad memory, diabetes, consumption, asthma, renal colic, rheumatism, ear, eye, nose troubles, etc.	Siddhasana, sirshasana, sarvangasana, matsyasana or ardha matsyendrasana.
3. Amenorrhoea, dysmenorrhoea, leucorrhoea, uterine and ovarine diseases.	Sarvangasana, salabhasana, paschimottanasana and bhujangasana (during pregnancy these asanas should not be done).
4. Chronic bronchitis.	Matsyasana and salabhasana.
5. Digestion.	Sarvangasana, vajrasana, paschimottanasana and baddha padmasana.
6. Liver and spleen enlargements.	Sarvangasana, halasana, mayurasana and baddha padmasana.

7. Chronic constipation.	Halasana, mayurasana, dhanurasana, matsyasana and padahastasana.
8. Hydrocele, elephantiasis, shortness of legs and arms.	Garudasana, trikonasana and utkasana.
9. Piles.	Siddhasana, paschimottan-asana, sirshasana, gomuk-hasana and maha mudra.
10. Dysentery.	Baddha padmasana and kukkutasana.
11. Myalgia and rheumatism.	Vrischikasana, sirshasana, paschimottanasana, sarvang-asana, etc.
12. Leprosy.	Sirshasana and maha mudra.
13. Relaxation.	Savasana.
14. Destroyer of all diseases and bestower of long life.	Padmasana, sirshasana, sarvangasana and paschimottanasana.

N.B. If you are suffering from some chronic disease you will have to combine mudras, pranayama and japa also. If a particular item is not suitable to your system, you can consult your spiritual guide. You will have to practise them with sincerity and patience for a long time.

Schedules for Practice

Elementary Course 'A' for Busy People

	From:	To:
Japa and meditation: 45 mins	4 a.m.	4.45 a.m.
Sirshasana: 5 mins)		
Sarvangasana: 5 mins)		
Matsyasana: 3 mins)		
Paschimottanasana: 5 mins)		
Other asanas: 5 mins)		
Savasana: 2 mins)	4.45 a.m.	5.10 a.m.
Rest: 15 mins	5.10 a.m.	5.25 a.m.
Bhastrika pranayama: 5 mins)		
Other pranayamas: 5 mins)	5.25 a.m.	5.35 a.m.
Rest: 5 mins	5.35 a.m.	5.40 a.m.
Study (svadhyaya): 45 mins	5.40 a.m.	6.25 a.m.
Morning walk: 35 mins	6.25 a.m.	7.00 a.m.
Asanas, pranayama, japa, meditation: 1½ hours	6.15 p.m.	7.45 p.m.
Bhajan (kirtan): 30 mins	7.45 p.m.	8.15 p.m.
Meals and rest: 15 mins	8.15 p.m.	8.30 p.m.
Study: 1 hour	8.30 p.m.	9.30 p.m.
Sleep: 6 hours	9.30 p.m.	3.30 a.m.

Advanced Course 'B' For Busy People

Japa and meditation: 1½ hours	3.30 a.m.	5.00 a.m.
Sirshasana: 30 mins	5.00 a.m.	5.30 a.m.
Sarvangasana, Mayurasana, Paschimottanasana, etc: 30 mins	5.30 a.m.	6.00 a.m.
Bhastrika and the other pranayamas: 30 mins	6.00 a.m.	6.30 a.m.
Study: 30 mins	6.30 a.m.	7.00 a.m.
Asanas, pranayama, japa and meditation: 3 hours	6.15 p.m.	9.15 p.m.
Meals: 15 mins	9.15 p.m.	9.30 p.m.
Study: 30 mins	9.30 p.m.	10 p.m.
Sleep: 5 hours	10 p.m.	3.00 a.m.

Course 'C' for Whole-Time Aspirants

Japa and meditation: 3½ hours	3.30 a.m.	7.00 a.m.
Asanas and pranayama: 2 hours	7.00 a.m.	9.00 a.m.
Asanas and pranayama: 2 hours	5.00 p.m.	7.00 p.m.
Japa and Meditation: 2 hours	7.00 p.m.	9.00 p.m.
Bhajan: 1 hour	9.00 p.m.	10 p.m.
Sleep: 5 hours	10 p.m.	3 a.m.

Common Routine for 'A' and 'B' Courses

Rest, small snack or cup of milk: 15 mins	7.00 a.m.	7.15 a.m.
Nishkama karma and household duties: 1¼ hours	7.15 a.m.	8.30 a.m.
Bathing, washing, breakfast, etc.: 1 hour	8.30 a.m.	9.30 a.m.
Office: 3 hours	1 a.m.	1 p.m.
Lunch, writing letters and interviews: 1 hour	1 p.m.	2 p.m.
Office: 3 hours	2 p.m.	5 p.m.
Evening tiffin and rest: 15 mins	5 p.m.	5.15 p.m.
Evening walk (two miles) and satsang: 1¼ hours	5.15 p.m.	6.30 p.m.

During other times mauna, nishkama karma, chanting, study, bath, meals, etc. must be nicely arranged.

Aspirants should have their own routine according to their growth, capacity and convenience.

GLOSSARY

Adharma: All that is contrary to righteousness
Adhikari: Qualified person
Ahimsa: Non-injury in thought, word and deed
Ajna chakra: The chakra situated at the space between the bushy eyebrows
Akasha: Space
Anahata: The fourth chakra, situated opposite the heart; mystical sounds
Ananda: Bliss
Apana: The down-going breath
Aparigraha: Non-covetousness
Artha: Meaning; sense; purpose; wealth
Asteyam: Non-stealing
Asana: Yoga posture
Atman: The Self
Atma-chintana: Reflection on the Self
Atma-jnana: Direct knowledge of the Self
Avidya: Ignorance; nescience
Ayurveda: A branch of Indian medicine

Bandha: A certain class of exercises in hatha yoga
Bhakta: Devotee
Bhava samadhi: Superconscious state attained by bhaktas or devotees through intense divine emotion
Bija mantra: The seed-letter in which there is latent power
Brahmacharya: Celibacy; the first stage of the Hindu's life, viz. celibate student's life
Brahmarandhra: The fontanelle
Brahman: The Absolute Reality
Brahmi amla: A medicinal oil made from the amla fruit
Buddhi: Intellect; understanding; reasoning

Chakra: Plexus; centre of psychic energy in the human system
Chin mudra: A position of the hand where the thumb and forefinger are touching and the other three fingers are outstretched.

Dama: Control of the outer senses
Devas: Gods
Dharma: Righteousness

Ekadasi: Eleventh day of the Hindu lunar fortnight

Gayatri mantra: One of the most sacred Vedic mantras
Guna: Quality born of nature
Guru: Teacher; preceptor

Ishtam: The particular form of God that one is devoted to

Japa: Repetition of God's name again and again
Jiva: Individual soul with ego
Jivanmukta: One who is liberated in this life
Jnana: Knowledge; wisdom of the Reality or Brahman the Absolute

Kaivalya: Transcendental state of absolute independence; moksha, final liberation; emancipation
Kama: Desire; passion; lust
Kanda: The egg-shaped centre of nerves located below the region of the navel
Karma: Action; the law of cause and effect
Kaya siddhi: Perfection of the body through yoga
Kirtan: Singing the name and glory of God
Kriya: Particular exercises in hatha yoga
Kumbhaka: Breath retention
Kundalini: The primordial cosmic energy located in the individual

Mala: Impurity of the mind
Mala: Beads used for counting the mantras when practising japa
Mantra: Sacred syllable or word or set of words through the reflection and repetition of which one attains perfection
Maya: The veiling and the projecting power of the universe
Moha: Infatuation; false identification and deluded attachment
Moksha: Liberation
Mudra: A certain class of exercise in hatha yoga

Nadi: Psychic channel
Nasikagra drishti: Gaze at the tip of the nose
Nirguna: Without attribute
Nirvana: Liberation
Nirvikalpa samadhi: The superconscious state where there is no mind or the triad (viz. knower, known and knowledge) or any idea whatsoever
Nishkama karma: Action without expectation of fruits
Niyama: The second step in raja yoga

Ojas shakti: Spiritual energy created through celibacy
OM: The sacred syllable symbolising Brahman

Para shakti: Supreme power
Prana: Vital energy; life-breath; life-force
Pranayama kosha: One of the sheaths of the Self, consisting of the pranas and the organs of action
Pranayama: Control of prana
Pratyahara: Sense control
Puraka: Inspiration; inhalation

Raja yogi: One who follows the path of raja yoga
Rajas: The principle of dynamism; one of the three gunas
Rechaka: Exhalation of the breath
Riddhi: Minor power
Rishi: A sage

Sadhana: Spiritual practice
Saguna: With qualities
Sahasrara: A region in the top of the head in the form of a

thousand petalled lotus, where kundalini shakti unites with Lord Shiva

Sakara: Having form

Sama: Tranquillity; control of mind

Samadhi: The state of super-consciousness where absoluteness is experienced attended with all-knowledge and joy

Samsara: Worldly existence

Samskara: Impression, pre-natal tendency

Samyama: Perfect restraint; concentration, meditation and samadhi

Sannyasin: A monk; one who has embraced the life of complete renunciation.

Satchidananda: Existence-knowledge-bliss absolute

Satsang: Association with the wise (good)

Sattva: Light, purity, reality

Satyam: Truth

Savikalpa samadhi: Samadhi with the triad of knower, knowledge and known

Shakti: Power; energy; force; the absolute power or cosmic energy

Shanti: Peace

Siddhi: Psychic power

Siva: Hindu god, Lord of yogis

Sushumna: The most important nadi which extends from the base of the spine to the top of the head, and through which kundalini is made to rise through the process of yoga

Tamas: Ignorance, inertia, darkness

Tapas: Purificatory action; austerity

Tratak: Steady gazing at a fixed point

Vasana: Subtle desire

Veerya: Seminal energy; strength; power

Vibhuti: Manifestation; the special forms in which the Lord exhibits Himself

Vichara: Enquiry into the nature of the Self

Vritti: Thought-wave; mental modification

Yama: One of the steps in raja yoga

TWENTY IMPORTANT SPIRITUAL INSTRUCTIONS

By

H.H. Sri Swami Sivanandaji Maharaj

1. ***BRAHMA-MUHURTA:*** Get up at 4 a.m. daily. This is Brahmamuhurta which is extremely favourable for meditation on God.
2. ***ASANA:*** Sit on Padma, Siddha or Sukha Asana for Japa and meditation for half an hour, facing the east or the north. Increase the period gradually to three hours. Do Sirshasana and Sarvangasana for keeping up Brahmacharya and health. Take light physical exercises as walking, etc., regularly. Do twenty Pranayamas.
3. ***JAPA:*** Repeat any Mantra as pure Om or Om Namo Narayanaya, Om Namah Sivaya, Om Namo Bhagavate Vasudevaya, Om Saravanabhavaya Namah, Sita Ram, Sri Ram, Hari Om, or Gayatri, according to your taste or inclination, from 108 to 21,600 times daily.
4. ***DIETETIC DISCIPLINE:*** Take Sattvic food, Suddha Ahara. Give up chillies, tamarind, garlic, onion, sour articles, oil, mustard, asafoetida. Observe moderation in diet (Mitahara). Do not overload the stomach. Give up those things which the mind likes best for a fortnight in a year. Eat simple food. Milk and fruits help concentration. Take food as medicine to keep the life going. Eating for enjoyment is sin. Give up salt and sugar for a month. You must be able to live on rice, Dhal and bread without any Chutni. Do not ask for

extra salt for Dhal and sugar for tea, coffee or milk.

5. ***MEDITATION-ROOM:*** Have a separate meditation-room under lock and key.
6. ***CHARITY:*** Do charity regularly, every month, or even daily according to your means, say six Paisa per rupee.
7. ***SVADHYAYA:*** Study systematically the Gita, the Ramayana, the Bhagavata, Sri Vishnu-Sahasranama, Lalita-Sahasranama, Aditya Hridaya, the Upanishads or the Yoga Vasishtha, the Bible, the Zend Avesta, the Koran, the Tripitakas, the Granth Sahib, etc., from half an hour to one hour daily and have Suddha Vichara.
8. ***BRAHMACHARYA:*** Preserve the vital force (*Veerya*) very, very carefully. Veerya is God in motion or manifestation—Vibhuti. Veerya is all power. Veerya is all money. Veerya is the essence of life, thought and intelligence.
9. ***PRAYER SLOKAS:*** Get by heart some prayer-Slokas, Stotras and repeat them as soon as you sit in the Asana before starting Japa or meditation. This will elevate the mind quickly.
10. ***SATSANGA:*** Have Satsanga. Give up bad company, smoking, meat and alcoholic liquors entirely. Do not develop any evil habits.
11. ***FAST ON EKADASI:*** Fast on Ekadasi or live on milk and fruits only.
12. ***JAPA MALA:*** Have a Japa Mala (rosary) round your neck or in your pocket or underneath your pillow at night.
13. ***MOUNA:*** Observe Mouna (vow of silence) for a couple of hours daily.

14. ***SPEAK THE TRUTH:*** Speak the truth at all cost. Speak a little. Speak sweetly.

15. ***PLAIN LIVING:*** Reduce your wants. If you have four shirts, reduce the number to three or two. Lead a happy, contented life. Avoid unnecessary worry. Have plain living and high thinking.

16. ***NEVER HURT ANYBODY:*** Never hurt anybody *(Ahimsa Paramo Dharmah)*. Control anger by love, Kshama (forgiveness) and Daya (compassion).

17. ***DO NOT DEPEND UPON SERVANTS:*** Do not depend upon servants. Self-reliance is the highest of all virtues.

18. ***SELF-ANALYSIS:*** Think of the mistakes you have committed during the course of the day, just before retiring to bed (self-analysis). Keep daily diary and self-correction register. Do not brood over past mistakes.

19. ***FULFIL DUTIES:*** Remember that death is awaiting you at every moment. Never fail to fulfil your duties. Have pure conduct (*Sadachara*).

20. ***SURRENDER TO GOD:*** Think of God as soon as you wake up and just before you go to sleep. Surrender yourself completely to God (Sharanagati)

Om Santih Santih Santih!

This is the essence of all spiritual Sadhanas.
This will lead you to Moksha.
All these Niyamas or spiritual canons must be rigidly observed. You must not give leniency to the mind.